CANCER OF THE GENITOURINARY TRACT

The University of Texas System Cancer Center
M. D. Anderson Hospital and Tumor Institute
23rd Annual Clinical Conference on Cancer

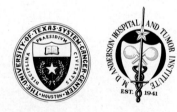

Published for
The University of Texas System Cancer Center
M. D. Anderson Hospital and Tumor Institute
Houston, Texas, by Raven Press, New York

The University of Texas System Cancer Center
M. D. Anderson Hospital and Tumor Institute
23rd Annual Clinical Conference on Cancer (23rd :

Cancer of the
Genitourinary Tract

Edited by

Douglas E. Johnson, M.D.
Department of Urology

Melvin L. Samuels, M.D.
Department of Medicine

The University of Texas System Cancer Center
M. D. Anderson Hospital and Tumor Institute
Houston, Texas

Raven Press ■ New York

Raven Press, 1140 Avenue of the Americas, New York, New York 10036

Library of Congress Cataloging in Publication Data

Clinical Conference on Cancer, 23d, Anderson Hospital
   and Tumor Institute, 1978.
   Cancer of the genitourinary tract.

   Includes bibliographies and index.
   1. Genito-urinary organs--Cancer--Congresses.
I. Johnson, Douglas E. II. Samuels, Melvin L.
III. Anderson Hospital and Tumor Institute, Houston,
Tex. IV. Title. [DNLM: 1. Urogenital neoplasms--
Congresses. W3 C162H 23d 1978c / WJ160 C641 1978c]
RC280.G4C58 1978   616.9'94'6   79-2070
ISBN 0-89004-383-3

This volume is a compilation of the proceedings of The University of Texas System Cancer Center M. D. Anderson Hospital and Tumor Institute 23rd Annual Clinical Conference on Cancer, held November 2 and 3, 1978, in Houston, Texas.

The material contained in this volume was submitted as previously unpublished material, except in the instances in which credit has been given to the source from which some of the illustrative material was derived.

Great care has been taken to maintain the accuracy of the information contained in the volume. However, the Editorial Staff and The University of Texas System Cancer Center cannot be held responsible for errors or for any consequences arising from the use of the information contained herein.

Preface

Cancers of the urinary system and male genital tract account for 16% of all malignant diseases. While the overall incidence of cancer has decreased slightly in the past quarter-century, the number of new cases of genitourinary cancer has continued to rise. Prostatic carcinoma has increased in incidence by more than 20% in the past 25 years, and remains the second most common cancer in men. Two percent of the male population in the U.S. can eventually expect to die from this neoplasm. The increased incidence of bladder cancer is presumably due to greater exposure to occupational and environmental carcinogens; this disease accounts for more deaths than carcinoma of the uterine cervix. Although the figures are not so striking for renal and testicular malignant diseases, these also have not decreased in incidence.

Fortunately, lessened reluctance on the part of patients to seek medical attention (due largely to greater public education) and improved methods of diagnosis are allowing earlier detection and institution of treatment for patients with these diseases. In the past the physician's armamentarium was severely restricted, but recent developments and improvements in therapy have provided multiple treatment options and are producing striking results.

The development of integrated therapy for patients with invasive bladder carcinoma using preoperative irradiation followed by radical cystectomy has more than doubled the five-year survival rate. The recent availability of active chemotherapy programs for this disease should further increase the number of patients saved. The use of any of several methods of irradiation (limited field, extended field, interstitial ^{125}I implantation, or combination interstitial and external radiation therapy) for patients with well-differentiated adenocarcinoma of the prostate who have disease localized to the pelvis has provided life expectancies similar to those of the age-adjusted population without prostatic cancer. The outlook for patients with testicular carcinoma has dramatically improved over the past five years with the development and refinement of active drug programs. In the past, the outlook for patients with metastatic renal carcinoma has been very poor, but the use of percutaneous renal artery occlusion followed by nephrectomy and progestin therapy is producing the first encouraging results, presumably by altering the immune response.

The successful treatment of a patient with a genitourinary tumor begins with a careful multidisciplinary evaluation that requires close cooperation between the primary care physician, urologist, pathologist, diagnostic radiologist, radiotherapist, and medical oncologist. Treatment today seldom is limited to a single specialty, and because active treatment programs using surgery, radiotherapy, or chemotherapy alone or in combination are readily available, they must be

v

chosen carefully. Therapy must be individualized for each patient and selected only after all factors have been considered.

The purpose of this book is to provide the clinician with a compendium of current and sometimes controversial treatment options available for managing the more common genitourinary tumors. We hope that it will be used by busy clinicians seeking a summary of the "state of the art" in the management of these tumors, as well by students and practitioners alike who wish to examine and evaluate the limitations, complications, and results that may be expected with the varying treatment modalities. If clinicians keep abreast of the moving edge of therapeutic investigation, we believe the patient will derive the ultimate benefit—improved therapy with reduced risks.

The Editors

Acknowledgments

We would like to extend our appreciation to all those who made possible the 23rd Annual Clinical Conference and the publication of this monograph, particularly the National Cancer Institute and the American Cancer Society, Texas Division, Inc.

Our special thanks go to the following members of the staff of M. D. Anderson Hospital, who organized the conference: Douglas E. Johnson and Melvin L. Samuels (cochairmen), Alberto G. Ayala, Liam Boyle, Emil J Freireich, David H. Hussey, Joseph G. Sinkovics, Andrew C. von Eschenbach, and Sidney Wallace.

Finally, we are grateful once again to the Publications Office of the Department of Information and Publications, M. D. Anderson Hospital, for their editorial assistance, and especially to Diane L. Culhane, Editor, for compiling and editing this volume.

Contents

Contributors

James A. Anderson, Ph.D.
Department of Diagnostic Radiology
The University of Texas System Cancer
  Center
M. D. Anderson Hospital and Tumor
  Institute
Houston, Texas 77030

Malcolm A. Bagshaw, M.D.
Division of Radiation Therapy
Department of Radiology
Stanford University School of Medicine
Stanford, California 94305

Marc T. Barrett, M.D.
Division of Urology
Baylor College of Medicine
Houston, Texas 77030

Thomas Bartholomew, M.D.
Division of Urology
Baylor College of Medicine
Houston, Texas 77030

Mostafa Batata, B.Ch., D.M.R.
Department of Radiation Therapy
Memorial Sloan-Kettering Cancer
  Center
New York, New York 10021

Prince D. Beach, M.D.
Section of Urology
Veterans Administration Hospital and
Baylor College of Medicine
Houston, Texas 77030

William R. Berry, M.D.
Department of Medicine
Duke University Medical Center
Durham, North Carolina 27710

Gerald P. Bodey, M.D.
Department of Developmental Therapeu-
  tics
The University of Texas System Cancer
  Center
M. D. Anderson Hospital and Tumor
  Institute
Houston, Texas 77030

R. Bruce Bracken, M.D.
Department of Urology
The University of Texas System Cancer
  Center
M. D. Anderson Hospital and Tumor
  Institute
Houston, Texas 77030

Barry Brown, Ph.D.
Department of Biomathematics
The University of Texas System Cancer
  Center
M. D. Anderson Hospital and Tumor
  Institute
Houston, Texas 77030

C. Eugene Carlton, Jr., M.D.
Division of Urology
Baylor College of Medicine
Houston, Texas 77030

Gerardo Chica, M.D.
Department of Urology
The University of Texas System Cancer
  Center
M. D. Anderson Hospital and Tumor
  Institute
Houston, Texas 77030

Vincent Chuang, M.D.
Department of Diagnostic Radiology
The University of Texas System Cancer
  Center
M. D. Anderson Hospital and Tumor
  Institute
Houston, Texas 77030

Edwin B. Cox, M.D.
Department of Medicine
Duke University Medical Center
Durham, North Carolina 27710

Lawrence H. Einhorn, M.D.
Department of Medicine
Indiana University School of Medicine
Indianapolis, Indiana 46202

Anne Ersil, B.Sc.
Department of Epidemiology
Queen's University
Kingston, Ontario, Canada

Fuad S. Freiha, M.D.
Division of Urology
Department of Surgery
Stanford University School of Medicine
Stanford, California 94305

Barry Green, M.D.
Department of Diagnostic Radiology
The University of Texas System Cancer
Center
M. D. Anderson Hospital and Tumor
Institute
Houston, Texas 77030

William Graham Guerriero, M.D.
Division of Urology
Baylor College of Medicine
Houston, Texas 77030

Evan M. Hersh, M.D.
Department of Developmental Therapeu-
tics
The University of Texas System Cancer
Center
M. D. Anderson Hospital and Tumor
Institute
Houston, Texas 77030

Robert C. Hickey, M.D.
Executive Vice President
The University of Texas System Cancer
Center
Director, Professor of Surgery
M. D. Anderson Hospital and Tumor
Institute
Houston, Texas 77030

Basil Hilaris, M.D.
Department of Radiation Therapy
Memorial Sloan-Kettering Cancer
Center
New York, New York 10021

Philip D. Hudgins, M.D.
Department of Radiology
The Methodist Hospital
Houston, Texas 77030

David H. Hussey, M.D.
Department of Radiotherapy
The University of Texas System Cancer
Center
M. D. Anderson Hospital and Tumor
Institute
Houston, Texas 77030

Douglas E. Johnson, M.D.
Department of Urology
The University of Texas System Cancer
Center
M. D. Anderson Hospital and Tumor
Institute
Houston, Texas 77030

John Laszlo, M.D.
Department of Medicine
Duke University Medical Center
Durham, North Carolina 27710

Charles A. LeMaistre, M.D.
President
The University of Texas System Cancer
Center
Houston, Texas 77030

John G. Maier, M.D., Ph.D.
Department of Radiation Oncology
The Fairfax Hospital
Falls Church, Virginia 22046

Lowell S. Miller, M.D.
Division of Therapeutic Radiology
Department of Radiology
Duke University Medical Center
Durham, North Carolina 27710
Present address: Department of Radio-
therapy
Park Plaza Hospital
Houston, Texas 77004

Alvaro Morales, M.D.
Department of Urology
Queen's University
Kingston, Ontario, Canada

Manuel E. Moran, M.D.
Department of Medicine
The University of Texas System Cancer
Center
M. D. Anderson Hospital and Tumor
Institute
Houston, Texas 77030

F. K. Mostofi, M.D.
Department of Genitourinary Pathology
Armed Forces Institute of Pathology
Washington, D.C. 20306

Gerald P. Murphy, M.D., D.Sc.
Director, Roswell Park Memorial Institute
Buffalo, New York 14263

David F. Paulson, M.D.
Department of Urologic Surgery
Duke University Medical Center
Durham, North Carolina 27710

David A. Pistenma, M.D.
Division of Radiation Therapy
Department of Radiology
Stanford University School of
Medicine
Stanford, California 94305

Carl Plager, M.D.
Department of Medicine
The University of Texas System Cancer
Center
M. D. Anderson Hospital and Tumor
Institute
Houston, Texas 77030

Naguib A. Samaan, M.D., Ph.D.
Department of Medicine
The University of Texas System Cancer
Center
M. D. Anderson Hospital and Tumor
Institute
Houston, Texas 77030

Melvin L. Samuels, M.D.
Department of Medicine
The University of Texas System Cancer
Center
M. D. Anderson Hospital and Tumor
Institute
Houston, Texas 77030

Joseph G. Sinkovics, M.D.
Department of Medicine
The University of Texas System Cancer
Center
M. D. Anderson Hospital and Tumor
Institute
Houston, Texas 77030

William J. Staubitz, M.D.
Department of Urology
State University of New York
Buffalo, New York 14214

David A. Swanson, M.D.
Department of Urology
The University of Texas System Cancer
Center
M. D. Anderson Hospital and Tumor
Institute
Houston, Texas 77030

Andrew C. von Eschenbach, M.D.
Department of Urology
The University of Texas System Cancer
Center
M. D. Anderson Hospital and Tumor
Institute
Houston, Texas 77030

Sidney Wallace, M.D.
Department of Diagnostic Radiology
The University of Texas System Cancer
Center
M. D. Anderson Hospital and Tumor
Institute
Houston, Texas 77030

Willet F. Whitmore, M.D.
Urologic Service
Memorial Sloan-Kettering Cancer
Center
New York, New York 10021

Alan Yagoda, M.D.
Department of Medicine
Memorial Sloan-Kettering Cancer
Center
New York, New York 10021

Introduction

Charles A. LeMaistre, M.D.

President, The University of Texas System Cancer Center

The subject of this clinical conference, cancer of the genitourinary tract, was previously addressed during the Sixth Annual Clinical Conference, in 1961. Some of the program participants for this conference also served on that program. No monograph was produced that year, but the proceedings of the conference were reviewed in *The Cancer Bulletin* in the spring of the following year.

In 1961 much less was known about genitourinary cancers than is known today, and the range of diagnostic and therapeutic tools was considerably smaller. As is true to a certain extent today, there was considerable disagreement over what types of therapy should be administered, to whom, and at what stages of disease.

Although participants in the 1961 conference concluded that "combined therapies offer the best hopes of cure," the following statements were also made: "After castration and estrogen administration [for cancer of the prostate] . . . , other therapeutic means are rarely of great help"; "In advanced, inoperable, or disseminated disease, both radioactive elements and chemical agents have been used with some degree of success to reduce suffering, prolong life, and, at least temporarily, to arrest further spread. These media are, *of course,* utilized *only when conventional therapy is ineffective or impossible,* and they do not supplant surgical removal or hormonal control"; and "The fact that five-year survival rates are approximately 30 to 40 percent with orchiectomy and hormonal therapy [for stage C prostatic cancer] discourages much use of the radical procedures."

With reference to radiotherapy, one author observed in a 1960 issue of *The Cancer Bulletin,* "new developments in supervoltage roentgenotherapy have occurred with such rapidity that a certain amount of confusion about the therapeutic value is understandable. . . . Appraisal of curative results by use of the five-year survival measurement is almost impossible in supervoltage roentgenography, because many series are small and the follow-up period is short."

Obviously, although we still are searching for a clearer understanding of the various cancers and better methods of diagnosing and staging, as well as treatment, we have made much progress. "What is past is but prologue," as Shakespeare wrote, but we might more aptly say of this subject, "You ain't seen nothin' yet!"

We wish to thank the participants in this program for accepting our invitations, and to express gratification for the high level of interest in the subject of genitourinary cancer, reflected in the highest preregistration enrollment figure in the history of the M. D. Anderson Annual Clinical Conferences, more than 750 physicians. We also express our gratitude to the cochairmen of the program committee, Drs. Douglas E. Johnson and Melvin L. Samuels, for their efforts during the past two years to organize this conference, and to the other members of the committee for their time and good advice.

This Twenty-third Annual Clinical Conference is made possible through the support of the Texas Division of the American Cancer Society, Inc., and the National Cancer Institute. And, of course, without the unstinting encouragement of The University of Texas System Board of Regents and the endorsement of the Texas Cancer Coordinating Commission, we could not reach out to so many physicians and steadily improve treatment for cancer patients everywhere.

A most important portion of our total program is the Eleventh Annual Special Pathology Conference. We are very fortunate to have as our featured speaker Dr. F. K. Mostofi, from the Armed Forces Institute of Pathology, Georgetown University Medical Center, and Johns Hopkins University School of Medicine. This pathology conference is presented by the M. D. Anderson Hospital Department of Pathology and is cosponsored by the Texas Society of Pathologists.

HEATH MEMORIAL AWARD LECTURE

Cancer of the Genitourinary Tract, edited by
D. E. Johnson and M. L. Samuels.
Raven Press, New York © 1979.

Introduction of Heath Memorial Award Recipient

Robert C. Hickey, M.D.

*Executive Vice President, The University of Texas System Cancer Center, and Director,
M. D. Anderson Hospital and Tumor Institute, Houston, Texas*

On behalf of my colleagues at M. D. Anderson Hospital and Tumor Institute, the Division of Continuing Education of the Graduate School of Biomedical Sciences, and The University of Texas Medical School, it is my very pleasant task to introduce the 1978 Heath Memorial Award recipient, Dr. Gerald P. Murphy. A man of tremendous energy and great mental and physical resources, Dr. Murphy is director of one of the three original comprehensive cancer centers, the Roswell Park Memorial Institute in Buffalo, New York.

A native of Montana, Dr. Murphy received his bachelor of science degree from Seattle University in 1955 and his M.D. degree from the University of Washington in 1959. He completed his internship and residency training at the Johns Hopkins Hospital in surgery and urology.

Dr. Murphy holds several honorary degrees and is a member of numerous professional organizations, including the American Urological Association and the American Surgical Association. He is secretary-general of the International Union Against Cancer and recently helped organize the very successful XIIth International Cancer Congress in Argentina.

Dr. Murphy has served on the National Cancer Advisory Board of the National Cancer Institute and served as chairman for the Commission on Cancer of the American College of Surgeons. He is also chief of the department of experimental surgery at Roswell Park Memorial Institute, professor of surgery at the State University of New York at Buffalo, professor of biology at Niagara University, consultant to the departments of urology of the Sisters of Charity Hospital and Millard Fillmore Hospital, and research professor of experimental pathology in the Graduate School of the State University of New York at Buffalo.

By reviewing Dr. Murphy's impressive list of publications, one can easily trace his professional career. Like all good urologists, Dr. Murphy began by studying renal stone formation, with and without infection, then turned his attention to renal physiology, surgical metabolism, anatomy, endocrinology, and renal transplantation in primates. The use of urea to reduce central nervous system edema caused by hyperosmolarity was popular at one time, but in 1960 Dr. Murphy warned the surgical world of the urinary electrolyte loss and deranged metabolism that could accompany this practice.

Dr. Murphy became involved in surgical physiology in 1962, when he became research associate and chief of the department of surgical physiology at the Walter Reed Army Institute of Research. Throughout the 1960s, Dr. Murphy published articles on cancer of the genitourinary tract, and the early 1970s saw many excellent contributions on cancer and related phenomena.

As well as being a prolific writer, Dr. Murphy is an editorial consultant to several medical and scientific journals and serves as editor-in-chief for the *Journal of Surgical Oncology* and *International Advances in Surgical Oncology.*

Dr. Murphy is a dedicated educator, researcher, and physician who has contributed significantly in each of these areas to the care and treatment of cancer patients. It is for these reasons that we honor him today by presenting to him the Heath Memorial Award.

Cancer of the Genitourinary Tract, edited by
D. E. Johnson and M. L. Samuels.
Raven Press, New York © 1979.

Prostatic Cancer: Perspectives on Progress

Gerald P. Murphy, M.D., D.Sc.

National Prostatic Cancer Project, Roswell Park Memorial Institute, Buffalo, New York

In the evolution of our knowledge about the origins and diagnosis of urologic cancer and the treatment and continuing care of patients with this disease, some major contributions have been acknowledged by all. We have an opportunity today to assess a different sort of collective progress that has greatly improved our approach, and that eventually will affect the outcome in our management of prostatic cancer.

It is a great privilege to present this brief material in the Heath Memorial Award Lecture. During these proceedings, I am sure many will acknowledge that the progress we have made together has been influenced greatly by institutions such as M. D. Anderson Hospital, and particularly by those people who have participated in clinical and scientific research.

The past decade has seen an increased and appropriate emphasis on comprehensive cancer centers. As an early prototype, M. D. Anderson Hospital's approach and concern are frequently replicated. There can be no higher tribute than the mere statement of this well-known fact, which I have seen evidence of throughout the world.

Within this same decade, efforts have focused on certain cancers, and the application of new techniques and scientific knowledge to the treatment of urologic cancer has progressed at an unprecedented rate. No one person or even institution is responsible for this progress. With this in mind, let us examine where we are going in the treatment of prostate cancer, what major improvements have been developed, and which of those are most likely to result in major benefits.

ENZYMES AND CANCER MARKERS

For decades, the key to both the diagnosis of prostatic cancer and the clinical assessment of prostatic cancer patients has been acid phosphatase activity and other enzymatic determinations. We live in a world of change and these assessments, our ability to apply them, and prospects for current improvement have changed indeed.

Since the early report of Gutman and co-workers (1936) of elevated serum acid phosphatase activity in prostatic cancer patients, particularly those with bony metastases, indirect measurement of this enzyme has been employed as a biochemical aid in diagnosis. Acid phosphatases are a group of enzymes that optimally hydrolyze esters of orthophosphoric acid in the pH range of 4.8 to 6.0. They were first identified in human erythrocytes in 1924 (Martland et al. 1924), and in this form have been found throughout the body in platelets, leukocytes, reticuloendothelial cells, the liver, the spleen, and the kidneys. The highest amounts of activity, however, are found in the epithelial cells and secretions of the prostate.

By conventional indirect substrate biochemical methods, prostatic acid phosphatase (PAP) is not usually detected in sera of healthy subjects. It has been felt in some cases of infiltrating tumors and metastatic disease of the prostate that the normal acinar connections to prostatic ducts do not develop. Thus, in those proliferating cells in which some of the synthesizing and secretory integrity of prostatic epithelium continues, there is an accumulation of PAP that diffuses into adjacent interstitial compartments and enters the bloodstream. In addition, some cells are believed to degenerate as a result of their outgrowing the nutrient blood supply, and the accumulated intracellular products are released directly to vascular channels to ultimately appear as an elevated blood level of PAP. In prostatic cancer cases, an elevation of serum acid phosphatase correlates with an advanced stage of the disease. For example, elevated levels have been reported in about 5% of those patients whose disease is confined to the prostate (Huggins and Hodges 1941), and the percentages increase dramatically to 20% and 80%, respectively, in cases in which there is extracapsular extension of the tumor or clinical disease metastatic to the bone (Woodard 1959, Sodeman and Batsakis 1977, Murphy et al. 1969).

No fewer than eight different substrates have been widely used to measure serum acid phosphatase. Unfortunately, they vary in terms of sensitivity, specificity, or both, for PAP and other serum phosphatases (Yam 1974). Moreover, the acid phosphatase activity values reported in the literature, resulting from the spectrophotometric analysis of the inorganic phosphate or organic moieties released from the particular substrate added to the serum, can differ even within the same sample when test conditions such as substrate concentration and degree of serum acid phosphatase elevation vary.

Inhibitors have been used to determine the activity of a specific enzyme in serum samples. Of the various compounds available, tartrate was considered the most useful clinically for prostatic cancer (Murphy et al. 1969), since it inhibits over 90% of prostatic acid phosphatase activity. However, tartrate also inhibits, without distinction, the hepatic, splenic, and renal sources of this enzyme, so the procedure can also produce misleading results if elevated serum acid phosphatase is due to altered output from these organs.

Additional sources of error include variation in pH, which affects the stability of acid phosphatase, substrate acidity, and storage temperature. In normal subjects, serum acid phosphatase levels do not exhibit a detectable circadian variation, in contrast to the well-defined diurnal pattern exhibited by patients with prostatic cancer (Batsakis et al. 1970). There are many other extraneous factors.

With advanced technology, new methods for identifying and measuring the isoenzymatic forms of PAP have been sought in recent years. This intense research effort has resulted in the development of several highly specific and extremely sensitive assays that hold great promise for screening for and early detection of prostatic cancer. A successful national trial in 32 states and the District of Columbia has been completed under the sponsorship of the American Cancer Society Task Force on Prostate Cancer.

Among the first significant improvements reported were descriptions of new methods that combined the specificity of immunologic methodology with the sensitivity of radioisotopic techniques (Foti et al. 1975b, Cooper and Foti 1974). Such methods are capable of detecting human PAP in a normal range in human male subjects of 0.5 to 7.2 ng/100 μl. This radioimmunoassay (RIA) is four to five times more sensitive than the enzymatic method using p-nitrophenyl-phosphate as a substrate. In the presence of intracapsular prostatic malignancy and in advanced extracapsular disease, such RIA techniques were twice as sensitive (Cooper et al. 1978a). However, false-positive results were recorded in 5.6% of the normal male controls. In a recent report in which a double-antibody radioimmunoassay was used to measure PAP, normal values fell within the range of 1.6 $\pm$ 0.8 ng/100 μl and levels higher than 4.0 ng/100 μl were found in patients with prostatic cancer (Choe et al. 1978).

There is no doubt, however, that the RIA techniques offer extreme sensitivity, high specificity, quantifiable results, and even the capability for determining "inactivated" PAP. Nevertheless, these procedures are complex and require a considerable degree of technical expertise to perform correctly. Other drawbacks include a 98-hour period to perform the test, instability of the isotopically labelled PAP, the use of radioactive materials requiring much precaution, and the average cost of $20 to $50 per assay.

Another immunoassay for PAP is counter-immunoelectrophoresis (CIEP), described by Chu and co-workers (1976). CIEP, after careful evaluation and comparison with RIA (McDonald et al. 1978, Chu et al. 1978), is favored for its relative simplicity, high sensitivity (comparable to that of RIA), and low cost ($3 per assay). Of particular importance in clinical application is the short period required to complete a test (two hours). In an early clinical trial (Chu et al. 1978), positive results were obtained on sera from patients with surgically staged prostatic carcinoma (6/20 stage B patients, 27/49 stage C, and 98/125 stage D). For some patients, measurements were obtained while they were undergoing treatment, which explains in part why some expected elevations did not occur within this period. Equally impressive was the fact that sera from 19 patients with benign prostatic hypertrophy (BPH), 89 patients with nonprostatic tumors, 12 patients with Gaucher's disease, 107 healthy volunteers, and 50 normal age-matched men all gave negative results (Chu et al. 1978).

The need for more clinical data and comparisons of RIA and CIEP in many laboratories in the United States led to a recent national field trial (August

Table 1. *Results of Acid Phosphatase Tests Performed by Individual Hospitals: Biochemical and CIEP Methods*

Stage	No. of Samples Tested	Percent Positive	
		Biochemical*	CIEP
A	64	12	38
B	178	11	35
C	235	17	49
D	485	51	69
Total	962	33	56

* Substrate method.

1978) coordinated by the National Prostatic Cancer Project and sponsored by the American Cancer Society (Tables 1 and 2). The specificity, reproducibility, and accuracy of these methods were verified by data contributed by over 25 institutions. The results with CIEP revealed a high rate of positive PAP tests in the early stages of prostate cancer, when elevations of serum acid phosphatase using conventional tests are rarely found (Woodard 1959). Moreover, other studies have shown that bone marrow acid phosphatase levels are of no added value (Cooper et al. 1978b, Belville et al. 1978, Sadlowski 1978, Boehme et al. 1978, Catane et al. 1978), regardless of the test used.

The advantages and disadvantages of the CIEP and RIA procedures may soon be irrelevant, as an even newer generation of assays is being developed. One such method (Lee et al. 1978) is a new solid-phase immunofluorometric assay that has a sensitivity of 60 pg/ml PAP, which is about 1,000 times more sensitive than RIA or CIEP. One distinctive advantage of this procedure is that the antibody can be reused in subsequent assays. Sera of patients (men and women) with nonprostatic cancer had normal serum acid phosphatase levels, which in healthy males averaged 5.619 ng/ml PAP (range = 1.399 to 9.839 ng/ml). However, patients with early stages of documented, surgically staged prostatic cancer exhibited elevated levels of serum PAP. Encouraging data such as these and those anticipated from other groups developing improved assays for serum PAP indicate that routine screening for prostatic cancer will soon be possible.

We observed in an earlier study that human PAP seems to have a different

Table 2. *Results of the CIEP Test in Pilot Study Performed at Roswell Park Memorial Institute*

Stage	No. of Samples Tested	Percent Positive
A	—	—
B	30	20
C	56	54
D	183	85
Total	269	71

site for its antibody bindings than for its enzyme activity (Chu et al. 1978). Foti and co-workers (1975a) have reported a similar observation. This is the basis for development of the CIEP technique, as well as for solid-phase fluorescent immunoassay of this clinically important enzyme. Anti-PAP (in the IgG fraction) is conjugated to Sepharose 4B to form a solid phase that specifically binds acid phosphatase of prostate origin. This solid-phase anti-PAP antibody not only separates PAP from other phosphatases and serum proteins, but also stabilizes the enzyme. Subsequently, the activity of PAP is measured by the hydrolyzed product, α-naphthol, which is fluorogenic and can be quantitated by spectrophotofluorometry with great sensitivity (Lee et al. 1978).

While progress has been made in determining the specificity of acid phosphatase, improved clinical applications for other isoenzymes, such as serum alkaline phosphatase, have been achieved. These results, while perhaps not as striking because of current technical limitations, nevertheless have provided an additional means of objectively evaluating patients with advanced disease. We have found them of particular value in patients undergoing chemotherapy at the various National Prostatic Cancer Project participating institutions, including M. D. Anderson Hospital.

Figure 1 shows the relationship between initial levels of total and bone alkaline

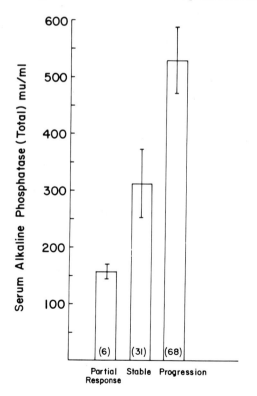

Figure 1. Relationship between initial levels of total and bone alkaline phosphatase and three categories of clinical response.

( ) Number of patients

phosphatase and three categories of clinical response (partial regression, stable disease, and progression), regardless of the treatment given. The patients with the lowest total or bone alkaline phosphatase level, or both, at the beginning of treatment achieved the best clinical response. Those with high levels of the enzyme at the start of therapy did not frequently respond to treatment. The differences in the enzyme levels in these three groups of patients were statistically significant at the level of $p < 0.01$. These measurements may have some prognostic value.

A significant number of patients had more than 25% reduction in the enzyme level when they obtained a partial response or when the disease had stabilized (Table 3). Of 22 patients with progression of disease, 20 (91%) did not show reduction in the total alkaline phosphatase level. The differences between partial response and progression groups were statistically significant. A decrease in the bone alkaline phosphatase level was found in 17 of 24 patients (71%) with partial response or with stabilization of disease (Table 4). Of the 22 patients who failed to respond to treatment, 16 (73%) did not show a decrease in the enzyme level.

The alkaline phosphatase levels also were analyzed in another group of patients participating in the National Prostatic Cancer Project. In 357 patients with proven bone metastases, 305 (85%) had elevated total alkaline phosphatase levels, mainly owing to elevation of the bone isoenzyme fraction. Fifty-two patients (15%) had normal levels of total alkaline phosphatase, despite having widespread bone metastases; however, 22 of these 52 patients also had abnormally high levels of bone alkaline phosphatase. In 12 of 17 patients, no liver involvement was found at autopsy and the mean total alkaline phosphatase level was elevated (233 mU/ml), owing to an increase in the bone isoenzyme fraction. The liver isoenzyme was normal, with a mean value of 46.3 mU/ml. In the five patients with proven liver metastases, the elevation of alkaline phosphatase was mainly due to an increased liver isoenzyme fraction with a mean value of 309 mU/ml. In three patients, no clinical suspicion of liver metastases was encountered and the elevation of the liver alkaline phosphatase could have been the first clue to liver involvement.

Table 3. *Total Alkaline Phosphatase at Time of Response*

Clinical Status*	No. of Pts. With More Than 25% Decrease	No. of Pts. With Less Than 25% Decrease	Totals
Partial response	4	1	5
Stable disease	8	11	19
Progression	2	20	22
Total	14	32	46

$p < 0.003$, partial response versus progression group and stable disease versus progression group.
* Schmidt et al. (1976).

Table 4. *Bone Alkaline Phosphatase at Time of Response*

Clinical Status	No. of Pts. With More Than 25% Decrease	No. of Pts. With Less Than 25% Decrease	Totals
Partial response	5	0	5
Stable disease	12	7	19
Progression	6	16	22
Total	23	23	46

$p < 0.01$, partial response versus progression group; $p < 0.03$, stable disease versus progression group.

Liver metastases in prostatic cancer patients were found in only 20% at autopsy. When recognized clinically, such metastases generally have indicated a poor prognosis and short life expectancy.

THE HISTOPATHOLOGY OF PRIMARY PROSTATIC CANCER

There can be no evaluation of end results nor application of new treatments in urologic oncology without a histologic diagnosis that provides a common language for describing prognosis, or at least a common means of assessing treatment results in patients who have undergone new treatments for cure or palliation. The histology of prostatic cancer has, regrettably, lacked a universal language, as well as, perhaps, any agreement on the essentials. However, in the past year, something remarkable has transpired. I would like to share the contributing events with you, while reemphasizing that they were made possible by many participating in this symposium, as well as others throughout the United States and elsewhere.

During 1978, a series of workshops was held to evaluate four major systems for the histologic grading of prostatic cancer at Fairview Hospital (Minneapolis), the Armed Forces Institute of Pathology, the Mayo Clinic and Foundation, and Roswell Park Memorial Institute (Murphy and Whitmore 1978). These conferences were designed to be multidisciplinary, including urologists (27), pathologists (24), radiotherapists (7), scientists (9), and biostatisticians and clinicians (5 each). They reviewed four currently employed, well-known systems of histologic classification against the background of available patient survival data, and included objective critiques by individuals not necessarily identified with any particular classification. Finally, all conferees attended a review and summary session sponsored by the American Cancer Society in June 1978 at Roswell Park Memorial Institute.

The Veterans Administration Cooperative Urological Research Group (VACURG) for prostatic cancer has evolved since 1966 a system for the histologic grading of prostatic cancer (Gleason 1966, 1977). The Gleason system is based upon the degree of glandular differentiation and the growth pattern of the tumor in relation to the prostatic stroma (Figure 2). The pattern may vary from a well-formed and questionably malignant grade 1 to an undifferentiated grade 5. The Gleason system assigns a histologic grade both to the predominant primary pattern and to any secondary pattern (Gleason 1966, 1977). In this regard it differs from all other systems, which judge the histologic grade on the basis of the most undifferentiated portion or the most representative (largest) portion of the material examined. Although the Gleason experience suggests that the histologic pattern of a tumor remains the same throughout the life of the host, the evidence is limited.

Experience within and outside of the workshops has demonstrated that the Gleason system is easily learned and reasonably reproducible. Although Dr. Gleason estimates his own reproducibility rate with this system to be 80%, in others' studies reproducibility has been approximately 70%. The margin of error of reproducibility from one institution to another could be as much as 50% and probably reflects the experience of and instruction given to the observer.

Although clinical staging information has been used in conjunction with the Gleason system to identify patient groups that correlate remarkably well with patient survival, it has generally been agreed that such combinations of histologic classification and clinical staging should not be universally adopted in evaluating histologic grading systems, since criteria of clinical staging vary in different places and at different times and since most reported systems of histologic grading have not incorporated such analyses.

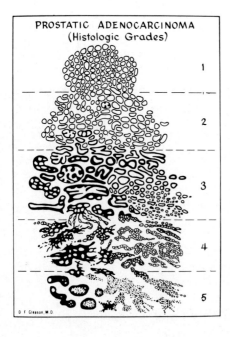

PROSTATIC ADENOCARCINOMA
(Histologic Grades)

Figure 2. Simplified drawing of histologic patterns, emphasizing degree of glandular differentiation and relation to stroma. Fundamental criteria for each grade include: (1) single, separate, uniform glands, tightly packed; (2) single, separate, uniform glands, loosely packed; (3) single, separate, varying glands, in varying distribution and/or smoothly or sharply circumscribed, papillary or cribriform masses; (4) raggedly infiltrating masses of fused glands (papillary, cribriform, or quite solid, dark or clear cells); (5) raggedly infiltrating anaplastic tumor and/or "comedocarcinoma." (Reproduced with permission from Gleason, D. F. 1977. *In* Tannenbaum, M. (ed.): Urologic Pathology: The Prostate. Lea & Febiger, Philadelphia, pp. 171–197.)

Needle biopsies were used in the Veterans Administration cooperative study in approximately 60% of 2,911 cases (Gleason 1966,1977). Although results with transurethral resection or open prostatectomy specimens were not necessarily superior to those with an adequate needle biopsy for purposes of histologic grading, the need for adequate and representative tissue sampling was repeatedly stressed.

Evaluation of the clinical relevance of the Gleason system, using cancer deaths as a reference point, has significant potential limitations in providing the clinician with prospective insights into tumor behavior, but all histologic grading systems reviewed share this limitation.

The system of grading primary prostatic cancer employed at the Armed Forces Institute of Pathology (Gleason and Mellinger 1974, Harada et al. 1977, Mellinger et al. 1967) depends primarily on two features: (1) the degree of nuclear anaplasia (slight, moderate, or marked), and (2) the pattern of glandular differentiation (large glands, small glands such as microacini or fused glands, cribriform appearance, and columns and cords). The latter feature corresponds to that used by Gleason. In fact, independent of the nuclear appearance in the primary tumor, a good correlation with the Gleason system was achieved by pathologists at the Armed Forces Institute of Pathology using glandular pattern as the principal grading criterion. In the Mostofi system (Mostofi 1975), the absence of a glandular pattern in any tumor, i.e., cords or sheets of cells, automatically implies a grade 3 lesion. Unlike the Gleason system, only one level of histologic grading is assigned by this system and that is based upon the predominant feature noted from inspection of all available material, although no attempt has been made to define what constitutes adequate material.

A classification system combining the histologic features of glandular pattern and nuclear cytology was presented by Dr. John Gaeta and has been used by the National Prostatic Cancer Project. The essential elements of this classification system are as follows:

Grade I—Glands well defined, medium and large. Separated by scant stroma. Cells uniform and normal size. Nucleoli may be present, but inconspicuous.

Grade II—Glands medium and small. Moderate amount of stroma. Cells slightly pleomorphic. Nucleoli predominant.

Grade III—Glands contain small acini. Frequent loss of glandular organization. Cribriform and scirrhous patterns. Cells show pronounced pleomorphism. Nuclei often vesicular. Acidorphilic nucleoli.

Grade IV—Glands contain round, expansile masses of tumor cells. No formation of glands. Cells small or large, uniform or pleomorphic, with significant mitotic activity.

This system was demonstrated to be simple, objective, and reproducible. In addition, retrospective studies demonstrated a good correlation between tumor grade and length of survival (Table 5).

The grading system used at the Mayo Clinic to classify prostatic cancer distin-

Table 5. *Correlation of Gaeta's Grades of Prostatic Carcinoma to Patient Survival Years*

Grade	No. of Patients	Total Years Surviving	No. Dead	No. Dead of Carcinoma	Correlation Between Grade and Years of Survival
1	6 (4%)	27.3	2	1 (50%)	0.036
2	43 (25%)	161.5	25	16 (64%)	0.099
3	83 (49%)	332.4	67	60 (89%)	0.180
4	37 (22%)	98.0	36	34 (94%)	0.346
Total	169	619.2	130	111	

guishes four grades on the basis of seven histologic criteria: (1) acinar structure, (2) individual cellular structure, (3) nuclear characteristics, (4) presence of nucleoli, (5) cytoplasmic characteristics, (6) mitotic activity, and (7) degree of invasiveness. This system has similarities to the Gleason, Mostofi, and Gaeta systems. Since it has fewer categories (four grades), it does not provide a greater degree of discrimination than the Gleason system. Like the Mostofi and Gaeta systems, it designates a tumor grade on the basis of predominant features and does not provide both a primary and secondary grade, as used by Gleason (Gleason 1966, 1977).

All classification systems have to deal with a number of basic considerations: (1) the tissue available for sampling, (2) the objective definability of grading criteria, (3) the degree of reproducibility of interpretation, (4) simplicity, and (5) the predictive value of the system relative to the biologic potential of the tumor. All the systems discussed meet these requirements equally well. Conventional systems of grading give some insight into local growth kinetics, i.e., the growth rate and ability of a tumor to infiltrate locally, and systemic growth kinetics, i.e., the tendency of a tumor to metastasize. However, at the present level of information, grading systems reliably predict neither the lethal potential of a tumor in an individual patient nor the responsiveness of an individual tumor to various forms of therapy. Caution must be exercised in using tumor grade in the individual patient as a basis for treatment selection.

The need for methods of determining the biologic potential of a tumor has repeatedly been emphasized. The nuclear and cytologic features of the tumor cell are potential sources of insight in this regard, and the usefulness of electron microscopy in such assessments also requires further study. The Gleason system does not use the cellular or nuclear features of tumors in classification, and prospective studies may profitably incorporate analysis of such characteristics in determining their potential clinical relevance.

Scattered observations suggest that the histologic appearance of metastatic prostatic lesions in the regional lymph nodes is similar to that in the primary tumors. However, more and better information is needed as to whether or not the histologic grade of a given tumor may change with time, treatment, or both. Evidence has been presented that patients with poorly differentiated prostatic tumors, as classified by the modified Mayo Clinic or Gleason system, generally have a greater frequency of increased serum acid phosphatase levels, a greater likelihood of positive pelvic lymph nodes, and an overall poorer survival than patients with better differentiated tumors.

The overall current consensus is that the Gleason system should tentatively be adopted as the pathologic reference point for classifying patients. This system can be used in conjunction with other systems. It seems definable, reproducible, and reasonably simple, and has clinical relevance, as judged by correlations with patient survival. Further study may demonstrate advantages from incorporation of the nuclear or cytologic characteristics of tumor cells into the Gleason system.

Thus, we can see there has been considerable progress in arriving at a consensus on the histological language of assessment of primary prostatic cancer. This useful concurrence will doubtless have a great impact on our evaluation of clinical trials and other modalities of assessment within the next few years.

RECEPTOR SITES

Unlike our colleagues in breast cancer treatment, we who have anticipated much in the prostatic cancer field have been hampered by methodological concerns in attempts to evaluate the presence of both androgenic and estrogenic receptors in human prostatic cancer. Within the past 24 months, developments in several laboratories have contributed to achievements in methodology and exchange of data that will now permit such progress. Early in 1979, an international workshop will contribute to further dialogue and presentation of very recent results. I would like to refer to the work in our own laboratories, briefly, to illustrate some of our basis for optimism today (Karr et al. 1978d).

Studies on cancer of the prostate have led to the characterization and measurement of androgen receptors in the human gland (Geller et al. 1975, Davies and Griffiths 1975, Rosen et al. 1975, Hawkins et al. 1977, Mobbs et al. 1977, Snochowski et al. 1977, Menon et al. 1977, 1978), but the case for the presence of estrogen receptors, to date, is not so well developed (Hawkins et al. 1975, 1976, Bashirelahi and Young 1976b, Bashirelahi et al. 1976). Measurement of specific estradiol-17β (E_2) and dihydrotestosterone (DHT) binding in the human prostate is complicated by the high affinity with which these steroids bind to intracellular receptors and sex hormone binding globulin (SHBG). High endogenous concentrations of DHT in the human prostate and lack of cellular and biologic uniformity in specimens analyzed has also increased the difficulty of assaying and interpreting human prostate receptor profiles.

With this background, we first characterized E_2 and DHT receptors in the baboon *(Papio anubis)* prostate (Figure 3). To obviate spurious findings resulting from the contamination of prostate cytosols with serum proteins, we used compounds that have negligible affinity for SHBG but compete selectively for E_2 and DHT receptors. This is an essential characteristic of nonradioactive competitors used in quantitative receptor assays in which the calculation of specific binding is based on the difference between total and nonspecific binding components. After demonstrating that diethylstilbestrol (DES) and cyproterone acetate

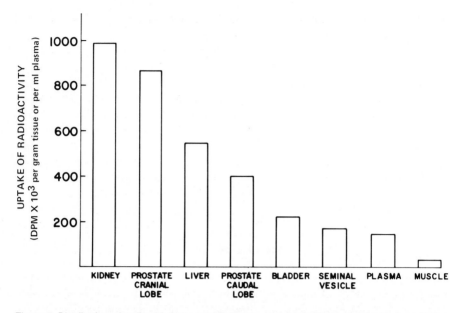

Figure 3. Distribution of radioactivity in various tissues and organs following the in vivo infusion of 1 mCi (^{3}H)-E_2 into each hypogastric artery of a male baboon. Except for the organs that metabolize and/or excrete E_2, the highest levels of radioactivity were present in the caudal and cranial lobes of the prostate.

(CA) are useful for this purpose, we measured E_2 and DHT receptors in the human prostate (Karr et al. 1978d).

These concentrations suggested the possibility of identifying an estrogen receptor in the baboon prostate. Subsequently, multiple point analyses of E_2 binding in cytosol from the caudal and cranial lobes of a baboon that had been castrated 40 hours previously were conducted following two-hour incubations at 4°C. These studies revealed a steroid binding protein that has a finite binding capacity (saturable) and strongly binds (high affinity) E_2.

Cytosols of two surgical specimens from prostatic cancer patients who were receiving DES therapy were analyzed for cytosol estrogen receptors. Multiple point analyses of E_2 binding following incubation (20 hours at 0–4°C) with decreasing concentrations of (^{3}H)-E_2 in the presence or absence of 100-fold molar excesses of DES yielded similar N and K_d values. In one 70-year-old patient, 3.2 femtomoles/mg cytosol protein were measured and the apparent K_d was 0.23×10^{-10} M. This tissue specimen had been frozen (<20°C) for 43 days prior to this analysis. Corresponding values for tissue obtained at transurethral resection of the prostate from a 64-year-old patient were 6.5 and 0.16 $\times 10^{-10}$ M. The tissues used in both analyses were taken from specimens that were poorly differentiated histologically (Karr et al. 1978d).

Initial results of steps taken to develop a single point measurement for E_2 binding in needle biopsy specimens are outlined in Table 6. The assay values

Table 6. Prostate Needle Biopsies: Bound Estradiol Displaced (%) by DES

Age of Patient	Endocrine Therapy*	Tissue Wt. (mg)	Concentration (^{3}H)-E$_2$ (nM) Incubated	% Competition	Histologic Differentiation	Treatment	6-Month Follow-up
64	None	13.7	0.5	54	Well	a,b	Stable disease
59	None	15.8	0.5	47	Moderately	♂-x†	—
62	Tace, ♂-x	27.7	0.5	43	Moderately	a,c	Objective remission
58	♂-x, 2 yr; Estracyt, 2 mo	19.9	0.5	28	Well	a,c	Objective remission
64	None	19.4	0.5	22	Moderately	b,d†	—
54	None	22.0	0.5	22	Moderately	a,c	Stable disease
76	None	16.6	0.5	22	Poorly	None	Stable disease
66	DES, ♂-x; Estracyt, 1 mo	22.2	1.5	15	Poorly	a,c	Progression
		11.2	1.5	10			
62	DES	12.9	0.5	5	Moderately	b†	—
71	Estracyt	7.0	1.5	0	Poorly	a,c	Progression
67	DES, ♂-x	13.1	1.5	0	Poorly	a,c	Progression

* At time of biopsy: 20-hour incubations in presence of 0.5 nM (^{3}H)-E$_2$; 2-hour incubations in presence of 1.5 nM (^{3}H)-E$_2$.
Treatment code: †, recommended; a, chemotherapy; b, DES; c, Estracyt; d, radiation.

are expressed as the percent reduction of (^3H)-E_2 binding in the presence of a 100-fold molar excess of DES. The average weight of the 12 specimens analyzed was 16.8 mg.

In contrast to our analyses of prostate tissue obtained at surgery, we were unable to demonstrate estrogen receptors in tissue obtained at various postmortem intervals that had been preserved ($<20°C$) from one day to 3.5 years (Table 7). Two of the 12 samples were BPH specimens, and the remaining 10 were from men ranging widely in age and without clinical or gross morphologic symptoms of prostatic cancer. However, in six of 10 specimens in which we also measured the androgen binding capacity of the cytosol, we were able to identify specific receptors for DHT (Karr et al. 1978d). The number of specific binding sites was lowest in the two BPH specimens (4.1 and 14.3 femtomoles) and the highest value measured (129.3 femtomoles) was from a specimen that had been excised at autopsy six hours after death and frozen for 10 days before the assay was conducted (Karr et al. 1978d).

The present study extends the findings of previous investigations, in which the affinity of SHBG for DES was reported to be negligible (Karr et al. 1978b, Gardner and Wittliff 1973). The capacities of the three natural and three synthetic steroids used in this study to bind with human SHBG and to compete with (^3H)-DHT for SHBG binding sites have previously been reported (Karr et al. 1978b), and revealed the same competitive ranking order as the present data determined for the baboon. A similar case for cyproterone acetate, a compound with known high affinity for androgen receptors, has also been documented for baboon (Karr et al. 1978a) and human serum SHBG (Davies and Griffiths 1975). The value of CA and DES as nonlabelled competitors in androgen and estrogen receptor analyses for use in prostate cytosol preparations contaminated with serum is thus apparent (Karr et al. 1978d).

Table 7. *Hormone Receptor Assays of Human Prostate*

Age of Patient	Postmortem Excision (hr)	Preservation $<-20°C$ (days)	DHT-R_c	
			N*	K_d
88[†]	6	1,436	4.1	$0.21 \times 10^{-9}M$
51[†]	1	29	14.3	$0.24 \times 10^{-9}M$
23	12	10	19.4	$0.99 \times 10^{-9}M$
55	5	28	40.1	$0.47 \times 10^{-9}M$
58	14	120	45.1	$1.0 \times 10^{-9}M$
28	12	1	49.6	$1.8 \times 10^{-9}M$
34	6	10	129.3	$4.0 \times 10^{-9}M$
40	1.5	911	0	0
43	10	7	—	—
57	8	14	—	—
58	5	1,095	0	0
64	1	1,095	0	0

* Femtomoles/mg cytosol protein.
† Benign prostate hypertrophy specimen.

Evaluation of the data showing competition by DES with (^3H)-E_2 for binding sites in cytosols from needle biopsy specimens suggests that those patients receiving hormonal therapy (DES or Estracyt) have fewer available binding sites for (^3H)-E_2. Whether these differences are due entirely to previous therapy or to tumor variation has yet to be investigated. Concurrent analysis of androgen receptor content in biopsy samples (Mobbs et al. 1978) would also allow us to predict more accurately the hormone dependency of a prostatic tumor in a manner analogous to the receptor profile analyses performed routinely on primary and metastatic tissue from breast cancer patients (Karr et al. 1978d).

Further study is required to obtain a better understanding of the relation of receptors to hormone responsiveness and differentiation of prostatic tissue, particularly since many factors are known to affect the measurement and interpretation of receptor data. Methodology is known to be a major variable (Menon et al. 1977). Other factors include age of patient, pathology, source of tissue, endocrine status of patient, previous and ongoing therapy, and method and duration of tissue preservation. Our data suggest that autopsy specimens are not ideal for E_2 receptor research. These (Karr et al. 1978d) and other studies (Karr et al. 1978c) suggest that a standard assay for hormone receptor profiles in human prostatic tissue may help clinicians select optimal therapeutic management of prostatic cancer patients in the near future.

These results are preliminary and related in part to developments in a small number of laboratories. There will certainly be further modifications and comments on specificity. Nevertheless, I am sure you share my great hope for an explosion of knowledge and its application and an improvement in our targeting of therapy for prostate cancer patients.

FUTURE PERSPECTIVES

Future perspectives in prostate cancer that may affect our concerns today have been summarized recently by Dr. Douglas Johnson, head of the Department of Urology of M. D. Anderson Hospital and Tumor Institute (Johnson 1978). This reference details additional factors that time will not permit me to summarize or allude to now. Fellow students of this disease process should refer to this important contribution.

We have reviewed the importance of the presence of endocrine receptors in human prostatic cancers. The development of agents to carry, as endocrine vehicles, a cytotoxic agent to such malignant tumors is still in its infancy (Kadohama et al. 1979), but these and other prototypes are currently undergoing preclinical, clinical, and randomized trial evaluation by the National Prostatic Cancer Project. I would be remiss not to acknowledge the many contributions this group has made towards the application of such agents. Although the study of this new class of drugs, their metabolism, and their primary site of action is still unfolding, these drugs are not envisioned as forms of palliation, but as adjuvant therapy and earlier forms of treatment. Figure 4 illustrates the mechanism of action of Estracyt, which can be summarized as follows:

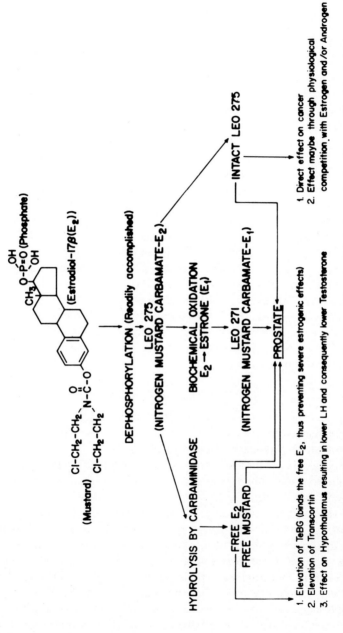

Figure 4. Schematic presentation of the mechanisms of action of Estracyt (nitrogen mustard carbamate-E₂-phosphate) in cancer of the prostate.

1. Dephosphorylation of Estracyt (i.e., removal of the phosphate group at position 17) is readily accomplished in all body tissues and fluids, yielding Leo 275.
2. Three different fates may befall Leo 275:
   a. Hydrolysis into its two constituents, estradiol-17β(E_2) and N-nitrogen mustard;
   b. Oxidation of the E_2 moiety to estrone (E_1), leading to Leo 271;
   c. Direct access of Leo 275 to tissues, including the prostate.
   These three events can all take place in the prostate.
3. The systemically liberated E_2 leads to the following:
   a. Evaluation of plasma testosterone-estradiol binding globulin, which binds the bulk of circulating E_2 (and T), possibly preventing excessive estrogenic effects;
   b. Elevation of plasma transcortin and cortisol concentrations due to the binding of the latter to the former;
   c. Decrease in circulating luteinizing hormone (probably through an effect at the pituitary-hypothalamic level), leading to decreased T production;
   d. Possible direct effect on the prostate.
4. The liberated N-nitrogen mustard may have a direct effect on the prostate.
5. Intact Leo 275 (and possibly 271) may physiologically compete with androgens and/or estrogens in the prostate, the effect depending on the concentration of the compound in the tissue (Muntzing, unpublished results). Also, Leo 275 may have a direct effect on cancerous cells of the prostate.

The effects of these agents have been demonstrated in vivo and in vitro (Kadohama et al. 1978), and the evidence confirms their primary cytotoxic action.

Adjuvant trials, however, are a problem (Higgins 1978). Clinical oncologic research has been primarily concerned with patients in the advanced stages of disease, when there is a high mortality and median survival is measured in months. The precise degree and meaning of responses in these patients can be difficult to determine (Higgins 1978). If a primary treatment modality produces a generally high or prolonged survival rate, large numbers of patients must be followed for a long period of time to detect the therapeutic benefit from the addition of the adjuvant therapy, and a therapeutic benefit may be impossible to detect with certainty. However, there are other ways to measure the treatment effect, such as disease-free interval, recurrence rate, and time from the appearance of metastatic disease.

We are entering an era in which biological benefit to patients can be measured by new treatments and unfolding techniques. Let us no longer speak of standard treatments and so-called proven results, but of these new techniques and treatments, which can only improve the prospects of patients with prostatic cancer.

It has been a privilege to share these viewpoints with you, and to present the Heath Memorial Award Lecture for 1978.

ACKNOWLEDGMENT

This investigation was supported by grant number 50175–04 awarded by the National Cancer Institute, Department of Health, Education and Welfare.

REFERENCES

Bashirelahi, N., J. H. O'Toole, and J. D. Young. 1976. A specific 17β-estradiol receptor in human benign hypertrophic prostate. Biochem. Med. 15:254–261.

Bashirelahi, N., and J. D. Young. 1976. Specific binding protein for 17β-estradiol in prostate with adenocarcinoma. Urology 8:553–558.

Batsakis, J. G., R. O. Briere, and S. F. Markel. 1970. Diagnostic Enzymology. American Society of Clinical Pathologists, Commission on Continuing Education, Chicago, pp. 1–231.

Belville, W. D., H. D. Cox, D. E. Mahan, J. P. Olmert, B. T. Mittemeyer, and A. W. Bruce. 1978. Bone marrow acid phosphatase by radioimmunoassay. Cancer 41:2286–2291.

Boehme, W. M., R. R. Augspurger, S. F. Wallner, and R. E. Donohue. 1978. Lack of usefulness of bone marrow enzymes and calcium in staging patients with prostatic cancer. Cancer 41:1433–1439.

Catane, R., S. Madajewicz, Z. L. Wajsman, T. M. Chu, A. Mittelman, and G. P. Murphy. 1978. Prostatic cancer: Immunochemical detection of prostatic acid phosphatase in serum and bone marrow. N.Y. State J. Med. 78:1060–1061.

Choe, B. K., E. J. Pontes, M. K. Morrison, and N. R. Rose. 1978. Human prostatic acid phosphatases. II. A double-antibody radioimmunoassay. Arch. Androl. 1:227–233.

Chu, T. M., M. C. Wang, R. Kajdasz, E. A. Barnard, R. Kucil, and G. P. Murphy. 1976. Prostate specific acid phosphohydrolase in the diagnosis of prostatic cancer. (Abstract) Proc. Am. Assoc. Cancer Res. 17:191.

Chu, T. M., M. C. Wang, W. W. Scott, R. P. Gibbons, D. E. Johnson, J. D. Schmidt, S. A. Loening, G. R. Prout, and G. P. Murphy. 1978. Immunochemical detection of serum prostatic acid phosphatase: Methodology and clinical evaluation. Invest. Urol. 15:319–323.

Cooper, J. F., and A. Foti. 1974. A radioimmunoassay for prostatic acid phosphatase. I. Methodology and range of normal male serum values. Invest. Urol. 12:98–102.

Cooper, J. F., A. Foti, H. H. Herschman, and W. Findle. 1978a. A solid phase radioimmunoassay for prostatic acid phosphatase. J. Urol. 119:386–391.

Cooper, J. F., A. G. Foti, and P. W. Shank. 1978b. Radioimmunochemical measurement of bone marrow prostatic acid phosphatase. J. Urol. 119:392–395.

Davies, P., and K. Griffiths. 1975. Similarities between 5α-dihydrotestosterone-receptor complexes from human and rat prostatic tissue: Effects on RNA polymerase activity. Mol. Cell. Endocrinol. 3:143–164.

Foti, A. G., M. M. Glovsky, and J. F. Cooper. 1975a. The effect of antibody on human prostatic acid phosphatase activity. I. Temperature and pH stabilization of acid phosphatase enzyme activity by rabbit antibody to acid phosphatase. Immunochemistry 12:131–136.

Foti, A., H. Herschman, and J. F. Cooper. 1975b. A solid-phase radioimmunoassay for human prostatic acid phosphatase. Cancer Res. 35:2446–2452.

Gardner, D. G., and J. L. Wittliff. 1973. Specific estrogen receptors in the lactating mammary gland of the rat. Biochemistry 12:3090–3096.

Geller, J., T. Cantor, and J. Albert. 1975. Evidence for a specific dihydrotestosterone-binding cytosol receptor in the human prostate. J. Clin. Endocrinol. Metab. 41:854–862.

Gleason, D. F. 1966. Classification of prostatic carcinomas. Cancer Chemother. Rep. 50:125–128.

Gleason, D. F. 1977. Histologic grading and clinical staging of prostatic carcinoma, in Urologic Pathology: The Prostate, M. Tannenbaum, ed. Lea & Febiger, Philadelphia, pp. 171–197.

Gleason, D. F., and G. T. Mellinger. 1974. Veterans Administration Cooperative Urological Research Group: Predictions of prognosis for prostatic adenocarcinoma and combined histological grading and clinical staging. J. Urol. 111:58–64.

Gutman, E. B., E. E. Sproul, and A. B. Gutman. 1936. Significance of increased phosphatase activity of bone at the site of osteoplastic metastases secondary to carcinoma of prostate gland. Am. J. Cancer 28:485–495.

Harada, M., F. K. Mostofi, D. K. Corle, D. P. Byar, and B. F. Trump. 1977. Preliminary studies of histologic prognosis in cancer of the prostate. Cancer Treat. Rep. 61:223–225.

Hawkins, E. F., M. Nijs, and C. Brassinne. 1976. Steroid receptors in the human prostate. 2. Some properties of the estrophilic molecule of benign prostatic hypertrophy. Biochem. Biophys. Res. Commun. 70:854–861.

Hawkins, E. F., M. Nijs, and C. Brassinne. 1977. Steroid receptors in the human prostate: Detection of tissue-specific androgen binding in prostatic cancer. Clin. Chim. Acta 75:303–312.

Hawkins, E. F., M. Nijs, C. Brassinne, and H. J. Tagnon. 1975. Steroid receptors in the human prostate. I. Estradiol-17β binding in benign prostatic hypertrophy. Steroids 26:458–469.

Higgins, G. A., Jr. 1978. Special problems in the evaluation of results in adjuvant trials of cancer treatment. J. Surg. Oncol. 10:321–326.

Huggins, C., and C. V. Hodges. 1941. Studies on prostatic cancer. I. The effect of castration, of estrogen and of androgen injection on serum phosphatases in metastatic carcinoma of the prostate. Cancer Res. 1:293–297.

Johnson, D. E. 1978. Carcinoma of the prostate: An editorial. Cancer Bull. 30:111.

Kadohama, N., R. Y. Kirdani, S. Madajewicz, G. P. Murphy, and A. A. Sandberg. 1979. Metabolic pattern of estramustine in human blood and prostatic tissue. N.Y. State J. Med. (in press).

Karr, J. P., R. Y. Kirdani, G. P. Murphy, and A. A. Sandberg. 1978a. Androgen binding in the baboon prostate. Arch. Androl. (in press).

Karr, J. P., R. Y. Kirdani, G. P. Murphy, and A. A. Sandberg. 1978b. Sex hormone globulin and transcortin in human and baboon males. Arch. Androl. 1:123–129.

Karr, J. P., and Sandberg, A. A. 1978c. Steroid receptors and prostatic cancer, in Prostatic Cancer, G. P. Murphy, ed. Publishing Scientists Group Inc., Littleton, Mass., pp. 49–74.

Karr, J. P., Z. Wajsman, S. Madajewicz, R. Y. Kirdani, G. P. Murphy, and A. A. Sandberg. 1978d. Steroid hormone receptors in the prostate. J. Urol. (in press).

Lee, C., M. C. Wang, G. P. Murphy, and T. M. Chu. 1978. A solid-phase fluorescent immunoassay for human prostatic acid phosphatase. Cancer Res. 38:2871–2878.

Martland, M., F. Hausman, and R. Robinson. Phosphoric esterase of blood. Biochem. J. 18:1152–1160, 1924.

McDonald, I., N. R. Rose, E. J. Pontes, and B. K. Choe. 1978. Human prostatic acid phosphatases. III. Counterimmunoelectrophoresis for rapid identification. Arch. Androl. 1:235–239.

Mellinger, G. T., D. F. Gleason, and J. Bailar, III. 1967. The histology and prognosis of prostatic cancer. J. Urol. 97:331–337.

Menon, M., C. E. Tananis, L. L. Hicks, E. F. Hawkins, M. G. McLoughlin, and P. C. Walsh. 1978. Characterization of the binding of a potent synthetic androgen, methyltrienolone (R 1881) to human tissues. J. Clin. Invest. 61:150–162.

Menon, M., C. E. Tananis, M. G. McLoughlin, and P. C. Walsh. 1977. Androgen receptors in human prostatic tissue: A review. Cancer Treat. Rep. 61:265–271.

Mobbs, B. G., I. E. Johnson, J. G. Connolly, and A. F. Clark. 1977. Evaluation of the use of cyproterone acetate competition to distinguish between high-affinity binding of (^{3}H)-dihydrotestosterone to human prostate cytosol receptors and to sex hormone-binding globulin. J. Steroid Biochem. 8:943–947.

Mobbs, B. G., I. E. Johnson, J. G. Connolly, and A. F. Clark. 1978. Androgen receptor assay in human benign and malignant prostatic tumour cytosol using protamine sulphate precipitation. J. Steroid Biochem. (in press).

Mostofi, F. K. 1975. Grading of prostatic carcinoma. Cancer Chemother. Rep. 59:111–117.

Murphy, G. P., G. Reynoso, G. M. Kenny, and J. F. Gaeta. 1969. Comparison of total and prostatic fraction serum acid phosphatase levels in patients with differentiated and undifferentiated prostatic carcinoma. Cancer 23:1309–1314.

Murphy, G. P., and W. F. Whitmore, Jr. 1978. A report of the workshops on the current status of the histologic grading of prostate cancer. Cancer (in press).

Rosen, V., I. Jung, E. E. Baulieu, and P. Robel. 1975. Androgen-binding proteins in human benign prostatic hypertrophy. J. Clin. Endocrinol. Metab. 41:761–770.

Sadlowski, R. W. 1978. Early stage prostatic cancer investigated by pelvic lymph node biopsy and bone marrow acid phosphatase. J. Urol. 119:89–93.

Schmidt, J. D., D. E. Johnson, W. W. Scott, R. P. Gibbons, G. R. Prout, and G. P. Murphy. 1976. Chemotherapy of advanced prostatic cancer: Evaluation of response parameters. Urology 7:602–610.

Snochowski, M., A. Pousette, P. Ekman, D. Bression, L. Andersson, B. Hogberg, and J. A. Gustafsson. 1977. Characterization and measurement of the androgen receptor in human benign prostatic hyperplasia and prostatic adenocarcinoma. J. Clin. Endocrinol. Metab. 45:920–930.

Sodeman, T. M., and J. C. Batsakis. 1977. Acid phosphatase, *in* Urologic Pathology—The Prostate, M. Tannenbaum, ed. Lea & Febiger, Philadelphia, pp. 129–139.

Woodard, H. Q. 1959. The clinical significance of serum acid phosphatase. Am. J. Med. 27:902–910.

Yam, L. T. 1974. Clinical significance of the human acid phosphatases: A review. Am. J. Med. 56:604–616.

MANAGEMENT OF METASTATIC RENAL CARCINOMA

Cancer of the Genitourinary Tract, edited by
D. E. Johnson and M. L. Samuels.
Raven Press, New York © 1979.

The Role of Nephrectomy in Metastatic Renal Carcinoma

Douglas E. Johnson, M.D., and David A. Swanson, M.D.

Department of Urology, The University of Texas System Cancer Center M. D. Anderson Hospital and Tumor Institute, Houston, Texas

Renal carcinoma accounts for approximately 2% of all cases of malignant disease and will be diagnosed in over 15,000 Americans this year, over half of whom will die from it. Metastases will be clinically evident in 25–57% of these patients when the primary renal tumor is diagnosed (Skinner et al. 1971, Lokich and Harrison 1975). In 642 patients with renal carcinoma seen at M. D. Anderson Hospital, sites of clinically determined metastases were distributed as follows: lung, 69%; bone, 43%; liver, 14%; brain, 7%; lymph node, 5%; skin, 4%; and thyroid, spermatic cord, vagina, breast, and nasopharynx combined less than 1%.

Patients who present with metastatic disease from a recently diagnosed but untreated primary renal adenocarcinoma pose complex therapeutic problems for the urologic surgeon and medical oncologist. Until recently, it was standard medical practice to recommend surgical exploration in an attempt to surgically remove the primary tumor prior to instituting local and/or systemic therapy for metastatic disease. Some of the major arguments advanced for performing nephrectomy in patients with metastatic disease have included: (1) alleviation of symptoms referable to the local lesion (hematuria, pain, fever, hepatopathy, anemia, erythrocytosis, hypercalcemia, etc.); (2) reduction of the likelihood of further dissemination of the disease; (3) prolongation of life with or without spontaneous regression of metastases; (4) enhancement of hormonal or drug therapy by removal of the bulk of the tumor; and (5) reduction of the psychological impact on the patient by removal of the primary tumor.

Although palliation can be achieved in selected instances, the rarity of tumor regression, coupled with the limited usefulness of adjuvant hormonal and drug therapy, has resulted in poor overall survival for these patients, with the majority dying within two years. Consequently, the removal of the primary tumor as part of an aggressive therapeutic approach ("adjunctive nephrectomy") has come under attack, but in the absence of randomized prospective clinical studies, the results remain conflicting and the therapy controversial. In an effort to better define the role of nephrectomy in these situations, we have reviewed both our own experience and that reported in the literature in treating patients with renal carcinoma who present with metastatic disease.

PALLIATION

Analysis of patients in whom nephrectomy has not been performed suggests that local symptoms seldom become severe enough to require a palliative nephrectomy. No differences in the quality of survival have been reported between nephrectomy and non-nephrectomy patients with metastatic disease treated at either M. D. Anderson Hospital (Johnson et al. 1975) or the Cleveland Clinic (Montie et al. 1977). Symptoms, such as flank pain, hematuria, fever, and malignant hypercalcemia, that could have been attributed to the primary lesion posed no greater problem in patients not subjected to nephrectomy. In addition, many of the systemic symptoms, such as hypercalcemia, hepatic dysfunction, and erythrocytosis, could be produced by the metastases. Less radical means that may be preferable for alleviating specific symptoms include administration of indocin, 25 mg p.o. t.i.d., for fever reduction; administration of mithramycin, 25 μg/kg i.v., for correction of hypercalcemia; and percutaneous renal artery occlusion for control of hematuria and pain.

ENHANCEMENT OF HORMONAL OR DRUG THERAPY

For years oncologists have argued that, by first removing the bulk of the tumor through nephrectomy, drug therapy could more effectively combat metastatic disease. To date, however, there has been little clinical evidence to support this premise. In 1975, we reported our experience with chemotherapy in the management of 80 patients with metastatic renal carcinoma (Johnson and Samuels 1975). In 22 instances, nephrectomy was performed prior to the institution of chemotherapy. The median survival for the group treated without nephrectomy was 5.5 months, compared to 6.0 months for the group subjected to nephrectomy prior to institution of chemotherapy. An additional 33 patients underwent nephrectomy prior to the discovery of metastases and, while there were seven objective responses in this group, the median survival was only eight months. Differences in survival time distributions among these three groups were not statistically significant at the 0.5 level. Other investigators have also reported that adjunctive nephrectomy does not appear to improve survival (Montie et al. 1977, Middleton 1967). These results are not surprising since no chemotherapeutic agent, used alone or in combination, has demonstrated consistent activity in this disease (Johnson and Samuels 1975, Woodruff et al. 1967, Talley 1973, Hrushesky and Murphy 1977).

Klugo and associates (1977), however, have recently reported that nephrectomy performed in the presence of metastatic disease combined with hormonal and nonhormonal chemotherapy significantly improves median survival as well as three-year survival rates. In a retrospective review of 101 patients, all of whom received medroxyprogesterone acetate initially, followed by androgens and cytotoxic drugs for progressive disease, they found that the median survival for patients treated without undergoing nephrectomy was 4.5 months, compared to 15.0 months for those treated with combined nephrectomy and hormonal chemotherapy. The three-year survival rate was 31% and the five-year survival rate was 13.7% for the 29 patients who underwent nephrectomy, as opposed to 9% and 3%, respectively, for the 64 patients treated without nephrectomy. These differences in survival are difficult to understand, since tumor regression was documented so infrequently (4%). Interestingly, the four responses were noted only in patients subjected to nephrectomy. In addition, survival in male patients treated by nephrectomy and medroxyprogesterone acetate was significantly better (median 36 months) than in females treated with the same program (4.5 months) or in males treated with hormonal chemotherapy alone (6.5 months). Montie and associates (1977) reported similar findings, with objective responses occurring only in male patients with pulmonary metastases treated by nephrectomy and parenteral medroxyprogesterone acetate.

The role the nephrectomized state played in the responses recorded in these series is uncertain, but these reports suggest a need for careful patient stratification in evaluating responses, especially with regard to sex, site of metastases, and previous management of the primary tumor. Currently, however, there are insufficient data to suggest any real enhancement of hormonal or cytotoxic chemotherapy by adjunctive nephrectomy.

IMPROVEMENT IN SURVIVAL

The major reason for considering nephrectomy in the face of metastatic disease has remained the unshakable belief that surgical extirpation of the primary tumor would enhance subsequent therapy and thereby prolong survival. Unfortunately, there have been few differences in overall survival rates between patients subjected to nephrectomy and those not undergoing surgery. Middleton (1967) reported that none of his 141 patients with metastatic disease was known to have survived two years, despite nephrectomy being performed on 33 occasions. Similarly, in a review of 93 consecutive patients presenting untreated with metastatic disease at M. D. Anderson Hospital, little difference in survival was noted between the 43 patients subjected to nephrectomy prior to institution of hormonal or cytotoxic chemotherapy (11.3 months) and 50 patients started on therapy without undergoing nephrectomy (7.9 months) (Johnson et al. 1975). While overall survival rates have not been improved by nephrectomy performed in the presence of metastatic disease, there is cumulative evidence to suggest that factors such as the site of metastatic disease and the number of metastases may alter these findings.

Site of Metastasis

The site of metastasis is an important factor in prognosis and needs to be taken into consideration when nephrectomy is being contemplated. While ne-

Table 1. *Survival According to Site of Metastasis**

Site of Metastasis	Number of Patients	Median Survival (months)
Lung	45	6
Liver	6	3
Brain	4	2.5
Bone	15	15

* Modified from Johnson and Samuels (1975).

phrectomy has not appreciably altered survival for patients with pulmonary or visceral metastases, patients with osseous metastases undergoing surgery have shown improvement (Table 1). Five of 14 patients (36%) with osseous metastases subjected to nephrectomy at the Cleveland Clinic were alive longer than one year, compared to only six of 33 (18%) with metastases at other sites (Montie et al. 1977). Four of the patients with osseous metastases lived longer than three years. Seven patients in the same series had pulmonary metastases only, with one patient living longer than one year (dead at 35 months) and one remaining alive with stable disease at 10 months. Our experience (Johnson et al. 1975) also originally suggested prolongation of survival following nephrectomy for patients with exclusive osseous metastases. Fifteen patients undergoing nephrectomy in the presence of osseous metastases achieved an adjusted median survival of 16.1 months, compared to 10.6 months for their 12 counterparts not undergoing nephrectomy. Nephrectomy did not appear to significantly alter survival when pulmonary or soft tissue metastases were present, with a median survival of 7.9 months for those undergoing nephrectomy and 5.4 months for those not undergoing surgery. Whether or not patients with osseous metastases alone represent a select group with a potential for extended survival, due perhaps to a slower growth rate of bony metastases, remains speculative (Montie et al. 1977). These findings, however, require further investigation, since other series have suggested that survival for patients with pulmonary metastases is no worse than that for those with osseous disease (Klugo et al. 1977).

Number of Metastases

Although metastatic disease is evident in 25–57% of patients with renal carcinoma at the time of diagnosis, a solitary metastasis is present in only 1–3% (Skinner et al. 1971, Middleton 1967, Tolia and Whitmore 1975). Treatment in these situations should be individualized, but aggressive surgical therapy appears to prolong survival in selected patients, with five-year survival rates reportedly ranging from 30% to 50%. Although our previous investigations (Johnson et al. 1975) suggested that osseous disease alone conferred a better prognosis, a recent review of 43 patients presenting with exclusively osseous metastases prior to treatment has suggested that the differences in survival are probably a reflection of the number of metastases present (Swanson and Johnson, unpublished data). All 17 patients with single osseous metastases underwent nephrectomy, with a median survival of 21 months. This represents a definite improvement over the 14 patients with multiple metastases who underwent nephrectomy with a median survival of only 9.5 months, a figure not significantly different from the survival of 10.6 months for the 12 patients with multiple osseous metastases who did not undergo a nephrectomy.

SPONTANEOUS REGRESSION

Renal carcinoma has been considered one of the more common types of malignant disease that undergoes spontaneous regression, but in only 51 cases has this occurred after nephrectomy (Freed et al. 1977). The rarity of this phenomenon has been emphasized by the finding of Montie and associates (1977) that only four cases occurred after nephrectomy in 474 patients with metastatic disease, an incidence of 0.8%. Since the operative mortality rate following nephrectomy performed in patients with metastatic disease ranges from 2.3% to 10% (Skinner et al. 1971, Johnson et al. 1975), there appears to be no justification for performing the procedure in the hope of effecting a spontaneous regression.

CONCLUSIONS

Nephrectomy performed in the presence of multiple metastatic deposits has neither enhanced hormonal or drug therapy nor affected the quality of survival. Overall survival rates remain poor, with few patients surviving two years. Adjunctive nephrectomy appears to be best reserved for patients with solitary metastases, in whom prolonged survival may be expected.

REFERENCES

Hrushesky, W. J., and G. P. Murphy. 1977. Current status of the therapy of advanced renal carcinoma. J. Surg. Oncol. 9:277–288.
Johnson, D. E., K. E. Kaesler, and M. L. Samuels. 1975. Is nephrectomy justified in patients with metastatic renal carcinoma? J. Urol. 114:27–29.
Johnson, D. E., and M. L. Samuels. 1975. Chemotherapy for metastatic renal carcinoma, *in* Cancer Chemotherapy—Fundamental Concepts and Recent Advances (Proceedings of The University of Texas System Cancer Center M. D. Anderson Hospital and Tumor Institute 19th Annual Clinical Conference on Cancer, 1975). Year Book Medical Publishers, Inc., Chicago, pp. 493–503.
Klugo, R. C., M. Detmers, R. E. Stiles, R. W. Talley, and J. C. Cerny. 1977. Aggressive versus conservative management of stage IV renal cell carcinoma. J. Urol. 118:244–246.
Lokich, J. J., and J. H. Harrison. 1975. Renal cell carcinoma: Natural history and chemotherapeutic experience. J. Urol. 114:371–374.
Middleton, R. G. 1967. Surgery for metastatic renal cell carcinoma. J. Urol. 97:973–977.
Montie, J. E., B. H. Stewart, R. A. Straffon, L. H. W. Banowsky, C. B. Hewitt, and D. K. Montague. 1977. The role of adjunctive nephrectomy in patients with metastatic renal cell carcinoma. J. Urol. 117:272–275.

Skinner, D. G., R. B. Colvin, C. D. Vermillion, R. C. Pfister, and W. F. Leadbetter. 1971. Diagnosis and management of renal cell carcinoma: A clinical and pathologic study of 309 cases. Cancer 28:1165–1177.

Talley, R. W. 1973. Chemotherapy of adenocarcinoma of the kidney. Cancer 32:1062–1065.

Tolia, B. M., and W. F. Whitmore, Jr. 1975. Solitary metastasis from renal cell carcinoma. J. Urol. 114:836–838.

Whitmore, W. F. 1967. Discussion, *in* Renal Neoplasia, J. S. King, Jr., ed. Little, Brown and Co., Boston, pp. 521–532.

Woodruff, M. W., D. Wagle, S. D. Gailani, and R. Jones. 1967. The current status of chemotherapy for advanced renal carcinoma. J. Urol. 97:611–618.

Cancer of the Genitourinary Tract, edited by
D. E. Johnson and M. L. Samuels.
Raven Press, New York © 1979.

Diagnostic Radiology in Renal Carcinoma

Sidney Wallace, M.D., Vincent Chuang, M.D., Barry Green, M.D.,
David A. Swanson, M.D.,* R. Bruce Bracken, M.D.,*
and Douglas E. Johnson, M.D.*

*Departments of Diagnostic Radiology and *Urology, The University of Texas System Cancer Center M. D. Anderson Hospital and Tumor Institute, Houston, Texas*

The diagnosis and staging of a renal carcinoma are primarily the responsibility of the diagnostic radiologist, who has recently become more involved in the therapeutic management of both primary and secondary renal neoplasms by means of transcatheter intra-arterial embolization (Wallace 1976). This presentation will describe the diagnostic approach and experience at M. D. Anderson Hospital in the management of 102 patients with renal carcinoma (Bracken et al. 1975, Goldstein et al. 1975, Johnson et al., in press).

DIAGNOSIS

The approach to the diagnosis of a renal mass used at M. D. Anderson Hospital is summarized in Figure 1. Pulmonary and osseous metastases are relatively common and are demonstrated by chest radiograms and radionuclide bone scans. Chest tomograms and specific views of the skeleton further define suspicious areas. Percutaneous biopsy of these lesions may be necessary for histologic confirmation (DeSantos et al. 1978, Zornoza et al. 1977).

Ultrasonography and computed tomography have radically altered the diagnostic evaluation of the patient with a renal mass.

Ultrasonography

Ultrasonography has the advantage of presenting the information in two planes, transverse and sagittal, which better defines the extent of disease, an essential aspect in determining resectability. Renal carcinoma is usually depicted by ultrasound as a solid mass containing multiple internal echoes with an irregular posterior wall (Figure 2). Complex patterns with cystic and solid components may be seen in necrotic or hemorrhagic tumors, as well as multiloculated or infected cysts, abscesses, etc. Further evaluation by computed tomography, angiography, and percutaneous puncture is usually necessary to establish a specific diagnosis (Goldstein et al. 1978). Extension of the neoplasm into the renal vein and inferior vena cava and metastases to the retroperitoneal lymph nodes,

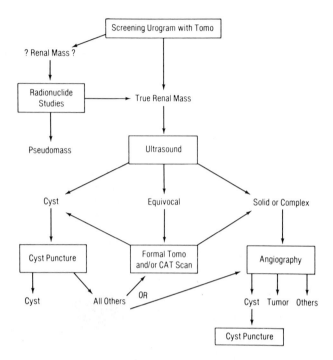

Figure 1. Approach to evaluation of renal mass lesions.

adrenal gland, and liver can be defined by ultrasonography, i.e., renal pansonography (Green et al., in press).

A significant shortcoming of ultrasonography is the fact that it is made uninterpretable by abdominal gas. On the other hand, a decided advantage is the fact that each unit at our institution performs 10 to 15 examinations each day at a cost approximately one third that with computed tomography.

Computed Tomography

The presence, nature, and extent of renal carcinoma are, on the whole, better defined by computed tomography (CT) (Sagel et al. 1977). Renal neoplasms are usually depicted as areas of decreased attenuation (Figure 3). There may be irregular zones of lower attenuation within the mass, presumably representing necrosis. Extension beyond the capsule into the renal vein or the inferior vena cava (Steele et al. 1978) and retroperitoneal lymph node metastases are readily demonstrated. Involvement of the liver is better determined by CT than by ultrasonography and radionuclide studies. The combination of ultrasonography and radionuclide hepatic scanning, however, detects the presence of hepatic abnormalities at a rate almost equal to that with CT alone at a combined cost two thirds that with CT (Snow, Goldstein, and Wallace, unpublished observations).

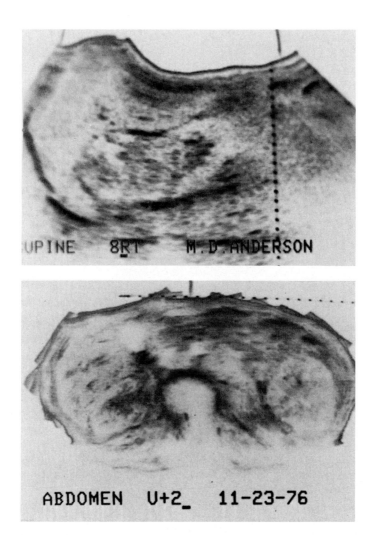

Figure 2. Renal carcinoma disclosed by ultrasonography. Top, Longitudinal section, right renal carcinoma. Solid mass in the upper pole of the right kidney is revealed by the multiple internal echoes. The renal carcinoma is readily separated from the liver. Bottom, Transverse section, left renal carcinoma. Echogenic mass replacing left kidney. Retroperitoneal metastasis, presumably in lymph node, is displacing the renal shadow.

Angiography

Angiography is now the last technique employed when the nature and extent of disease are still unresolved or preparations are being made for therapeutic management (Green, in press). This evaluation includes aortography, bilateral selective renal arteriography, selective hepatic arteriography, inferior venacavography, and sometimes renal venography.

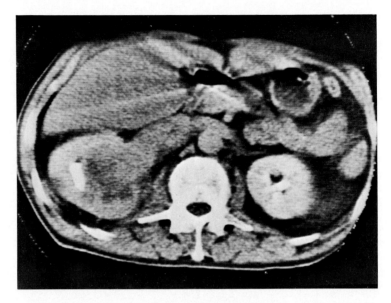

Figure 3. Renal carcinoma disclosed by computed tomography. The right renal carcinoma is an area of decreased attenuation in the medial aspect of the kidney, distorting the collecting system. The neoplasm extends into the renal vein and inferior vena cava. Note another small area of decreased attenuation along the lateral cortex, which proved to be a benign cyst.

Renal carcinomas are hypervascular in 65% of cases, isovascular in 20%, and hypo- or avascular in 15% (Folin 1967). The vascularity of the metastases usually mimics that of the primary neoplasm. Liver metastases occur in 10–15% of cases and are better defined by angiography because of their vascularity. Hypervascular metastases as small as 5 mm in diameter can be detected, but hypovascular metastases less than 2 cm in diameter are easily overlooked. The left lobe of the liver is difficult to evaluate by angiography and is better evaluated by radionuclide scanning, ultrasonography, or computed tomography (Snow, Goldstein, and Wallace, unpublished observations) (Figure 4 left).

At autopsy, approximately 6% of patients with renal carcinoma are found to have had neoplasm in the opposite kidney. Although this is less common at the time of presentation with a renal carcinoma, the necessity of establishing the status of the "normal" kidney prior to nephrectomy is obvious (Figure 4 right).

Inferior venacavography will delineate tumor projection into the lumen, as well as extrinsic compression by the neoplasm or lymph node metastases.

The entire evaluation usually requires approximately 300 cc of contrast material 60–76% meglumine diatrizoate. Attempts at management are delayed for at least one day because of the increase in complications when diagnosis and embolization are performed at the same time.

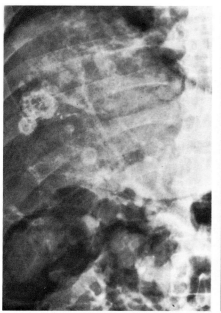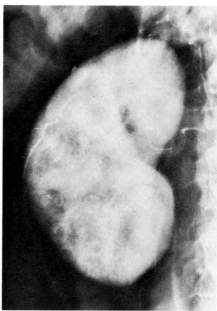

Figure 4. Metastatic renal carcinoma disclosed by angiography. Left, Hepatic metastases as small as 5 mm in diameter, when hypervascular, are best demonstrated by selective hepatic arteriography. Right, Renal metastases discovered only after selective renal arteriographic examination of a supposedly normal kidney.

MANAGEMENT

The diagnostic radiologist, extending his angiographic techniques, has taken an active role in conjuntion with the urologist in managing patients with primary and secondary renal carcinoma. Transcatheter intra-arterial embolization of the neoplasms was initially suggested by Lalli, Peterson, and Bookstein in 1969. Lang (1971), employing radioactive gold grains as emboli, noted a decrease in the size of renal carcinomas in 20 patients, while Almgard et al. (1973) reported encouraging results after autologous muscle tissue embolization of renal neoplasms. At M. D. Anderson Hospital and Tumor Institute, 102 patients with renal carcinoma have undergone transcatheter intravascular tumor embolization as part of the therapeutic management utilizing Gelfoam and Gianturco stainless steel coils since 1974 (Wallace et al. 1978).

Technique

The materials embolized have included autologous clot and tissue (Reuter and Chuang 1974), clot modified with thrombin, amicar, Gelfoam, Oxycel, and Ivalon (Tadvarthy et al. 1975), silastic spheres (Hilal et al. 1970), silicone rubber (Doppman et al. 1971), cyanoacrylates (Dotter et al. 1975), balloon catheters

(Wholey et al. 1970), and mechanical devices such as the stainless steel coil (Gianturco et al. 1975, Wallace et al. 1978, Anderson, Wallace, Gianturco, and Gerson, unpublished observations), and brush (Gomes et al. 1978). The autologous clot is effective for hours to days, until it lyses or recanulates. The clot may be modified, but its life-span is still limited. Gelfoam serves as a framework for additional thrombus formation and the occlusion usually lasts weeks or even months (Barth et al. 1977) (Figure 5 left). Histologic sections of arteries occluded by Gelfoam have shown an intense acute arteritis characterized by polymorphonuclear cells infiltrating the vessel wall and the immediate perivascular tissues. Because of the temporary nature and unpredictability of such occlusion, these measures suffice only for short-term preoperative management. However, when there is a need for more complete obstruction preoperatively or for palliative intravascular occlusion, a more permanent agent is employed. The stainless steel coil with attached wool or Dacron threads, as described by Gianturco et al. (1975), has been extremely effective for large vessel occlusion (Figure 5 right).

The combination of Gelfoam particles for the peripheral arterial bed and the stainless steel coil for central vascular obstruction is used in most of our patients (Figure 6) because of our familiarity with these materials and certain theoretical advantages (Anderson et al. 1977). Presumably, the occlusion of the peripheral vessels decreases collateral circulation. The interruption of the major vessel with coils acts like an internal ligature, which is safer than attempting to fill the major vessel with particles. This complete occlusion of the artery allows the surgeon to approach the renal veins directly. The embolized tumor is left in situ for 2 to 10 days, especially in patients with metastases, to stimulate an immune response to the ischemic neoplasm.

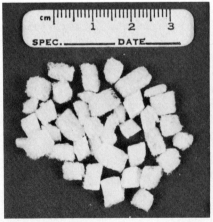 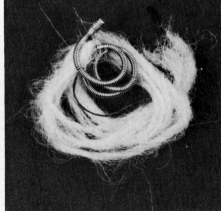

Figure 5. Embolic materials. Left, Gelfoam, 3 mm cubes. Right, Gianturco stainless steel coil with attached Dacron strands.

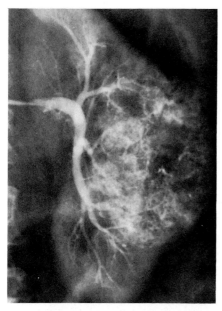
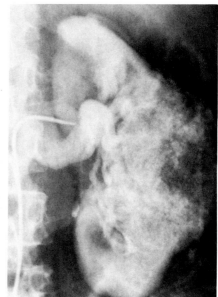
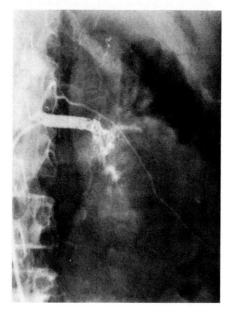

Figure 6. Transcatheter arterial occlusion for renal carcinoma. Renal angiography demonstrates a hypervascular carcinoma, (top left) arterial phase and (top right) venous phase. Bottom, Renal artery occlusion. Gelfoam embolization was followed by coil occlusion.

Indications

This procedure is indicated (1) preoperatively to shorten surgery and decrease blood loss, (2) to control hemorrhaging and alleviate pain, (3) to reduce tumor bulk in conjunction with chemotherapy in patients with inoperable disease, and (4), theoretically, to stimulate an immune response (Swanson, in press).

Complications

Virtually all patients undergoing renal arterial occlusion experience flank *pain* of 24 to 48 hours' duration requiring narcotics for relief. The narcotics are given intravenously in aliquots of 25 mg of Demerol during embolization. *Fever* up to 40° C almost always accompanies the pain, lasting as long as five days, but antibiotics are seldom needed. *Anorexia, nausea,* and *vomiting* may occur for three to five days, requiring symptomatic management. In a few patients *paralytic ileus* may require nasogastric suction and intravenous fluids. *Hypertension* occurs in many patients during embolization and lasts two to four hours. No patient has experienced persistent hypertension.

Major complications have been relatively few. *Renal failure* occurred early in the series in two patients, in one of whom it was irreversible. This was believed to be related to the large volume of contrast material used (300 cc), and to the infarction that was performed at the same time. In the last 80 patients, these two events have been separated by at least 24 hours without another episode of failure. *Renal abscess* complicated occlusion in two patients, with one fatality due to gram-negative septicemia. A preexisting pyuria was held responsible. Consequently, in the presence of a urinary tract infection, antibiotics are given one week before and after embolization. *Unintentional embolization* of the Gelfoam and steel coils is always a potential complication. A balloon catheter has been used by some to minimize the likelihood of escape of Gelfoam emboli. This has not been employed in this series because the Gelfoam emboli are used only to occlude the tumor. Central occlusion is accomplished with a coil. Loss of a coil into the aorta occurred in one patient. Chuang (unpublished data) has developed a method for extracting the errant stainless steel coil.

Clinical Material

One hundred two patients with renal carcinoma were managed in part by transcatheter intra-arterial embolization of the neoplasm. In 72 patients the embolization was employed in conjunction with nephrectomy. Twenty-three of these patients had regional disease, while 49 had metastases, usually to the lung or bone. Infarction alone was the palliative treatment for 25 patients. Hormonal therapy with Depo-Provera was part of the therapeutic protocol, especially in the presence of metastatic disease. Secondary foci of renal carcinoma were embolized in seven patients, in the lumbar spine and pelvis in five, and in the base of the skull and the liver in one each. The renal artery was occluded in 97 patients, the internal iliac artery in four, and the lumbar arteries, the hepatic artery, and the external carotid artery in one each.

RESULTS AND DISCUSSION

When technically feasible, the patient with a renal carcinoma is treated by a transabdominal radical nephrectomy. No additional assistance is required in removing renal carcinomas of small or moderate size localized within the capsule (stage I). The five-year survival rate of patients with stage I disease is approximately 60%. It is not now considered advantageous to subject these patients to the morbidity associated with embolization. Removal of larger stage I tumors, which are frequently hypervascular, is facilitated by renal artery occlusion.

Stage II neoplasms include those extending through the capsule into the perinephric fat. The presence of regional lymph node metastases or a tumor thrombus in the renal vein or inferior vena cava signifies stage III disease. The five-year survival rate for patients with stage II or III renal carcinomas ranges from 30% to 35%. In cases involving these advanced tumors, especially if they are hypervascular, dilated tortuous veins usually cover the surface of the neoplasm and the renal hilum. Regional lymph node metastases and a tumor thrombus in the renal vein or inferior vena cava may impede access to the renal artery. Preoperative renal artery occlusion with Gelfoam and stainless steel coils can help facilitate the nephrectomy. Occlusion should be performed 48 to 72 hours prior to surgery for optimum effect. The collateral circulation is kept to a minimum. With the decrease in the arterial inflow, the veins collapse. The occluded renal artery containing the steel coils, with its associated inflammatory response, is readily palpated in the hilum and is, in essence, preligated. The major hilar renal veins are approached and ligated first. In the presence of tumor thrombus, the hazards of tumor embolization are reduced and the thrombectomy is facilitated. The infarcted neoplasm is smaller and the kidney is edematous, creating a more definable plane between the neoplasm and the renal bed. These factors decrease blood loss and reduce the time required for surgery.

Approximately 25–40% of patients with renal carcinoma present with metastatic disease. This group has a median survival of six months, regardless of whether treatment consists of nephrectomy, chemotherapy, hormonal therapy, immune therapy or a combination of these. The occurrence of spontaneous remission of metastases after nephrectomy has been widely publicized, but only approximately 50 cases have been reported. In a review of 641 cases of renal carcinoma at M. D. Anderson Hospital, Sternberg (personal communication) found only five involving spontaneous remission of metastases after nephrectomy. The median survival of 5.9 months with pulmonary metastases was not statistically altered by nephrectomy or hormonal therapy (Johnson and Samuels 1975). With osseous metastases, median survival following nephrectomy was extented from 10 to 16 months (Johnson et al. 1975). However, it must be appreciated that patients undergoing nephrectomy usually have less extensive disease. Patients with hepatic or cerebral metastases were not subjected to nephrectomy because of their four-month median survival.

Infarction With Nephrectomy

Of the 102 patients in this series, 49 presenting with metastases were treated by occlusion, nephrectomy, and hormonal therapy. The interval between occlusion and nephrectomy was usually 2 to 10 days, with 10 months being the longest interval. Since a response to this combined regimen is usually observed within 4.5 months and may continue for 12 to 14 months, responses are not evaluated until the patient has survived at least 4.5 months. Therefore, of these 49 patients, only 36 are currently evaluable.

In this group of 36 patients with pulmonary metastases, the median survival thus far is 17 months, in contrast to 6 months for a control group. A response was noted in 21 of the 36 patients (58%). Six responses were complete, with disappearance of pulmonary metastases for 6 to 18 months and survival as long as 30 months. Five patients had partial responses (50% or more reduction). In one case involving a mixed response, the pulmonary lesions decreased more than 50% while the osseous metastases progressed. Nine patients experienced measurable regression of less than 50% or stabilization for more than 12 months. Of the responders, nine are still alive with a median follow-up of 20 months.

Infarction Without Nephrectomy

Twenty-five patients were treated by embolization without nephrectomy. These patients were not candidates for surgery because of their general medical condition or the extent of tumor involvement. One patient with apparent contiguous growth of tumor into the liver underwent infarction without nephrectomy and is still alive without demonstrable metastases 48 months later. He experienced immediate and permanent relief of pain. Twenty other patients survived one week to 11 months (median survival four months) and one patient is alive with progressive metastatic disease five months after infarction.

Examination of one patient 80 years of age for hematuria (L. Gomez, personal communication) revealed a left renal carcinoma with a large hypervascular retroperitoneal metastasis. After treatment by embolization of the renal tumor alone, the patient experienced no further hematuria, but died eight months later from an unrelated cerebrovascular accident. At autopsy, no viable tumor was noted in the renal or retroperitoneal masses. Ring reported control of renal carcinoma in a solitary kidney in three patients treated by segmental embolization (personal communication). The remainder of the kidneys adequately sustained urinary function.

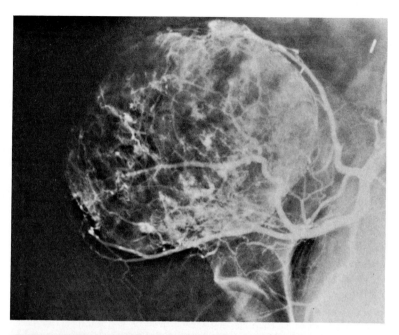

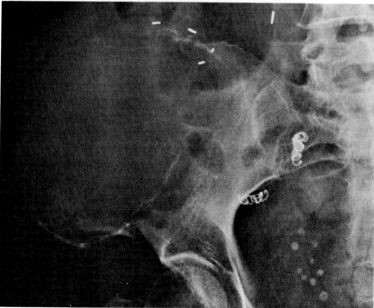

Figure 7. Transcatheter occlusion for metastatic renal carcinoma. Top, Hypervascular metasta-sis to the right ilium. Bottom, Occlusion of right internal iliac artery with Gelfoam and steel coils alleviating pain for nine months.

Occlusion of Metastases

Metastatic foci were embolized in eight patients (Wallace et al., in press). In seven of these, embolization was used to relieve bone pain previously uncontrolled by radiation therapy, surgery, or chemotherapy. Most of the vascular supply to the metastases was occluded by Gelfoam and coils. Pain relief was accomplished in five of the seven for three to eight months (Figure 7). Embolization of liver metastases was attempted in one patient with no obvious response.

CONCLUSIONS

Transcatheter embolization offers some promise, especially when combined with nephrectomy and chemo- or hormonal therapy, in the management of patients with metastatic renal carcinoma. Preoperative transcatheter embolization of the renal neoplasm is undoubtedly of assistance to the surgeon. Further investigation is necessary to determine the optimal interval between occlusion and nephrectomy and the place of chemotherapy, hormonal therapy, and immunotherapy in this therapeutic approach.

REFERENCES

Almgard, L. E., I. Fernstrom, M. Haverling, and A. Ljungqvist. 1973. Treatment of renal adenocarcinoma by embolic occlusion of the renal circulation. Br. J. Urol. 45:474–479.

Anderson, J. H., S. Wallace, and C. Gianturco. 1977. Transcatheter intravascular coil occlusion of experimental arteriovenous fistulas. Am. J. Roentgenol. 129:795–798.

Barth, K. H., J. D. Strandberg, and R. I. White. 1977. Long term follow-up of transcatheter embolization with autologous clot, Oxycel and Gelfoam in domestic swine. Invest. Radiol. 12:273–280.

Bracken, R. B., D. E. Johnson, H. M. Goldstein, S. Wallace, and A. G. Ayala. 1975. Percutaneous transfemoral renal artery occlusion in patients with renal carcinoma: A preliminary report. Urology 6:6–10.

DeSantos, L. A., J. Lukeman, S. Wallace, J. A. Murray, and A. G. Ayala. 1978. Percutaneous needle biopsy of bone in the cancer patient. Am. J. Roentgenol. 130:641–649.

Doppman, J. L., W. Zapol, and J. L. Pierce. 1971. Transcatheter embolization with a silicone rubber preparation—Experimental observations. Invest. Radiol. 6:304–309.

Dotter, C. T., M. L. Goldman, and J. Rosch. 1975. Instant selective arterial occlusion with isobutyl-2-cyanoacrylate. Radiology 114:227–230.

Folin, J. 1967. Angiography in renal tumours—Its value in diagnosis and differential diagnosis as a complement to conventional methods. Acta Radiol. [Suppl.] (Stockh.) 267:7–91.

Gianturco, C., J. H. Anderson, and S. Wallace. 1975. Mechanical devices for arterial occlusion. Am. J. Roentgenol. 124:428–435.

Goldstein, H. M., B. Green, and R. M. Weaver. 1978. Ultrasonic detection of renal tumor extension into the inferior vena cava. Am. J. Roentgenol. 130:1083–1085.

Goldstein, H. M., H. Medellin, T. Beydoun, S. Wallace, Y. Ben-Menachem, R. B. Bracken, and D. E. Johnson. 1975. Transcatheter embolization of renal cell carcinoma. Am. J. Roentgenol. 123:557–562.

Gomes, A. S., J. A. Rysavy, C. A. Spadaccini, P. Probst, V. D'Souza, and K. Amplatz. 1978. The use of the bristle brush for transcatheter embolization. Radiology 129:345–350.

Green, B. 1979. Pelvic ultrasonography, in Ultrasound Atlas, D. A. Sarti and F. Sample, eds. G. K. Hall & Co., Boston (in press).

Green, B., H. M. Goldstein, and R. M. Weaver. 1979. Abdominal pansonography in the evaluation of renal cancer. Radiology (in press).

Hilal, S., L. Mount, and J. Correll. 1970. Therapeutic embolization of vascular malformation of the external carotid circulation: Clinical and experimental results. IX. Symposium Neuroradiologicum, Goteburg, Sweden, Aug. 24–29.

Johnson, D. E., R. B. Bracken, D. A. Swanson, and S. Wallace. 1979. Arterial occlusive techniques in the management of renal diseases, *in* Urology Update Series, Vol. I, lesson 37. Biomedia, Inc., Princeton, N.J. (in press).

Johnson, D. E., K. E. Kaesler, and M. L. Samuels. 1975. Is nephrectomy justified in patients with metastatic renal carcinoma? J. Urol. 114:27–29.

Johnson, D. E., and M. L. Samuels. 1975. Chemotherapy for metastatic renal carcinoma, *in* Cancer Chemotherapy—Fundamental Concepts and Recent Advances. Year Book Medical Publishers, Inc., Chicago, pp. 495–503.

Lalli, A. F., N. Peterson, and J. J. Bookstein. 1969. Roentgen-guided infarctions of kidneys and lungs: Potential therapeutic technic. Radiology 93:434–435.

Lang, E. K. 1971. Superselective arterial catheterization as vehicle for delivering radioactive infarct particles to tumors. Radiology 98:391–399.

Reuter, S. R., and V. P. Chuang. 1974. Control of abdominal bleeding with autogenous embolized material. Radiologie 14:68–91.

Sagel, S. S., R. J. Stanley, R. G. Levitt, and G. Geisse. 1977. Computed tomography of the kidney. Radiology 124:359–370.

Steele, J. R., P. J. Sones, and L. T. Heffner. 1978. The detection of inferior vena caval thrombosis with computed tomography. Radiology 128:385–386.

Swanson, D. A. 1979. The current immunologic status of renal carcinoma. Cancer Bull. (in press).

Tadvarthy, S. M., J. H. Moller, and K. Amplatz. 1975. Polyvinyl alcohol (Ivalon)—A new embolic material. Am. J. Roentgenol. 125:609–616.

Wallace, S. 1976. Interventional radiology. Cancer 37:517–531.

Wallace, S., M. Granmayeh, L. A. DeSantos, J. A. Murray, M. M. Romsdahl, R. B. Bracken, and K. Jonsson. 1979. Arterial occlusion of pelvic bone tumors. Cancer (in press).

Wallace, S., D. E. Schwarten, D. C. Smith, L. P. Gerson, and L. J. Davis. 1978. Intrarenal arteriovenous fistulas: Transcatheter steel coil occlusion. J. Urol. 120:282–286.

Wholey, M. H., R. Stockdale, and T. K. Hung. 1970. A percutaneous balloon catheter for the immediate control of hemorrhage. Radiology 95:65–71.

Zornoza, J., J. Snow, J. M. Lukeman, and H. I. Libshitz. 1977. Aspiration needle biopsy of discrete pulmonary lesions using a new thin needle: Report of the first 100 cases. Radiology 123:519–520.

Cancer of the Genitourinary Tract, edited by
D. E. Johnson and M. L. Samuels.
Raven Press, New York © 1979.

Immunological Studies in Human Urological Cancer

Evan M. Hersh, Sidney Wallace,* Douglas E. Johnson,† and R. Bruce Bracken†

*Departments of Developmental Therapeutics, *Diagnostic Radiology, and †Urology, The University of Texas System Cancer Center M. D. Anderson Hospital and Tumor Institute, Houston, Texas*

Immunological factors play an important role in almost all human malignant diseases. Immunological testing, evaluation, and, more recently, therapy have become important in diagnosis, staging, management, and treatment, at least in the experimental setting. In most human cancers, tumor antigens and immune responses to these antigens have been described. Furthermore, a variety of non-immunologically specific host defense mechanisms, such as the activity of natural killer cells and activated macrophages in the destruction of tumor cells, have been recognized in recent years as important to the overall host control of tumor growth and dissemination. The relationship between the stage of disease and the level of immunological reactivity strongly suggests a suppressive effect of the tumor on host defense mechanisms. Indeed, it has been demonstrated unequivocally in recent years that tumors produce a variety of immuno-suppressive factors that circulate in the blood. In addition, there is a strong re-lationship between immunocompetence and prognosis, so that at every stage of the disease immunocompetent patients have a better prognosis than immunoin-competent patients. Finally, evidence is increasing in almost every human ma-lignant disease that active nonspecific, active specific, adoptive, or immunore-storative immunotherapy can prolong remission duration and survival after conventional therapy.

In this paper we will attempt to accomplish several objectives. We will review various immunological aspects of urological cancer, emphasizing the relationship between the stage of the disease and the immunological reactivity of the subject, the relationship between immunocompetence and prognosis, the immuno-suppressive activity of the tumor, and the presence of specific tumor immunity. We will also outline various approaches to the assessment of both general immu-nocompetence and specific tumor immunity in cancer, with special reference to urological cancer. Finally, we will review some immunological studies con-ducted in our institution on patients undergoing renal infarction. Emphasis will be placed on three major types of urological cancer—renal, bladder, and prostate carcinoma.

IMMUNOLOGICAL EVALUATION IN UROLOGICAL CANCER

The approaches to the evaluation of general immunocompetence and of non-tumor-specific host defense mechanisms that have been applied to patients with urological cancer are outlined in Table 1. These can be viewed broadly as tests of cellular or serological mechanisms. In regard to cellular mechanisms studied in vivo, we can measure the size of the cutaneous inflammatory response to the topical application of croton oil or the cellular response to the abrasion of the skin in the skin window technique. We can measure recall antigen delayed hypersensitivity to antigens to which individuals are commonly exposed, such as dermatophytin, *Candida* organisms, streptokinase-streptodornase, or mumps. We can also measure the development of primary delayed hypersensitivity after immunization with haptens, such as dinitrochlorobenzene (DNCB), or to protein antigens, such as keyhole limpet hemocyanin.

In recent years, measurement of circulating leukocyte levels has been reemphasized in response to reports of a relationship between the level of circulating lymphocytes and the prognosis of the cancer patient. Recently we have developed the ability to measure T and B lymphocytes, as well as certain of their subpopulations. These measurements have provided interesting information on the immunological aspects of human malignant disease.

Recent data suggesting that macrophages and the reticuloendothelial system are important in host defense against cancer also indicate that measurement of circulating monocyte levels could be important.

During the last decade, our ability to study lymphocyte function in vitro

Table 1. *Evaluation of Nonspecific Host-Defense Mechanisms in Human Urological Cancer*

Cellular mechanisms
  In vivo
    Inflammatory response
    Recall delayed hypersensitivity
    Primary delayed hypersensitivity
    Circulating leukocyte levels
      Lymphocytes
      T + B cells
      Monocytes
  In vitro
    Lymphocyte blastogenesis
    Lymphocyte mediator production (lymphokines)
    Serum blocking factor analysis
  Other
    Lymph node morphology
Serologic mechanisms
  Immunoglobulin levels
  Antibody response
  Serum lysozyme level
  Immune complexes
  Other serum factors

has developed extensively. We can measure lymphocyte proliferative responses (lymphocyte blastogenesis) to a variety of stimulants, including T cell mitogens, such as phytohemagglutinin (PHA), and concanavalin-A and B cell mitogens, such as pokeweed mitogen. We can measure the production of mediators or lymphokines by stimulated lymphocytes and can use the lymphocyte proliferative response to measure a variety of blocking factors. It is also important, particularly in urological cancer, to evaluate the morphology of the lymphoid system. Thus, as will be described below, in some cases of urological cancer, lymphocyte depletion in regional lymph nodes has been an important marker of immune depression or depression of host defense mechanisms by tumor.

Serological mechanisms of nonspecific host defense in cancer have not received as much attention as cellular mechanisms. However, there are data indicating that immunoglobulin levels, the antibody response, the level of serum lysozyme, measurement of levels of circulating immune complexes, and various serum blocking factors that interfere with cell-mediated immunity have all been important in characterizing host defense and its failure in urological cancer.

The approaches to the evaluation of specific host defense mechanisms in human urological cancer are outlined in Table 2. Extensive progress has also been made in this area of clinical research. In terms of cellular mechanisms, we can measure lymphocyte blastogenic responses to autologous or allogeneic tumor cells or tumor antigen, as well as the lymphocyte mediator production response to these materials. Indirect approaches to the evaluation of mediator production, which have been used extensively in urological cancer, include the measurement of leukocyte migration inhibition and leukocyte adherence inhibition on exposure of patients' cells to antigen extracts of urological tumors.

We can also measure various effector mechanisms of cell-mediated cytotoxicity including T cell-mediated, K cell-mediated, and antibody-dependent cell-mediated cytotoxicity, as well as so-called natural killer cell activity to tumor cells. These can be measured by proliferation inhibition assays, chromium release

Table 2. *Specific Host-Defense Mechanisms in Human Urological Cancer*

Cellular mechanisms
  Lymphocyte responses
    Blastogenesis
    Mediator production
    Leukocyte migration inhibition
    Leukocyte adherence inhibition
  Effector mechanisms—cytotoxicity
    T cell-mediated
    Killer (K) cell-mediated
    Natural killer (NK) cell-mediated
Serologic mechanisms
  Cytotoxic antibody
  Antibody-dependent cell-mediated cytotoxicity (ADCC) antibody
  Blocking factors (specific)

assays, or assays in which residual tumor cells in microwells are counted after exposure to effector lymphocytes or monocytes.

Serological mechanisms are also important, but again have been less well studied. They are examined by measurements of cytotoxic antibody and of antibody active in ADCC, and evaluation of circulating specific blocking factors.

An important aspect of host defense and its failure in human cancer is the mechanism by which the tumor evades host control. Such mechanisms are outlined in Table 3. By means of antigenic modulation, the tumor cells no longer expose on their surface components that can be recognized by the host defense mechanisms. Antigenic modulation includes antigen masking, antigen internalization, and antigen loss. Tumors are known to produce circulating immunosuppressive factors, including factors that inhibit lymphocyte proliferation, chemotaxis, and the production of lymphokines. The antiproliferative factors produced by tumor cells also apparently inhibit leukocyte production in vivo. Thus, lymphopenia, monocytopenia, and lymph node lymphocyte depletion are common among patients with advancing malignant disease.

Another major mechanism by which tumors evade host control is through the release of blocking factors that impair effector cell attack against the tumor. They include soluble shed antigen, antigen-antibody complexes, and probably also blocking antibody. Certain products released from the tumor activate suppressor cells, including suppressor T cells, suppressor B cells, and suppressor monocytes. Finally, through mechanisms that are not yet understood, the tumor cells can release factors that activate lymphocytes, which in turn produce products that accelerate tumor proliferation and metastasis. Many of these mechanisms will be described below.

Table 3. *Mechanisms of Evasion of Host Control by Malignant Tumors*

Antigenic modulation-immunoresistance
Antigenic masking
Antigenic internalization
Antigen loss
Production of immunosuppressive factors
Lymphocyte proliferation inhibition
Chemotaxis inhibitory factor
Lymphokine production inhibition
Tumor-induced immunocytopenia
Lymphopenia
Monocytopenia
Lymph node lymphocyte depletion
Blocking of cell-mediated effector mechanisms
Soluble shed antigen
Antigen-antibody complexes
Blocking antibody (IgG$_2$)
Tumor-induced suppressor cells
T cells
B cells
Monocytes
Immunostimulation of tumor growth

RECENT STUDIES OF HOST DEFENSE IN UROLOGICAL CANCER

Both nonspecific and tumor-specific host mechanisms have been extensively studied in urological cancer. Almost all the factors outlined above have been described in this group of diseases. In the area of nonspecific host defense mechanisms, important relationships have been described in renal, bladder, and prostate cancer. In renal cancer, nonspecific tests such as lymphocyte blastogenic response to PHA and T lymphocyte levels in the peripheral blood correlate with tumor-specific immunity, and the combinations of results of tumor-specific immunity studies and nonspecific host defense studies correlate very well with the stage of disease (Kjaer and Thomsen 1976).

One of the most useful tests in evaluating host defense in renal cancer has been sensitization and subsequent skin testing with DNCB. For example, the conversion of DNCB skin tests from negative to positive has correlated well with spontaneous remission, and subsequent relapse has correlated well with positive-to-negative conversion of DNCB skin tests in at least one patient with renal cancer (Boasberg et al. 1976).

In bladder cancer (as well as prostate cancer, but not renal cancer), a variety of tests have shown a good correlation with the stage of disease (Fahey et al. 1977). Thus, the degree of DNCB negativity, recall antigen negativity, and lack of response to the cutaneous inflammatory agent croton oil increases with the stage of the disease. Also, there is a significant relationship between disease presence and immunodeficiency, and, conversely, disease absence and immunocompetence. Furthermore, DNCB-positive patients with bladder cancer have a good prognosis in terms of survival, while DNCB-negative patients have a poor prognosis. This is true both for patients with localized invasive disease and for those with advanced metastatic disease. One group has described a complex interrelationship between the grade of malignancy in bladder cancer and tumor stage. In grades I and II there is no correlation of DNCB response with stage, but in grades III and IV there is a highly significant correlation between advanced disease and DNCB negativity. This study involved more than 150 patients and the data are considered to be highly valid (Adolphs and Steffens 1977a).

Other parameters besides skin test reactivity and the cutaneous inflammatory response appear to be related to the presence of tumor or the stage of the disease in bladder cancer. Thus, one group measuring chemotaxis using the Boyden chamber method (Hausman and Brosman 1976) found a good correlation between impaired chemotaxis and the presence of tumor, and between normal chemotaxis and the absence of tumor. Furthermore, in patients studied before and after surgery, chemotaxis improved after the tumor was removed.

One mechanism of impaired host defense in bladder cancer may be related to the presence of suppressor cells. Thus, one group has reported that both peripheral blood leukocytes and lymph node lymphocytes from patients with malignant disease show low stimulation in the mixed lymphocyte culture (Herr 1977, Herr et al. 1976). This improves after surgical removal of the tumor.

Immunological relationships have also been described in patients with prostate carcinoma. Several investigators have reported an excellent correlation between increasing DNCB negativity and advancing grade or stage of disease (Fahey et al. 1977, Adolphs and Steffens 1977b). One group has proposed immunostaging of patients with prostate cancer (Ablin et al. 1976b). It studied 28 patients and included evaluation of immunoglobulin levels, presence of blocking factors, and presence of cell-mediated immunity as measured by delayed-hypersensitivity and lymphocyte blastogenic responses, and correlated the results of these tests with the stage of disease. There was an excellent correlation between the so-called immunostage and the clinical stage of disease, with a *p* value of .01.

Morphological and functional studies have been conducted on regional lymph nodes in patients with prostate cancer. The lymphocyte blastogenic responses of regional lymph node lymphocytes were found to be normal in cancer-bearing subjects, except when lymphocyte depletion was present morphologically in the lymph nodes. Under these circumstances, the blastogenic responses were approximately half the normal level (Herr 1978). The lymphocyte blastogenic responses to PHA of the peripheral blood lymphocytes of patients with prostate carcinoma apparently reflect the presence of circulating blocking factors. A blocking factor was found in the alpha-2-macroglobulin fraction. After cryosurgery for prostate carcinoma, there was an increase in lymphocyte blastogenic responses associated with a decrease in the level of serum alpha-2-macroglobulin in patients with a favorable outcome (Ablin 1977). Cryoprostatectomy apparently also has other immunological effects, including increasing the serum levels of IgM and IgG. This has been speculated to be related to the induction of antitumor antibody (Ablin et al. 1977).

The above outlined studies of nonspecific host defense mechanisms in cancer and specifically in urological cancer make clear that these relationships are quite important in estimating the stage of disease and the prognosis of the patient, and also in understanding the nature of the tumor-host interaction. As will be outlined below, these considerations become even more important when evaluated in terms of tumor-specific immunity.

Tumor-specific immunity has been rather extensively studied in urological cancer. One major approach to the evaluation of tumor immunity in urological cancer has been the use of lymphocyte cytotoxicity to tumor cells. In one study, lymphocyte cytotoxicity to allogeneic cultured tumor cells was studied in patients with various stages of renal carcinoma. Both peripheral blood lymphocytes and lymphocytes extracted from early-stage renal tumors showed high degrees of cytotoxicity to allogeneic cultured renal carcinoma cells. This contrasted with little or no reactivity in patients with stage IV disease (Bichler et al. 1975).

Another important technique that has been used to study tumor immunity in urological cancer patients has been leukocyte migration inhibition (LMI). In one study (Kjaer 1976a), antigen was extracted from autologous and allogeneic renal carcinoma, from normal renal tissue, and from fetal renal tissue. Overall,

50% of patients showed reactivity to autologous and allogeneic renal cancer and fetal renal tissue, but only 3% showed reactivity to normal adult renal tissue. Thus, this assay detects relatively tumor-specific immunity in these patients. Also of interest, a very low percentage of normal subjects showed reactivity to the specific tumor antigens. The reactivity to the appropriate antigens was higher in patients without distant metastases than in those with distant metastases. Also, patients with a vigorous LMI response survived longer than those with a low LMI response (Kjaer 1976a).

Apparently blocking factors play an important role in the modification of tumor-specific immunity in renal carcinoma. This role has been examined through leukocyte washing studies (Kjaer 1976b). Thus, in patients with advanced disease, leukocyte migration-inhibition responses are weak. However, after six washings of the leukocytes to remove surface-bound materials, leukocyte migration inhibition increases, and after 10 washings it increases further. Thus, there are blocking factors bound on the surface of the patients' leukocytes that can be removed by washing.

Some of the most extensive studies of tumor-specific immunity in urological cancer have been done in bladder cancer patients. The most important work has been done by O'Toole and co-workers (O'Toole et al. 1973, O'Toole 1977), who have used a cytotoxicity assay in which either residual tumor cells in microwells are counted after lymphocyte tumor cell interaction or a chromium release assay is used. The following observations have been made. Before treatment, most patients show positive cytotoxicity to allogeneic cultured bladder cancer cells with the degree of reactivity related to subsequent prognosis. All patients show negative reactions after radiotherapy. Reactivity returns quickly in patients with a good prognosis, but there is little or no return during the first year in those with a poor prognosis. In patients followed longer than a year, a return of vigorous reactivity against bladder cancer cells is associated with recurrence.

There is also some evidence that tumor-specific immunity exists in prostatic carcinoma and is related to stage and prognosis. Thus, a saline extract of prostate cancer was used to study leukocyte migration inhibition in 38 patients with prostate cancer (Ablin et al. 1976c). About 35% of the patients reacted, compared to 8% of normal controls. There was some correlation with stage and grade, but it was weak. The same investigators have also used leukocyte adherence-inhibition assays and blocking by autologous patient serum to show evidence for tumor-specific immunity (Ablin et al. 1976a).

Finally, the conventional immunodiagnostic approach of using tumor antigens may also be beneficial in urological cancer. For example, the carcinoembryonic antigen (CEA) assay has been used to follow patients with prostate cancer after surgery. There was an excellent correlation with clinical status of disease in 70% of patients, which was better than that with the acid phosphatase level (Kane et al. 1976).

Table 4. *Change in Delayed Type Hypersensitivity (DTH) After Renal Infarction With or Without Nephrectomy for Renal Carcinoma**

	Number of Patients With Change in DTH		Number of Skin Tests Showing Change	
Group	Increase	Decrease	Increase	Decrease
Infarction with or without nephrectomy	11	3	40	16
Infarction only	10	1	32	6

* Eighteen patients, 102 DTH skin tests.

IMMUNOLOGICAL STUDIES OF RENAL INFARCTION

In our own work, we have emphasized studies of general immunocompetence and immunodeficiency in patients undergoing infarction for renal carcinoma. We have studied delayed hypersensitivity to the recall antigens dermatophytin, *Candida,* varidase, and mumps, and in vitro lymphocyte blastogenic responses to the mitogens and antigens PHA, pokeweed mitogen (PWM), concanavalin-A (Con-A), and streptolysin O (SLO). Eighteen patients were evaluated before and approximately two weeks after renal infarction. Some patients subsequently underwent nephrectomy and others did not.

In terms of delayed hypersensitivity, an increase in immunocompetence was observed after the procedure. Thus, as shown in Tables 4 and 5, the number of patients showing a change in delayed hypersensitivity, the number of individual skin tests showing a change, and the mean diameters of delayed-hypersensitivity reactions all tended toward the positive. Eleven patients showed increases in reactivity (>100% in diameter) and three showed decreases (>50% in diameter), 40 skin test diameters increased and 16 decreased, and the mean and median diameters increased from 7.8 to 13.25 and from 5.0 to 13.27 mm, respectively. This is a clear indication that immunological reactivity improves after nephrectomy.

In contrast, as shown in Table 6, the results with lymphocyte blastogenesis are somewhat confusing. There was a decrease compared to simultaneously

Table 5. *Delayed Type Hypersensitivity in Patients With Renal Carcinoma Before and After Infarction With or Without Nephrectomy*

	Diameter of Values Showing Change (mm)	
Parameter	Pretherapy	Posttherapy
Mean	7.8	13.25
±S.D.	7.9	9.40
Median	5.0	13.27

Table 6. *Lymphocyte Blastogenesis in Patients With Renal Carcinoma Before and After Infarction With or Without Nephrectomy*

	Response* to							
	PHA		PWM		Con-A		SLO	
Group	Pre	Post	Pre	Post	Pre	Post	Pre	Post
Patients	53.8	20.2	37.8	21.8	11.5	16.7	19.3	12.7
Normal controls	34.4	35.0	26.0	30.5	18.1	21.4	27.2	29.1

* $Cpm/1.5\times10^5$ lymphocytes $\times\ 10^3$.

evaluated control subjects in PHA response, PWM response, and SLO response, and no significant change or a slight increase in the Con-A response in post- as compared to pre-therapy values. This suggests that some stress effect on circulating lymphocytes may be manifested by these depressed post-treatment values. Patients' lymphocytes were cultured in autologous and allogeneic serum and there appeared to be no major circulating serum factor that could account for post-therapy blastogenic responses.

CONCLUSIONS

Immunological factors are important in renal, bladder, and prostate cancer. The following conclusions can be drawn:

1. Tumor burden suppresses nonspecific host defense, which improves when the tumor is removed.

2. Good general immunocompetence correlates with good prognosis.

3. Tumor-specific immunity to these tumors is present.

4. Levels of tumor-specific immunity correlate with disease status. They are positive early in the disease, absent if the disease is extensive, and depressed by therapy. Good post-therapy reactions indicate a good prognosis.

5. Serum factors can block nonspecific or specific immunity.

There is evidence for a relationship between immunocompetence and prognosis, for a relationship between grade and stage of disease and prognosis, and for the release of immunosuppressive serum factors from the tumor. There is also strong evidence for tumor-specific immunity in all major types of urological cancer. Both tumor cells and tumor antigens are useful in immune assays, which include leukocyte migration inhibition and leukocyte adherence inhibition. Both nonspecific and tumor-specific approaches should be useful for staging disease, arriving at a prognosis, and monitoring therapy.

ACKNOWLEDGMENTS

This investigation was supported by grants CA-05831 and CA-14984, awarded by the National Cancer Institute, Department of Health, Education and Welfare.

REFERENCES

Ablin, R. J. 1977. Serum proteins in prostatic cancer. VI. Reduction of the suppressive ("blocking"?) properties of serum on in vitro parameters of cell-mediated immunologic responsiveness following cryosurgery. Urol. Int. 32:65–73.

Ablin, R. J., R. A. Bhatti, P. D. Guinan, and G. R. Bruns. 1976a. Evaluation of cellular immunologic responsiveness in the clinical management of patients with prostatic cancer. IV. Leucocyte adherence inhibition. Urol. Int. 31:459–469.

Ablin, R. J., P. D. Guinan, B. Sundar, and I. M. Bush. 1976b. "Immunostaging" of patients with prostatic cancer: Correlation of "immunostage" and clinical stage. An interim report. Curr. Ther. Res. 20:674–679.

Ablin, R. J., C. Marrow, P. D. Guinan, G. R. Bruns, N. Sadoughi, T. John, and I. M. Bush. 1976c. Urol. Int. 31:444–458.

Ablin, R. J., W. A. Soanes, and M. J. Gonder. 1977. Serum proteins in prostatic cancer. V. Alterations in immunoglobulins and clinical responsiveness following cryoprostatectomy. Urol. Int. 32:56–64.

Adolphs, H. D., and L. Steffens. 1977a. Evaluation of the immunocompetence of patients with transitional cell carcinoma of the bladder. Urol. Res. 5:29–33.

Adolphs, H. D., and L. Steffens. 1977b. Correlation between tumour stage, tumour grade, and immunocompetence in patients with carcinoma of the bladder and prostate. Eur. Urol. 3:23–25.

Bichler, K. H., W. Ax, and C. Tautz. 1975. Cell-mediated immunity in patients with renal adenocarcinoma. Eur. Urol. 1:231–234.

Boasberg, P. D., F. R. Eilber, and D. L. Morton. 1976. Immunocompetence and spontaneous regression of metastatic renal cell carcinoma. J. Surg. Oncol. 8:207–210.

Fahey, J. L., S. Brosman, and F. Dorey. 1977. Immunological responsiveness in patients with bladder cancer. Cancer Res. 37:2875–2878.

Hausman, M. S., and S. A. Brosman. 1976. Abnormal monocyte function in bladder cancer patients J. Urol. 115:537–547.

Herr, H. W. 1977. Suppressor cell activity in lymph nodes regional to bladder carcinoma. Surg. Forum 28:546–548.

Herr, H. W. 1978. Immune reactivity of lymph nodes regional to prostatic cancer. J. Surg. Res. 24:409–414.

Herr, H. W., M. A. Bean, and W. F. Whitmore. 1976. Decreased ability of blood leukocytes from patients with tumors of the urinary bladder to act as stimulator cells in mixed leukocyte culture. Cancer Res. 36:2754–2760.

Kane, R. D., D. D. Mickey, and D. F. Paulson. 1976. Serial carcinoembryonic antigen assays in patients with metastatic carcinoma of prostate being treated with chemotherapy. Urology 8:559–562.

Kjaer, M. 1976a. Prognostic value of tumour-directed, cell-mediated hypersensitivity detected by means of the leucocyte migration technique in patients with renal carcinoma. Eur. J. Cancer 12:889–898.

Kjaer, M. 1976b. Effect of leucocyte washings on cellular immunity to human renal carcinoma. Eur. J. Cancer 12:783–792.

Kjaer, M., and M. Thomsen. 1976. General immunocompetence and tumour-directed, cell-mediated hypersensitivity in vitro in patients with renal carcinoma. Acta Path. Microbiol. Scand. 84:403–413.

O'Toole, C. 1977. A ^{51}chromium isotope release assay for detecting cytotoxicity to human bladder carcinoma. Int. J. Cancer 19:324–331.

O'Toole, C., B. Unsgaard, L. E. Almgard, and B. Johansson. 1973. The cellular immune response to carcinoma of the urinary bladder: Correlation to clinical stage and treatment. Br. J. Cancer 28:266–275.

Cancer of the Genitourinary Tract, edited by
D. E. Johnson and M. L. Samuels.
Raven Press, New York © 1979.

Experimental Studies With Transcatheter Vascular Occlusion

James H. Anderson, Ph.D.,* Gerardo Chica, M.D.,† Sidney
Wallace, M.D.,* and Douglas E. Johnson, M.D.†

*Departments of * Diagnostic Radiology and † Urology, The University of Texas System
Cancer Center M. D. Anderson Hospital and Tumor Institute, Houston, Texas*

Transcatheter vascular occlusion is being used with increasing frequency to treat a wide variety of clinical conditions (Rosch et al. 1972, Wallace et al. 1976, Kerber et al. 1978, Walter et al. 1978). In the management of the renal cell carcinoma patient, the procedure has been used preoperatively to facilitate surgery by decreasing vascularity and as a nonoperative procedure when surgery is contraindicated (Almgard et al. 1973, Goldstein et al. 1975, Wallace and Goldstein 1976). Preliminary clinical data suggest that, in combination with nephrectomy, chemotherapy, or both, transcatheter vascular occlusion may provide better patient management than surgery or chemotherapy used alone or together. These results, as well as those by others reporting encouraging results following transcatheter vascular occlusion for the cancer patient (Feldman et al. 1975, Bree et al. 1976, Goldstein et al. 1976, Wallace and Goldstein 1976), have stimulated interest in animal research aimed at improving vascular occlusion methodology and extending its application. We wish to present the results of animal research studies conducted to examine techniques of transcatheter renal arterial occlusion and application of the procedure in an animal tumor model.

MATERIALS USED FOR VASCULAR OCCLUSION

A large number of materials have been employed for transcatheter vascular occlusion including autologous tissue and blood clot (Almgard et al. 1973, Reuter and Chuang 1974, White et al. 1974), metallic and plastic spheres (Kricheff et al. 1972), tissue adhesive (Kerber et al. 1978), Gelfoam (Bree et al. 1976, Wallace 1976), silicone rubber (Doppman et al. 1971), and stainless steel coils (Gianturco et al. 1975, Anderson et al. 1977a,b). The selection of materials depends on various factors, including the patient's clinical condition and the desired extent and duration of occlusion. In addition, technical factors relating to the procedure and local and regional hemodynamics, including the extent of collateral circulation, must be evaluated. In the renal cell carcinoma patient, one must consider whether the procedure is being employed as an adjuvant or an alternative to surgery.

Gelfoam has been used extensively in transcatheter vascular occlusions involving the kidney. The material is readily available from commercial sources. It can be cut into strips or small pieces, is highly compressible when wet with saline or contrast medium, and offers little resistance when injected through standard angiographic catheters (Figure 1). Individual pieces of Gelfoam can be loaded into a syringe immediately prior to catheter delivery, which allows some control over the degree of occlusion. Gelfoam occlusion is readily seen fluoroscopically as stasis of contrast medium in the renal vascular bed. Gelfoam has been used largely to control bleeding at sites unresponsive to vasoconstrictor therapy and to occlude the vascular supply of tumors.

Reports in the literature indicate that occlusion with Gelfoam cubes or strips lasts for days to months (Goldstein et al. 1976, Wallace 1976). This variability in duration of occlusion and a similar variability in degree have been attributed largely to recanalization. Our laboratory animal studies have confirmed this reported variability and have revealed additional factors of clinical importance. First, immediate postocclusion angiographic examination may not always give a true indication of the degree of occlusion. Angiographic studies performed in dogs three days to four weeks after renal arterial occlusion with Gelfoam cubes 2–3 mm in diameter have shown wide variability in the extent of occlusion (Figure 2). In many instances, angiographic studies performed several hours after occlusion have shown significant perfusion of vasculature that had previously been obviously occluded. It is unlikely that recanalization would account for the perfusion in this short period of time, and other factors may be involved. It is possible that, shortly after occlusion, the injected cubes of Gelfoam become distributed more distally within the vessels. This would seem most likely to occur at branching points of larger vessels, where proximal pressure in the main renal artery may force the larger Gelfoam pieces distally into one of the

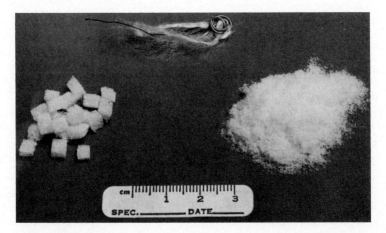

Figure 1. Occlusion materials employed in canine studies include Gelfoam cubes, Gelfoam powder (mixed with Renografin to create a suspension), and stainless steel coils.

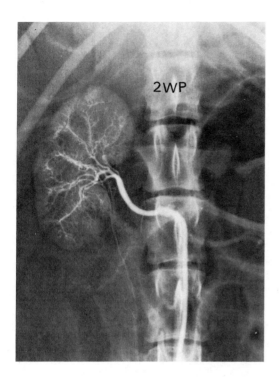

Figure 2. Renal arteriogram two weeks following occlusion with Gelfoam plugs. Recanalization of some previously occluded vessels has occurred. ("2WP" is experimental animal code number.)

branches, allowing blood to flow in the other. Second, vasospasm induced by the catheter may impede peripheral distribution of the Gelfoam. Subsequent relaxation after catheterization may allow more distal migration of the Gelfoam. With time, some degree of recanalization following Gelfoam occlusion can be expected, particularly if small particles of Gelfoam are used.

Transcatheter vascular embolization with small particles is useful when occlusion at the small vessel level is desired, as for control of small vessel bleeding or for tumor occlusion when extensive collateral circulation exists. In such situations, occlusion of only the primary or secondary vessels supplying the lesion may enhance blood flow through existing collaterals. This observation was clearly evident in previous animal studies relating to transcatheter vascular occlusion of the splenic arterial supply (Anderson et al. 1977a). The penetration of embolic material into small vessels supplying a lesion may reduce the potential functional capabilities of collateral circulation. In addition, the use of small-particle emboli usually provides a more homogeneous distribution of the material within the vascular supply of the lesion. However, embolization with small-particle material is accompanied by several potential complications, including passage of the material through arteriovenous shunts and reflux of the lighter, smaller particles into the aorta during the embolization procedure.

Figure 3 illustrates a canine renal arterial embolization using a suspension made from mixing 200 mg of Gelfoam powder in 10 cc of Renografin 76.

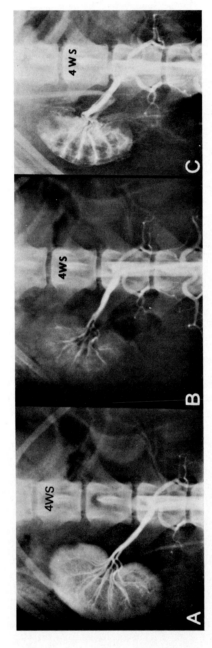

Figure 3. A, Preocclusion renal arteriogram. B, Arteriogram immediately following occlusion with Gelfoam powder–Renografin suspension. C, Arteriogram four weeks following occlusion. Note irregular vascular pattern and early venous filling. ("4WS" is experimental animal code number.)

The slurry is radiopaque, is easily injected through small catheters, and distributes evenly throughout the vascular supply, as evidenced during the occlusion procedure by a faint but persistent homogeneous opacity throughout the kidney. Three days after occlusion, angiographic examination revealed recanalization of the main renal artery, and at one week recanalization extended to the secondary and tertiary interlobar branches. Two and four weeks after occlusion, recanalization extended throughout the major portion of the renal vasculature except for the peripheral cortical vessels. Histologic examination showed the presence of Gelfoam particles in the smaller renal vessels with uniform extensive renal infarction.

Our laboratory experience with the Gelfoam-contrast slurry reveals a major contraindication to its use. If enough of the material is employed to occlude up to the distal one third of the main renal artery, turbulence created by blood flowing into the artery may cause reflux of the occluding material into the aorta, and the small Gelfoam particles could be easily drawn into the contralateral renal artery or the lumbar vessels. This observation, along with the potentially dangerous passage of the material through arteriovenous communications, raises serious questions concerning its clinical use.

Permanent occlusion of the main renal artery is best accomplished with stainless steel coils (Figure 4). The coils are made from 2-inch segments of 0.035-inch angiographic guide wire from which the internal mandril has been removed. The stainless steel coils are preshaped to form a helical configuration and woolen strands are attached to help induce thrombosis. They are easily passed through

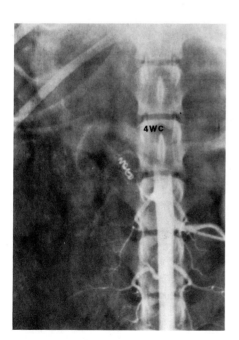

Figure 4. Aortogram showing completely occluded renal artery four weeks after occlusion with a stainless steel coil. ("4WC" is experimental animal code number.)

a 7 French Teflon angiographic catheter to form a mechanical block in the vessel immediately distal to the catheter tip. The principal advantage of the coil is that it provides large central vessel occlusion. Eventually the coil becomes fibrotically encased, ensuring permanent occlusion.

In dogs, stainless steel coil occlusion of the main renal artery provided a much different response than that seen with either Gelfoam cubes or the Gelfoam-contrast medium slurry. The coil produced total occlusion of the main renal artery with no evidence of recanalization. However, this type of occlusion by itself does not provide distribution of emboli into more peripheral portions of the renal vascular supply, which may be required when collateral circulation supplies the lesion, as is sometimes the case in hypervascular hypernephromas. In the normal dog kidney, collaterals mainly from the lumbar arteries serve as a source of blood following main renal arterial occlusion. Although kidneys occluded with the coil showed some renal function, as evidenced by caliceal opacification, occlusion of the main renal artery produced atrophic kidneys in four weeks. This may not be the case with highly vascular neoplasms, in which central blockage of the main arterial supply may simply enhance blood flow through extensive collateral channels.

There is no single occluding material that may be considered for transcatheter vascular occlusive therapy in all clinical conditions. Factors involving the clinical status of the patient and alternative modes of therapy must be considered. The choice of occluding materials depends in part on the degree and duration of occlusion desired and the anatomical characteristics of the main vascular supply and collateral circulation. Embolization into smaller vessels may be advantageous in highly vascular lesions, but the possibility of recanalization must be considered. Combined use of Gelfoam embolization and more central occlusion with the stainless steel coil may provide the most permanent form of occlusion. At M. D. Anderson Hospital and Tumor Institute, this combination occlusion procedure is used in renal cell carcinoma patients when transcatheter vascular occlusion procedures are indicated. In such cases, combination therapy including transcatheter vascular occlusion and nephrectomy, chemotherapy, or both, are employed.

VASCULAR OCCLUSION STUDIES IN AN ANIMAL TUMOR MODEL

A major problem relating to laboratory research in vascular occlusion for renal cell carcinoma is the lack of a large animal model, which is necessary to duplicate the clinical therapeutic approach using selective transcatheter occlusion procedures. In recent years, attention has been directed to a murine renal cell carcinoma model that has been reported to share some characteristics with human renal cell carcinoma, including its ability to metastasize to the lungs (Murphy and Hrushesky 1973) (Figure 5). The tumor originally arose spontaneously as a renal cortical adenocarcinoma in an inbred Balb/cCr mouse. Tumor-bearing and normal Balb/cCr mice are available from the West Seneca Labora-

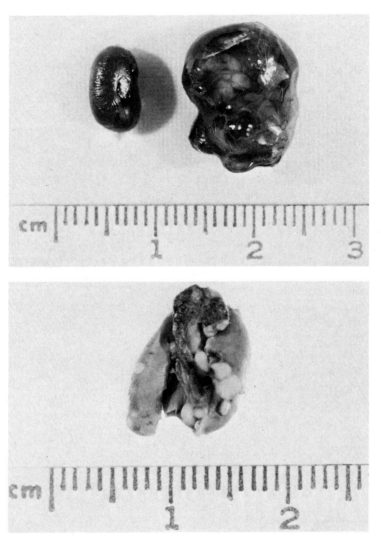

Figure 5. Top, Necropsy photograph showing primary renal tumor in Balb/cCr mouse kidney (right) 28 days following intrarenal injection of tumor cell suspension. The kidney on the left did not receive tumor cell injection and is normal in size. Bottom, Photograph of lungs showing metastatic lesions.

tory of Roswell Park Memorial Institute. The tumor model is currently being maintained in our laboratory by intrarenal transfer of a tumor cell suspension (prepared from tumor-bearing animals) into recipient Balb/cCr mice every 28 to 35 days. The model has been used to evaluate the effect of systemically administered chemotherapeutic agents on the primary renal tumor and its metastatic pulmonary lesions (Hrushesky and Murphy 1973, 1974, Murphy and Williams 1974).

Attempts in our laboratory to embolize the arterial supply to the renal tumor were unsuccessful because of technical problems associated with the size of the animal (25 gm). However, it is possible to surgically ligate the renal vascular pedicle and evaluate the therapeutic effects of this procedure.

Our laboratory experience using this model has indicated that ligation of the renal vasculature alone has little effect on the life span of renal tumor-bearing mice. For this preliminary study, the renal tumor was initiated in normal Balb/cCr mice by intrarenal subcapsular injection of a tumor cell suspension obtained from a tumor-bearing mouse donor. Animals receiving intrarenal tumor cell injections and no therapy died, on the average, 41 days following tumor induction, while those that underwent ligation of the renal vascular supply 14 days after tumor cell injection died, on the average, 48 days following tumor induction.

The murine renal cell carcinoma model employed has been used primarily to evaluate systemically administered chemotherapeutic drugs. However, several observations made during the study cast doubt on the use of this model to evaluate therapies that involve local manipulation of the primary tumor target site. Initiation of tumor growth is best achieved by intrarenal subcapsular injection of a tumor cell suspension. Although small-gauge (31-gauge) needles and small-volume (0.05-ml) injections are used, it is impossible to ensure that tumor cells do not leak from the kidney during or following subcapsular injection. Tumor growth often occurs not only at the primary site of injection, but also in perirenal regions. Therapeutic modalities aimed chiefly at the kidney as a target site, i.e., nephrectomy and ligation of the renal vasculature, may not affect the growth of tumors derived from leakage of cells during injection. For this reason, studies involving systemically administered agents may be more applicable to this model.

ACKNOWLEDGMENTS

This investigation was supported by grant number KO4-CA-00083–03 RAD, awarded by the National Cancer Institute, U.S. Department of Health, Education and Welfare. Research support was also provided by the George Alfred Cook Memorial Fund and the John S. Dunn Research Foundation.

REFERENCES

Almgard, L. E., I. Fernstrom, and M. Haverling. 1973. Treatment of renal adenocarcinoma by embolic occlusion of the renal circulation. Br. J. Urol. 45:474–479.

Anderson, J. H., A. VuBan, S. Wallace, J. P. Hester, and J. S. Burke. 1977a. Transcatheter splenic arterial occlusion: An experimental study in dogs. Radiology 125:95–102.

Anderson, J. H., S. Wallace, and C. Gianturco. 1977b. Transcatheter intravascular coil occlusion of experimental arteriovenous fistulas. Am. J. Roentgenol. 129:795–798.

Bree, R. L., H. M. Goldstein, and S. Wallace. 1976. Transcatheter embolization of the internal iliac artery in the management of neoplasms of the pelvis. Surg. Gynecol. Obstet. 143:597–601.

Doppman, J. L., W. Zapol, and J. Pierce. 1971. Transcatheter embolization with silicone rubber preparation: Experimental observations. Invest. Radiol. 6:304–309.

Feldman, F., W. J. Casarella, and H. M. Dick. 1975. Selective intraarterial embolization of bone tumors: A useful adjunct in the management of selective disease. Am. J. Roentgenol. 123:130–139.

Gianturco, C., J. H. Anderson, and S. Wallace. 1975. Mechanical devices for arterial occlusion. Am. J. Roentgenol. 124:428–435.

Goldstein, H. M., H. Medellin, M. T. Beydoun, S. Wallace, Y. Ben-Menachem, R. B. Bracken, and D. E. Johnson. 1975. Transcatheter embolization of renal cell carcinoma. Am. J. Roentgenol. 123:557–562.

Goldstein, H. M., S. Wallace, J. H. Anderson, R. L. Bree, and C. Gianturco. 1976. Transcatheter occlusion of abdominal tumor. Radiology 120:539–545.

Hrushesky, W. J., and G. P. Murphy. 1973. Investigation of a new renal tumor model. J. Surg. Res. 15:327–336.

Hrushesky, W. J., and G. P. Murphy. 1974. Evaluation of chemotherapeutic agents in a new murine renal carcinoma model. J. Natl. Cancer Inst. 52:1117–1122.

Kerber, C. W., L. D. Cromwell, and P. E. Sheptak. 1978. Intraarterial cyanoacrylate: An adjunct in the treatment of spinal/paraspinal arteriovenous malformations. Am. J. Roentgenol. 103:99–103.

Kricheff, I. I., M. Madayog, and P. Braunstein. 1972. Transfemoral catheter embolization of cerebral and posterior fossa arteriovenous malformation. Radiology 103:107–111.

Murphy, G. P., and W. J. Hrushesky. 1973. A murine renal cell carcinoma. J. Natl. Cancer Inst. 50:1013–1021.

Murphy, G. P., and P. D. Williams. 1974. Testing of chemotherapeutic agents in murine renal cell adenocarcinoma. Res. Commun. Chem. Pathol. Pharmacol. 9:265–277.

Reuter, S. R., and V. P. Chuang. 1974. Control of abdominal bleeding with autogenous embolized material. Radiologe 14:86–91.

Rosch, J., C. T. Dotter, and M. J. Brown. 1972. Selective arterial embolization. Radiology 102:303–306.

Wallace, S. 1976. Interventional radiology. Cancer 37:517–531.

Wallace, S., C. Gianturco, J. H. Anderson, H. M. Goldstein, L. J. Davis, and R. L. Bree. 1976. Transcatheter intravascular steel coil occlusion. Am. J. Roentgenol. 127:381–387.

Wallace, S., and H. M. Goldstein. 1976. Intravascular occlusive therapy. Postgrad. Med. 59:141–146.

Walter, J. F., J. J. Bookstein, R. A. Kramer, W. B. Connor, M. L. Trollope, and R. W. Jamplis. 1978. Therapeutic angiography. Arch. Surg. 113:432–439.

White, R. I., F. A. Giargiana, and W. Bell. 1974. Bleeding duodenal ulcer control: Selective arterial embolization with analogous blood clot. J.A.M.A. 229:546–548.

Cancer of the Genitourinary Tract, edited by
D. E. Johnson and M. L. Samuels.
Raven Press, New York © 1979.

Current Status of Chemotherapy in Metastatic Renal Carcinoma

Gerald P. Bodey, M.D.

*Department of Developmental Therapeutics, The University of Texas System Cancer Center
M. D. Anderson Hospital and Tumor Institute, Houston, Texas*

Because renal cell carcinoma is uncommon, few oncologists acquire extensive experience with this disease. Nevertheless, it is estimated that over 7,000 patients will die this year from renal carcinoma (Cancer statistics 1978, 1978). There are about 3.5 new cases per 100,000 people per year in this country, and they involve males nearly twice as frequently as females. Approximately 85% of all renal malignant tumors are adenocarcinoma, the remainder being tumors of the pelvis and renal capsule.

The most common signs and symptom of renal carcinoma are a palpable mass (in 50% of patients), hematuria (60%), and pain (50%). However, this "classic triad" has been found in as few as 9% of patients at diagnosis (Skinner et al. 1978). Other common systemic manifestations of malignant disease, such as weight loss, anemia, and fever, are detected in 20–30% of patients initially. Renal carcinoma is interesting because of its association with a variety of paraneoplastic syndromes. Polycythemia (2–10%), secondary hyperparathyroidism (3%), and hepatic abnormalities (15%) without liver metastases are recognized complications.

Skinner et al. (1978) reviewed 309 patients with renal cell carcinoma treated at the Massachusetts General Hospital during a 30-year period. One third of the patients had stage 1 disease and only one quarter had metastatic disease. Most of these patients were treated with simple or radical nephrectomy. The five-year survival rates with the two procedures were similar and correlated with stage of disease. Only six of 77 patients (8%) with stage 4 disease survived five years and five of these six underwent excision of solitary pulmonary nodules. Table 1 compares the survival rates in this series and that reported by Prout (1974). The extent of disease and survival were related to histologic grade in both series.

Common sites of metastases from renal carcinoma are the lung, bone, opposite kidney, and retroperitoneum. Although considerable interest has arisen over the disappearance of distant metastases, mainly in the lung, following surgical excision of the primary tumor, it occurred in less than 1% of cases in a large

Table 1. *Survival in Patients with Renal Carcinoma*

Stage	Prout Study*		Skinner Study†	
	5-Year	10-Year	5-Year	10-Year
1	66	60	65	56
2	64	67	47	20
3	42	38	51	37
4	11	0	8	7

* Prout 1974.
† Skinner et al. 1978.

series. However, surgical excision of a single distant metastasis has produced long-term survival in about 30% of patients (Skinner et al. 1978).

For many years, hormonal therapy has been advocated for patients with metastatic renal carcinoma. This therapy was based upon observations on stilbestrol-induced adenocarcinomas of the kidney in male golden hamsters (Bloom 1964). The removal of stilbestrol or administration of testosterone or progesterone halted the growth of these tumors. Hrushesky and Murphy (1977) have recently reviewed the results of progestational therapy of human renal carcinoma. Prior to 1971, about 17% of patients were reported to have demonstrated response to these agents (Table 2). However, criteria for response were poorly defined in most series. In more recent series, using stricter criteria for response, less than 5% of patients have responded to progesterone derivatives.

Most chemotherapeutic agents have not been very effective against renal carcinoma. Unfortunately, few investigators see a sufficient number of patients with this disease to gain much experience, so only a few drugs have been investigated thoroughly. Table 3 lists some of the important chemotherapeutic agents tested in patients with renal carcinoma. Only vinblastine has demonstrated substantial activity against this tumor. In a series reported by Hrushesky and Murphy (1977), a weekly dose of 0.1–0.3 mg/kg was generally used. Complete remissions were obtained in three of 135 patients, lasting up to four years. Twenty-three

Table 2. *Response of Patients to Progesterone Derivatives for Renal Carcinoma*

Series	Number of Patients	Percent Responding
Bloom (1971)	80	16
Wagle and Murphy (1971)	43	17
Samuels et al. (1968)	23	17
Alberto and Senn (1974)	58	0
Hahn and Brodovsky (1976)	166	0
Lokich and Harrison (1975)	73	0
Talley (1973)	98	7
1967–1971	228	17
1971–1976	415	2

Table 3. *Response of Patients to Single-Agent Chemotherapy for Renal Carcinoma*

Agent	Number of Patients Treated	Percent Responding
Vinblastine	135	25
MeCCNU	79	7
5-fluorouracil	51	5
Hydroxyurea	45	5
Cyclophosphamide	44	0
Nitrogen mustard	35	4
6-mercaptopurine	26	2
Mitomycin-C	26	11
Cis-platinum	20	0
Bleomycin	20	0
Adriamycin	15	0

patients obtained partial remissions and seven achieved lesser responses. It is interesting that the response rate for 39 patients who received 2–3 mg/kg/wk was 31%, whereas that for 96 patients who received <2 mg/kg/wk was only 15%, suggesting a correlation between dose and frequency of response.

Combination chemotherapy has been investigated in patients with renal carcinoma, primarily with combinations of vinblastine, nitrosoureas, and progestational agents (Table 4), but none of these regimens has demonstrated superiority to the high-dose vinblastine regimens. The best results reported recently were achieved with a combination of Adriamycin (75 mg/m^2 every three weeks), vincristine (2 mg weekly), medroxyprogesterone acetate (400 mg weekly), and bacillus Calmette-Guérin (BCG) (3–6×10^8 organisms weekly by scarification) (Ishmael et al. 1978). Ten of 31 patients achieved complete or partial remissions, but survival data were not reported. In eight of the 10 patients who responded, the primary tumor was resected before chemoimmunotherapy was administered. In a recent study of vinblastine plus chloroethyl cyclohexyl nitroso urea (CCNU), 120 mg/m^2 of CCNU was given on day 1 and 0.1 mg/kg of vinblastine on

Table 4. *Response of Patients to Combination Chemotherapy for Renal Carcinoma*

Regimen	Number of Patients	Percent Responding
VLB* + 5FU + medroxyprogesterone acetate	20	0
MeCCNU + medroxyprogesterone acetate	38	11
VLB + medroxyprogesterone acetate	38	8
MeCCNU + VLB	15	7
VLB + hydroxyurea	15	0
CCNU + VLB	29	24
Vincristine + Adriamycin + BCG + medroxyprogesterone acetate	31	33

* Vinblastine, velban, and vincaleukoblastine.

days 1 and 8 (or 15) of each 6- to 8-week cycle (Davis and Manalo 1978). A response rate of 24% was obtained in 29 patients. The two complete remissions persisted for 19+ and 24 months, while the five partial remissions lasted two to nine months.

Since currently available therapy is only marginally effective against advanced renal carcinoma, the investigation of new agents is of critical importance. Several agents appeared to be promising in early phase I clinical trials. Eagen et al. (1976) obtained partial remissions in two of five patients treated with dianhydrogalactitol, lasting 93+ and 203+ days. Both of these patients had failed on prior therapy with vinblastine. Unfortunately, in a larger series (Hahn 1977) the initial encouraging result was not confirmed.

Triazinate is a triazine folate antagonist that inhibits dihydrofolate reductase. It differs from methotrexate in that it does not need active enzymatic transport to penetrate the cell membrane. Since one mechanism of resistance to methotrexate is loss of membrane transport, triazinate was expected to be effective against tumors that might be resistant to methotrexate. In early phase II clinical trials with this drug, three of six patients with renal carcinoma achieved partial remissions (Rodriguez et al. 1977). Subsequent studies have failed to demonstrate any advantages for triazinate over methotrexate, but an extensive trial of this drug in renal carcinoma has not been undertaken.

Neocarzinostatin is an antitumor polypeptide obtained from *Streptomyces carzinostaticus* that selectively inhibits DNA synthesis. Initial Japanese studies indicated that it had activity against a variety of tumors, especially acute leukemia and gastric carcinoma. It was considered to be of potential value against renal carcinoma because after administration to rabbits, the drug concentrated in the kidney (Maeda et al. 1976). We have treated 19 patients with neocarzinostatin and five have had stabilization of previously progressive disease for two to over seven months.

Vindesine, or desacetyl vinblastine amide sulfate, is a new vinca alkaloid that is considerably more potent against tumor cell lines in vitro than vincristine or vinblastine, as well as less toxic in animals than vincristine. Several different schedules of drug administration are currently under investigation, but a frequent schedule is 4 mg/m^2 every 10 to 14 days. Major toxicities include myelosuppression, alopecia, phlebitis, constipation, and paralytic ileus. About 35% of patients receiving at least two courses develop paresthesia. In our initial phase I study, we observed one incomplete response, one case of stable disease, and five failures in seven patients treated. Other investigators have also observed minimal responses with vindesine in initial studies. Because of the activity of vinblastine in this disease, vindesine deserves further evaluation.

The likelihood of discovering a highly active antitumor agent for renal carcinoma is hampered by the scarcity of patients. Recent emphasis has been concentrated on adequately evaluating new agents in common tumors, and broad phase II studies have been discouraged. Thus, potentially active agents in uncommon tumors may be overlooked if they do not first show activity against common tumors. Several interesting new agents that are undergoing late phase I–early phase II clinical trials deserve investigation in renal carcinoma.

Bruceantin is one of a series of plant alkaloids derived from *Brucea antidysenterica* that have shown activity against a variety of animal tumors. Currently phase I studies are being completed and early phase II studies are being planned. We have used a five-day schedule at three-week intervals, and it appears that the optimum dose is 3.0–3.6 mg/m^2/day with this schedule. At this dose, toxicities include nausea and vomiting, hypotension, and fever. Although the antitumor activity of this agent has not yet been defined in humans, it is of interest because of its unique structure and in vitro activity.

4'-9-Acridinylamino-methane-sulfon-m-anisidide (AMSA) is one of a series of acridine derivatives currently undergoing phase II clinical trials. This drug intercalates with DNA and inhibits DNA polymerase. It is active against several animal tumors and produces long-term survivals in animals with B16 melanoma. It does not appear to produce any schedule dependency. We have used a three-day schedule with an optimum dose of 40 mg/m^2/day, and the major dose-limiting toxicity has been myelosuppression. One patient with renal carcinoma achieved a partial remission with AMSA and another maintained disease stabilization for more than eight weeks. In early phase II studies AMSA has been shown to have activity against acute leukemia and breast carcinoma, and it should be investigated in renal carcinoma.

Another new agent that has aroused considerable interest is N-phosphonacetyl-L-aspartate (PALA), a transition state inhibitor of aspartate transcarbamylase. There is an inverse correlation between drug efficacy and tumor ATCase levels. The drug is of special interest because it has produced complete, prolonged, unmaintained remissions in animals with Lewis lung carcinoma. Phase I studies are currently in progress with a dose of 5 gm/m^2 for one day at two-week intervals. The drug is not myelosuppressive and dose-limiting toxicities appear to be mucositis and dermatitis. Thus far, only one patient with renal carcinoma who has been treated with the drug has failed to respond.

Progress in the treatment of advanced renal carcinoma has been slow. Vinblastine is the most active chemotherapeutic agent of those tested adequately, but few patients have obtained prolonged complete remissions and more than 60% fail to obtain any meaningful response. No combination of drugs has produced results superior to those with vinblastine alone. Hence, if improvements are to be realized, emphasis must be placed on the evaluation of new drugs. It is hoped that, with an aggressive, concerted effort, effective agents will be discovered.

REFERENCES

Alberto, P., and H. J. Senn. 1974. Hormonal therapy of renal carcinoma alone and in association with cytostatic drugs. Cancer 33:1226–1229.

Bloom, H. J. G. 1964. Hormone treatment of renal tumors—Experimental and clinical observations, *in* Tumors of the Kidney and Ureter, E. W. Riches, ed. Williams & Wilkins Co., Baltimore, pp. 311–320.

Bloom, H. J. G. 1971. Medroxyprogesterone acetate (Provera) in the treatment of metastatic renal cancer. Br. J. Cancer 25:250–265.

Cancer statistics 1978. 1978. CA 28:17–32.

Davis, T. E., and F. B. Manalo. 1978. Combination chemotherapy of advanced renal cancer with CCNU and vinblastine (Abstract C-39). Proc. Am. Assoc. Cancer Res. Am. Soc. Clin. Oncol. 19:316.

Eagan, R. T., C. G. Moertel, R. G. Hahn, and A. J. Schutt. 1976. Brief communication: Phase I study of a five-day intermittent schedule for 1,2:5,6-dianhydrogalactitol (NSC-132313). J. Natl. Cancer Inst. 56:179–181.

Hahn, R. G. 1977. Megace, VP-16, Cytoxan and galactitol phase II treatment trials in advanced renal cell cancer (Abstract C-262). Proc. Am. Assoc. Cancer Res. Am. Soc. Clin. Oncol. 18:332.

Hahn, R. G., and H. Brodovsky. 1976. Methyl CCNU, Velban and Depo-Provera treatment trials in advanced renal cancer (Abstract C-38). Proc. Am. Assoc. Cancer Res. Am. Soc. Clin. Oncol. 17:246.

Hrushesky, W. J., and G. P. Murphy. 1977. Current status of the therapy of advanced renal carcinoma. J. Surg. Oncol. 9:277–288.

Ishmael, D. R., L. J. Burpo, and R. H. Bottomley. 1978. Combined therapy of advanced hypernephroma with medroxyprogesterone, BCG, Adriamycin and vincristine (Abstract C-403). Proc. Am. Assoc. Cancer Res. Am. Soc. Clin. Oncol. 19:407.

Lokich, J. J., and J. H. Harrison. 1975. Renal cell carcinoma: Natural history and chemotherapeutic experience. J. Urol. 114:371–374.

Maeda, H., N. Yamamoto, and A. Yamashita. 1976. Fate and distribution of [^{14}C] succinyl neocarzinostatin in rats. Eur. J. Cancer 12:865–870.

Prout, G. R., Jr. 1974. The kidney and ureter, *in* Cancer Medicine, J. F. Holland and E. Frei, III, eds. Lea & Febiger, Philadelphia, pp. 1655–1669.

Rodriguez, V., S. P. Richman, R. S. Benjamin, M. A. Burgess, W. K. Murphy, M. Valdivieso, R. L. Banner, J. U. Gutterman, G. P. Bodey, and E. J Freireich. 1977. Phase 2 study of Baker's antifol in solid tumors. Cancer Res. 37:980–983.

Samuels, M. L., P. Sullivan, and C. D. Howe. 1968. Medroxyprogesterone acetate in the treatment of renal cell carcinoma (hypernephroma). Cancer 22:525–532.

Skinner, D. G., R. B. Colvin, C. D. Vermillion, R. C. Pfister, and W. F. Leadbetter. 1978. Diagnosis and management of renal cell carcinoma. Cancer 28:1165–1177.

Talley, R. W. 1973. Chemotherapy of adenocarcinoma of the kidney. Cancer 32:1062–1065.

Wagle, D. G., and G. P. Murphy. 1971. Hormonal therapy in advanced renal cell carcinoma. Cancer 28:318–321.

Cancer of the Genitourinary Tract, edited by
D. E. Johnson and M. L. Samuels.
Raven Press, New York © 1979.

Paraneoplastic Syndromes Associated With Renal Carcinoma

Naguib A. Samaan, M.D., Ph.D.

Section of Endocrinology, Department of Medicine, The University of Texas System Cancer Center M. D. Anderson Hospital and Tumor Institute, Houston, Texas

Ectopic hormone production by nonendocrine tumors has been recognized with increasing frequency during the past decade (Omenn 1970). The substances these tumors secrete may be the same as natural hormones or chemically different from true hormones but capable of imitating them biologically.

Inclusion of a tumor within the ectopic hormone or paraendocrine syndrome requires the demonstration of one or more inappropriate hormones produced by the neoplasm, arising from cells not considered a normal source of that hormone. This is demonstrated by finding high levels of the hormone in the tumor compared with normal tissue, by examining arteriovenous differences in hormone levels across the tumor bed, or by observing that the hormone excess and its metabolic effects disappear once the tumor has been removed or arrested.

Accurate clinical knowledge of this syndrome is important for differential diagnosis and treatment. The proper management of the metabolic complications may be of more immediate importance than the management of the underlying malignant disease itself.

Perhaps the most interesting of the proposed hypotheses of ectopic hormone production by nonendocrine tumors is the so-called deletion defect theory of Gellhorn (1958). The hypothesis is based upon the concept that all body cells contain the general transformation necessary for the synthesis of all body proteins, including polypeptide hormones. The fact that only specific cells in an endocrine organ produce a hormone is presumably due to a suppression or deletion of genetic potential from all other body cells. Any factor that modifies or reduces this deletion should extend the biosynthesis of individual hormones to tissues and organs that are normally nonproducers. If the neoplastic process in the course of its chaotic protein metabolism suppresses the deletion phenomenon, we might have a reasonable explanation for the ectopic production of one or more polypeptide hormones. Unfortunately, this theory leaves many questions unanswered.

Azzopardi and Williams (1968) suggested that all tumors involved in the ectopic hormone syndromes are linked by a single progenitory cell type, which must be multipotential and migratory, normally associated with peptide production. The amine precursor uptake and decarboxylation (APUD) cell system was proposed by Pearse (1969), who postulated that the APUD cell system originates in the neural crest. It has been argued that the neural crest origin does not apply to the gastrointestinal APUD cells, and at least two distinct origins of APUD cells have been postulated.

The neuroectoderm is the source of pheochromocytoma and the thyroid C cells, but the endoderm is the more likely source of enterochromaffin and argentaffin/argyrophil cells of the gastrointestinal tract and pancreas (Andrews 1963, Lambert et al. 1970, Brown et al. 1971). The separation of APUD cells into two groups according to endodermal or neuroectodermal origin parallels the separation of familial multiple endocrine adenomatosis (MEA) into two types (Kaplan et al. 1970). The first, or MEA type I (Wermer 1963), is associated with endodermal derivation, and includes tumors of the carcinoid syndrome arising from enterochromaffin or argyrophil cells of the gastrointestinal tract and those of the Zollinger-Ellison syndrome, which arise in pancreatic islets. The second, or MEA type II, is associated with ectodermal derivation, and includes tumors of C cells or the parafollicular cells of the thyroid gland (medullary carcinoma of the thyroid) and the adrenal medulla (pheochromocytoma). Weichert (1970) developed a unified theory and concluded that the syndrome of multiple endocrine adenomatosis may simply be adysplasia of the neural ectoderm.

However, none of the above hypotheses completely explains the pathophysiology of the inappropriate hormone production by nonendocrine tumors, including the kidney.

Hypernephroma is one of the tumors that are known to produce ectopic hormones. The presence of hypercalcemia and hypophosphatemia associated with hypernephroma was first noted by Albright and Reifenstein (1948). Since that time, many cases of hypernephroma associated with hypercalcemia have been described.

The occurrence of hypercalcemia in patients with hypernephroma may be due to skeletal metastasis, ectopic hormone production, or prostaglandin secretion by the tumor.

We measured the immunoreactive parathyroid hormone (iPTH) level in the peripheral blood of 20 patients with hypernephroma. The method used for measurement of iPTH was that of Samaan et al. (1974) using Burroughs-Wellcome antiserum lot AS 211/32, which is predominantly directed to the aminoterminal region, where the biological activity of PTH molecules resides. Ten of these 20 patients had normal serum calcium and serum iPTH, five had high serum calcium and serum iPTH, and three had high serum calcium but normal serum iPTH. The remaining two patients had high serum iPTH but normal serum calcium (Table 1).

The presence of high serum calcium with normal serum iPTH may be explained by the fact that the antibody used is incapable of binding with the parathyroid hormonelike substance or iPTH fragments produced by the tumor

Table 1. *Calcium and iPTH Levels in 20 Patients with Renal Cell Carcinoma*

Patient	Calcium (mg%)	iPTH (ng/ml)
	Normal	*Normal*
1	9.1	0.5
2	9.8	0.4
3	8.7	0.1
4	9.5	0.5
5	9.6	0.5
6	9.2	0.6
7	10.3	0.9
8	9.3	0.4
9	9.0	0.6
10	10.2	0.3
	Elevated	*Elevated*
11	14.8	5.6
12	14.6	4.0
13	12.6	1.1
14	17.0	2.6
15	12.8	2.2
	Elevated	*Normal*
16	12.1	0.4
17	14.5	0.1
18	14.7	0.1
	Normal	*Elevated*
19	9.5	2.2
20	9.7	4.5

or that the hypercalcemia was produced by factors other than iPTH, such as prostaglandin. The high serum iPTH found in two patients with normal serum calcium may indicate that hormone production by the tumor precedes other biochemical and clinical changes.

The arteriovenous difference in iPTH was measured in two patients with hypercalcemia at the time of surgery. The serum iPTH level was higher in the venous blood draining the tumor than in the arterial blood. Following nephrectomy, the patients' serum calcium dropped to hypocalcemic levels and they required calcium administration to maintain normal serum calcium levels. These results indicate that the hypercalcemia found in these patients was due to production of parathyroid hormone by the tumor.

The kidney is capable of producing polypeptides such as erythropoietin (Rubin et al. 1975), prostaglandins (Zins 1975), and steroids such as 1,25-dihydroxycholecalciferol (DeLuca 1975). In view of the kidney's role in the synthesis of renin and erythropoietin, the levels of these hormones were studied in 57 patients with renal cell carcinoma by Sufrin et al. (1977). They found renin elevations in 37%, which were unrelated to blood pressure levels but were associated with high-grade, high-stage lesions of mixed histologic cell type and indicated a poor prognosis. Erythropoietin was raised in 63% of patients and was a more sensitive indicator than renin of the presence of renal adenocarcinoma. However, it was less specific than renin and did not correlate directly with tumor grade, stage, histologic type, prognosis, or hematocrit and hemoglobin levels. These authors concluded that renin and erythropoietin determinations may be of value as biochemical tumor markers in renal adenocarcinoma.

We measured plasma renin levels in 12 patients with renal carcinoma and found seven had significant elevations of plasma renin in the presence of normal blood pressure (Figure 1). The durations of survival in those seven patients were not significantly different from those with normal plasma renin levels.

Golde et al. (1974) reported one case of a patient with renal carcinoma who had high serum human chorionic gonadotropin (HCG). None of our 20 patients studied showed high beta-HCG, but two showed high alpha-HCG.

We also measured the basal serum prolactin (PRL), human placental lactogen (HPL), and calcitonin levels in the same 20 patients and found that serum PRL was abnormally elevated in eight patients, HPL in four, and immunoreactive calcitonin in two (Figure 2).

Two aspects of the relationship between hormones and the kidney merit consideration, the types of hormones that may be produced by adenocarcinoma of the kidney, and the role hormones might play in treating patients with extensive adenocarcinoma of renal origin.

Recently, suspicion has been raised that renal carcinoma is an endocrine-sensitive tumor. Vasquez-Lopez (1944) and Matthews et al. (1947) noted that estrogen administration to male hamsters consistently caused renal adenomas

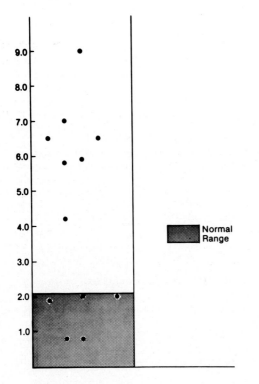

Figure 1. Plasma renin levels in 12 patients with renal carcinoma.

Normal Range

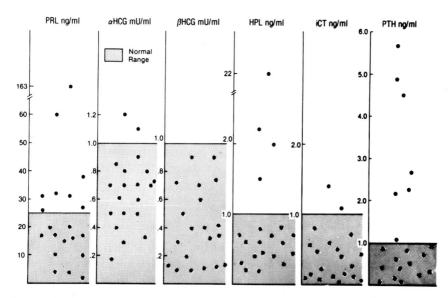

Figure 2. Basal serum prolactin, human placental lactogen, and calcitonin levels in 20 patients with renal carcinoma.

and metastatic carcinoma. A variety of estrogens were found to induce renal tumors in hamsters, but no tumor development was observed if progesterone or testosterone was administered simultaneously (Kirkman 1959a). In mature female hamsters, reduction of progesterone production rendered them susceptible to the carcinogenic effect of estrogen (Kirkman 1959b). Cortisone increased the incidence of primary tumors and of metastasis in estrogen-dependent transplants, but did not change the growth rate of these tumors (Kirkman 1959a).

Bloom et al. (1973) studied the effect of hormone therapy on patients with carcinoma of the kidney and reviewed the literature. They suggested that tumor regression can be induced by hormonal therapy in a limited number of patients with metastatic renal cancer. Subjective improvement occurred in about 50% of treated cases, but patients treated with progestins or androgens had an overall objective response rate of 15%. The authors concluded that, although the response is usually incomplete or of limited duration, hormone therapy may offer a new lease on life of two or three years to seriously ill and elderly patients.

The measurement of estrogen and progesterone receptors in renal cell carcinoma may offer us a tool for predicting the effect of hormone manipulation and therapy on metastatic renal carcinoma. The effect of estrogen-blocking agents such as tamoxifen also remains to be determined.

ACKNOWLEDGMENT

This investigation was supported by grant number CA-05831-17, awarded by the National Cancer Institute, Department of Health, Education, and Welfare, and grant ACS PDT-41F, awarded by the American Cancer Society.

REFERENCES

Albright, F., and E. C. Reifenstein, Jr. (eds.). 1948. The Parathyroid Glands and Metabolic Bone Disease: Selected Studies. Williams & Wilkins Co., Baltimore, pp. 393.

Andrews, A. 1963. A study of the developmental relationship between enterochromaffin cells and the neural crest. J. Embryol. Exp. Morphol. 11:307–327.

Azzopardi, J. G., and E. D. Williams. 1968. Pathology of "non-endocrine" tumors associated with Cushing's syndrome. Cancer 22:274–286.

Bloom, H. J. G. 1973. Hormone-induced and spontaneous regression of metastatic renal cancer. Cancer 32:1066–1071.

Brown, R. E., M. R. Schweisthal, and W. J. S. Still. 1971. Ultrastructural observations on the embryogenesis of islet cells in the rat pancreas in vitro. Proc. Soc. Exp. Biol. Med. 136:441–445.

DeLuca, H. F. 1975. The kidney as an endocrine organ involved in the function of vitamin D. Am. J. Med. 58:39–47.

Gellhorn, A. 1958. Recent studies on pathophysiologic mechanisms in human neoplastic disease. J. Chronic Dis. 8:158–170.

Golde, D. W., M. Schambelan, B. D. Weintraub, and S. W. Rosen. 1974. Gonadotropin secreting renal carcinoma. Cancer 33:1048–1053.

Kaplan, E. L., C. D. Arnaud, B. J. Hill, and G. W. Peskin. 1970. Adrenal medullary calcitonin-like factor: A key to multiple endocrine neoplasia, type 2. Surgery 68:146–149.

Kirkman, H. 1959a. Estrogen-induced tumors of the kidney. III. Growth characteristics in the Syrian hamster. Natl. Cancer Inst. Monogr. 1:1–58.

Kirkman, H. 1959b. Estrogen-induced tumors of the kidney. IV. Incidence in female Syrian hamsters. Natl. Cancer Inst. Monogr. 1:59–92.

Lambert, A. E., L. Orci, and A. E. Renold. 1970. Some factors controlling differentiation and/or modulation of rat pancreatic islet cells. Adv. Metab. Disord. (Suppl.) 1:35–43.

Matthews, V. S., H. Kirkman, and R. L. Bacon. 1947. Kidney damage in the golden hamster following chronic administration of diethylstilbestrol and sesame oil. Proc. Soc. Exp. Biol. Med. 66:195–223.

Omenn, G. S. 1970. Ectopic polypeptide hormone production by tumors. Ann. Intern. Med. 72:136–138.

Pearse, A. E. G. 1969. The cytochemistry and ultrastructure of polypeptide hormone-producing cells of the APUD series and the embryologic, physiologic, and pathologic implications of the concept. J. Histochem. Cytochem. 17:303–313.

Rubin, A. L., J. S. Cheigh, and K. H. Stenzel. 1975. Symposium on endocrine functions of the kidney. Am. J. Med. 58:1–3.

Samaan, N. A., R. C. Hickey, C. S. Hill, Jr., H. Medellin, and R. Gates. 1974. Parathyroid tumors: Preoperative localization and their association with other tumors. Cancer 33:933–939.

Sufrin, G., E. A. Mirand, R. H. Moore, T. M. Chu, and G. P. Murphy. 1977. Hormones in renal cancer. J. Urol. 117:433–438.

Vasquez-Lopez, E. 1944. The reaction of the pituitary gland and related hypothalamic centers in the hamster to prolonged treatment with estrogens. J. Pathol. Bacteriol. 56:1–3.

Weichert, R. F., III. 1970. The neural ectodermal origin of the peptide-secreting endocrine glands: A unifying concept for the etiology of multiple endocrine adenomatosis, and the inappropriate secretion of hormones by nonendocrine tumors. Am. J. Med. 49:232–241.

Wermer, P. 1963. Endocrine adenomatosis and peptic ulcer in a large kindred: Inherited multiple tumors and mosaic pleiotropism in man. Am. J. Med. 35:205–212.

Zins, G. R. 1975. Renal prostaglandins. Am. J. Med. 58:14–24.

BLADDER CARCINOMA

Cancer of the Genitourinary Tract, edited by
D. E. Johnson and M. L. Samuels.
Raven Press, New York © 1979.

Preoperative Irradiation for Bladder Cancer: The 2,000- Versus 5,000-Rad Controversy

Lowell S. Miller, M.D.

Division of Therapeutic Radiology, Duke University Medical Center, Durham, North Carolina

Preoperative irradiation for cancer dates back to October 27, 1913, when a Dr. Pinch made the first of five applications of a 100-mg radium source to a 73-year-old man with cancer of the rectum that was later excised perineally on April 1, 1914 (Symonds 1914). Whitmore et al. pioneered the use of preoperative irradiation for bladder cancer and recently recorded a crude five-year survival rate of 40% for patients with tumors in clinical stages B_2–C (1977a), in contrast to 16% in an earlier series in which patients were managed with radical cystectomy alone (1963). Significant evidence of the superiority of preoperative radiotherapy and radical cystectomy over unassisted radiotherapy has been reported based on experience at M. D. Anderson Hospital and Tumor Institute (Miller 1971).

There is fairly general agreement that irradiation should precede cystectomy, at least in cases of invasive disease, but opinion is divided on the dose that should be employed. There are several camps (Caldwell 1977, van der Werf-Messing 1978, Bloom 1978), but in this country the two principal positions are the low dose (2,000 rads/five fractions/one week, TDF 48), advocated by the Memorial Sloan-Kettering Cancer Center (MSK) group (Whitmore et al. 1977b), and the intermediate dose (5,000 rads/25 fractions/five weeks, TDF 82), recommended by workers at M. D. Anderson Hospital and Tumor Institute (MDAH) (Miller 1977). I shall attempt to compare results with these two dose levels.

In scholarly detail, Whitmore and his colleagues (1977b) have described 86 patients managed with 2,000 rads, cystectomy, and pelvic node dissection, and many of the parameters they employed can be compared with those in the MDAH experience. Through 1970, the latter includes 125 patients who received preoperative irradiation. Of these, 33 (26%) failed to undergo the intended cystectomy for the following reasons: the tumor was explored but found to be nonresectable in 10 cases, extrapelvic metastases were discovered in eight, there was intercurrent disease in six, the patient refused surgery in six, the tumor was inoperable on clinical reevaluation in two, and no gross residual tumor was found in one. Cystectomy specimens were evaluated microscopically in all but two of the remaining 92 cases, and the characteristics of these 90 cases will be compared to those in the MSK series. Among these 90, but also tabulated separately, are 30 similarly managed, more recent patients who participated in a randomized prospective trial comparing combined treatment with radiotherapy alone. Pelvic lymphadenectomy was not performed in any of the 90 MDAH cases.

There is no evidence that techniques or criteria for clinical staging have differed at the two institutions, classification at each depending upon correlation of the gross observations at endoscopy and bimanual palpation during anesthesia with microscopic assessment of depth of invasion in biopsy specimens. Through 1970, the most recent year for which analysis has been reported by either group, results of neither intravenous urography nor pedal lymphangiography were allowed to influence stage classification. In the absence of a clearly more valid common footing, it appears reasonable to compare results of the two regimens on the basis of clinical stage.

Table 1 shows that the MDAH series of 90 patients includes older cases, but inclusive dates for the 30 cases in the clinical trial series are similar to those for the MSK series. Median ages for these series are similar, but the explanation for the disparity in sex ratios is not readily apparent. It is noteworthy that a smaller percentage of MDAH patients had had earlier surgical treatment. That a higher proportion of MDAH tumors were bimanually palpable reflects the higher proportion of deeply invasive cancers. The slightly higher incidence of nontransitional carcinomas in the MDAH series may be due to different histologic criteria.

Both institutions have used megavoltage photons. Treatment fields recommended by the MDAH group have been smaller (Miller and Johnson 1973) than those advocated at MSK (Whitmore et al. 1977b). As seen in Figure 1,

Table 1. *Comparison of Memorial Sloan-Kettering and M. D. Anderson Hospital Series*

Variable	Memorial Sloan-Kettering Series	M. D. Anderson Hospital Series	
		Total Series	Clinical Trial
Inclusive dates	1966–1970	1955–1970	1964–1970
No. of patients	86	90	30
Median age (yrs.)	62	61	63.5
Male:female ratio	8:1	2.3:1	2:1
Prior therapeutic resect.	54 (63%)	26 (29%)	8 (27%)
Tumor bimanually palpable	57 (66%)	85 (94%)	30 (100%)
Clinical stage:			
O–A–B_1	29 (34%)	4 (4%)	0 (0%)
B_2–C	52 (60%)	78 (87%)	30 (100%)
D_1	5 (6%)	8 (9%)	0 (0%)
Transitional carcinoma	(93%)	(82%)	(90%)
Squamous carcinoma or adenocarcinoma	(7%)	(18%)	(10%)

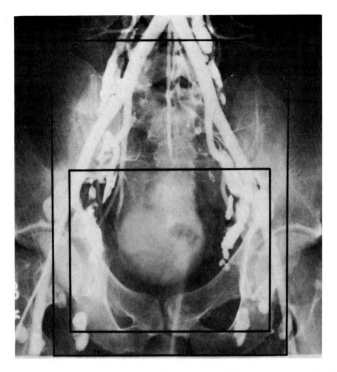

Figure 1. The larger rectangle represents the treatment field recommended at MSK, the contained smaller rectangle, that advocated at MDAH. (Slightly modified from Miller 1978, with permission of Biomedia, Inc.)

the tissue volume encompassed by the former is usually narrower and extends only from the caudal rim of the obturator foramina to the lower poles of the sacroiliac joints, omitting the less commonly involved (Whitmore et al. 1977b) common iliac and upper hypogastric lymph nodes in the interest of limiting the gut volume at risk. On the premise that the entire surgical field should be encompassed, the MSK portals (usually an opposed anteroposterior pair) are wider and extend from the bottom of the ischial tuberosities to the top of the fifth lumbar vertebra. Multifield or rotational techniques that aim at partial sparing of anterior abdominal wall and posterior rectum have been employed routinely by the MDAH group, but are used at MSK only for patients whose anteroposterior diameter exceeds 22 cm.

The mean tumor dose for the MDAH total series was 4,892 rads/34 days, for the 30 patients comprising the clinical trial series, 4,949 rads/34 days, and for the MSK series, 2,000 rads/seven days. Median interval between the end of pelvic irradiation and cystectomy for both MDAH series was 47 days, while the mean interval for the MSK series was just two days.

RESULTS

Clinical Stage

The M. D. Anderson Hospital experience with superficial tumors has been disappointing, but is too small to allow meaningful comparison with that at Memorial Sloan-Kettering. For fixed tumors, neither therapeutic regimen has met with any success.

In the broad sense, the two regimens have yielded identical crude five-year survival rates for patients with deeply invasive bladder tumors (Table 2), but the higher survival rate in the MDAH clinical trial series and the fact that it was more nearly synchronous with the MSK 2,000-rads series suggest that the 5,000-rads regimen is more effective.

Stage Reduction

Demonstration in the cystectomy specimen of a tumor stage lower than that clinically estimated prior to irradiation can largely be attributed (Whitmore et al. 1977b) to the impact of radiotherapy. This stand is bolstered by the fact that the incidence of stage reduction increases with radiation dose (Table 3). The higher incidence in the better studied MDAH clinical trial series suggests that the 48% recorded for the total series may be too low. The influence of dose is apparent also in the incidence of tumor-free cystectomy specimens. An important corollary to the relationship of dose to incidence of stage reduction and tumor-free cystectomy specimens is the increased five-year survival rate associated with each parameter (Table 4).

Gross Morphology

Our failure to record a substantial segment of the data for the MDAH experience precludes confident comparison with the better documented MSK series, but data for the more nearly synchronous and better studied clinical trial series (Table 5) suggest that grossly solid tumors are more effectively managed with the 5,000-rads regimen.

Table 2. *Crude Five-Year Survival*

Clinical Stage	Memorial Sloan-Kettering Series	M. D. Anderson Hospital Series	
		Total Series	Clinical Trial
O–A–B_1	15/29 (51%)	0/4 (0%)	—
B_2–C	21/52 (40%)	31/78 (40%)	16/30 (53%)
D_1	0/5 (0%)	0/8 (0%)	—

Table 3. *Comparison of Incidences of Pathologic and Clinical Stages*

Pathologic Stage	Memorial Sloan-Kettering Series	M. D. Anderson Hospital Series	
		Total Series	Clinical Trial
Lower than clinical*	27%	48%	73%
Same as clinical	31%	21%	13%
Higher than clinical	42%	8%	7%
Tumor present, stage unrecorded	—	23%	7%

* Includes those with no residual tumor—5% in MSK series, 29% in MDAH total series, and 43% in MDAH clinical trial.

Table 4. *M. D. Anderson Hospital Series, Influence of Stage Reduction on Crude Five-Year Survival*

Pathologic Stage	Total Series	Clinical Trial
No residual tumor	14/26 (54%)	9/13 (69%)
Lower than clinical but tumor in specimen	7/17 (41%)	4/9 (44%)
Same as clinical	8/19 (42%)	3/4 (75%)
Higher than clinical	0/7 (0%)	0/2 (0%)
Tumor present, stage unrecorded	2/21 (10%)	0/2 (0%)
Total	31/90 (34%)	16/30 (53%)

Table 5. *Influence of Gross Morphology on Crude Five-Year Survival*

Morphology	Memorial Sloan-Kettering Series	M. D. Anderson Hospital Series	
		Total Series	Clinical Trial
Papillary	16/35 (46%)	0/4 (0%)	—
Solid ± papillary	20/51 (39%)	22/54 (41%)	15/27 (56%)
Not recorded	—	9/32 (28%)	1/3 (33%)

Excretory Urography

Upper urinary tract obstruction had the expected adverse effect on prognosis at both institutions (Table 6). The lower incidence of obstruction in the MDAH clinical trial series (23%, as compared to 36% in the MSK series and 44% in the MDAH total series) reflects the absence of stage D_1 tumors.

Table 6. *Influence of Excretory Urographic Findings on Crude Five-Year Survival*

Finding	Memorial Sloan-Kettering Series	M. D. Anderson Hospital Series	
		Total Series	Clinical Trial
Hydronephrosis or nonfunctioning kidneys, unilateral or bilateral	9/31 (29%)	9/40 (23%)	3/7 (43%)
Normal	27/55 (49%)	22/49 (45%)	13/23 (57%)
Not recorded	—	0/1 (0%)	—

Failure

Rates of failure to control local and distant tumors (Table 7) are remarkably similar for the three series, but suggest a slight advantage for the 5,000-rads regimen. Intercomparison by clinical stage (Table 8) has been possible only on an all-sites basis (local and distant sites combined) and again provides only slight support for the higher dose treatment. Because only three of the 90 MDAH patients were irradiated through fields as large as 15×15 cm (Table 9), no evidence can be offered to confirm or refute the MSK suggestion that larger treatment fields are beneficial.

Table 7. *Sites of Failure and Failure Rates*

Site	Memorial Sloan-Kettering Series	M. D. Anderson Hospital Series	
		Total Series	Clinical Trial
Pelvic	15 (17%)	14 (16%)	4 (13%)
Alone	12 (14%)	8 (9%)	3 (10%)
With extrapelvic	3 (3%)	6 (7%)	1 (3%)
Extrapelvic only	19 (22%)	18 (20%)	6 (20%)
Undetermined	2 (2%)	—	—
Total	36/86 (42%)	32/90 (36%)	10/30 (33%)

Table 8. *Influence of Clinical Stage on Total Incidence of Failure (All Sites)*

Clinical Stage	Memorial Sloan-Kettering Series	M. D. Anderson Hospital Series	
		Total Series	Clinical Trial
O–A–B$_1$	11/29 (38%)	2/4 (50%)	—
B$_2$–C	21/52 (40%)	26/78 (33%)	10/30 (33%)
D$_1$	4/5 (80%)	4/8 (50%)	—
Total	36/86 (42%)	32/90 (36%)	10/30 (33%)

Table 9. *Influence of Field Size on Total Incidence of Failure (All Sites)*

Field Size	Memorial Sloan-Kettering Series	M. D. Anderson Hospital Series	
		Total Series	Clinical Trial
≥15 × 15 cm	4/14 (29%)	1/3 (33%)	—
< 15 × 15 cm	32/72 (44%)	31/87 (36%)	10/30 (33%)
Total	36/86 (42%)	32/90 (36%)	10/30 (33%)

Complications

The data in Table 10 differ from those previously reported (Miller 1977) in that the 33 patients who did not undergo cystectomy have been excluded, minor complications have been omitted, and there have been a few reclassifications. For the MDAH total series of 90 patients, the incidence of major and fatal complications remains very high: 85 complications (involving 49, or 54%, of the patients), including 20 fatalities (22%). Not surprisingly, many of these complications resulted from treatment in the early years of the program. For the 30 patients in the more recent clinical trial series, there were 17 complications (involving 12, or 40%, of the patients), including three fatalities (10%). The latter rate closely approximates the eight fatalities out of 86 patients (9%) in the MSK series. The MDAH decreases in incidence of complications, especially pyelonephritis, bowel obstruction, peritonitis, and rectal injury, are tributes to the growing skill of our surgical colleagues.

Table 10. *Major and Fatal Complications (Preoperative and Postoperative) in M. D. Anderson Hospital Series*

Type of Complication	Number of Complications (Fatal)	
	Total Series	Clinical Trial
Wound infection and/or dehiscence	13	2
Bowel fistula	12 (3)	2 (1)
Ureteroileal obstruction or leak	12 (1)	3
Cardiovascular-pulmonary obstruction	8 (6)	2 (2)
Pyelonephritis	8 (2)	1
Bowel obstruction	8 (1)	1
Stomal stenosis	7	4
Peritonitis	5 (3)	—
Rectal injury	5	—
Renal lithiasis	3 (1)	2
Hemorrhage	2 (2)	—
Septicemia	1 (1)	—
Hemorrhagic cystitis	1	—
Total	85 (20)	17 (3)

CONCLUSIONS

The higher dose regimen appears on first appraisal to be less cost effective. However, a comparison of reasonably contemporaneous 2,000- and 5,000-rads series on the basis of clinical stage suggests that the MDAH experience (containing a higher proportion of women and patients with nontransitional carcinomas, a lower proportion of patients with superficial tumors and previous surgical treatment, and employing a higher dose of preoperative irradiation through smaller fields without resort to pelvic node dissection), especially that experience derived from the clinical trial series, demonstrates:

1. in stages B_2–C, a higher crude five-year survival rate;
2. a sharply higher incidence of stage reduction and tumor-free cystectomy specimens, together with higher crude five-year survival rates for patients in these categories;
3. a suggestively higher crude rate of five-year survival for patients with grossly solid tumors;
4. a questionably lower rate of failure to control or prevent pelvic and extrapelvic tumor; and
5. a decreasing incidence of major and fatal complications of treatment with increasing radiotherapeutic and surgical experience.

REFERENCES

Bloom, H. J. G. 1978. The local, regional and systemic attack on bladder cancer. Int. J. Radiat. Oncol. Biol. Phys. 4:533–537.

Caldwell, W. L. 1977. The role of irradiation in the management of clinical stage B_1 (grades II and III) and stages B_2 and C bladder cancer. Cancer Res. 37:2759–2763.

Miller, L. S. 1971. Clinical evaluation and therapy for urinary bladder: Radiotherapy, *in* Oncology 1970, vol. IV. Year Book Medical Publishers, Inc., Chicago, pp. 283–290.

Miller, L. S., and D. E. Johnson. 1973. Megavoltage irradiation for bladder cancer: Alone, postoperative, or preoperative? *in* Seventh National Cancer Conference Proceedings. American Cancer Society, Inc., New York, pp. 771–782.

Miller, L. S. 1977. Bladder cancer: Superiority of preoperative irradiation and cystectomy in clinical stages B_2 and C. Cancer 39:973–980.

Miller, L. S. 1978. Radiotherapy of bladder cancer. Weekly Urology Update Series, Lesson 27, 1:2–7.

Symonds, C. J. 1914. Cancer of rectum: Excision after application of radium. Proc. R. Soc. Med. 7:152.

van der Werf-Messing, B. H. 1978. Cancer of the urinary bladder treated by interstitial radium implant. Int. J. Radiat. Oncol. Biol. Phys. 4:373–378.

Whitmore, W. F., R. F. Phillips, H. Grabstald, E. L. Bronstein, A. R. Mackenzie, and O. Hustu. 1963. Experience with preoperative irradiation followed by radical cystectomy for the treatment of bladder cancer. Am. J. Roentgenol. 90:1016–1022.

Whitmore, W. F., M. A. Batata, M. A. Ghoneim, H. Grabstald, and A. Unal. 1977a. Radical cystectomy with or without prior irradiation in the treatment of bladder cancer. J. Urol. 118:184–187.

Whitmore, W. F., M. A. Batata, B. S. Hilaris, G. N. Reddy, A. Unal, M. A. Ghoneim, H. Grabstald, and F. Chu. 1977b. A comparative study of two preoperative radiation regimens with cystectomy for bladder cancer. Cancer 40:1077–1086.

Cancer of the Genitourinary Tract, edited by
D. E. Johnson and M. L. Samuels.
Raven Press, New York © 1979.

Preoperative Irradiation With Cystectomy for Bladder Cancer

Willet F. Whitmore, Jr., M.D., and Mostafa A. Batata, B.Ch., D.M.R.

Urologic Service, Department of Surgery, and Department of Radiation Therapy, Memorial Sloan-Kettering Cancer Center, New York, New York

Explorations of integrated radiotherapy and cystectomy for bladder cancer patients began approximately 20 years ago because of (1) dissatisfaction with the results of radiation therapy or surgery alone in the management of such patients, coupled with evidence that each approach controlled some bladder cancers, (2) clinical evidence (Barnes et al. 1946, Emmett and Winterringer 1955, Riches 1960, and Magri 1962) that irradiation enhanced the results of surgery, and (3) experimental evidence that preoperative irradiation may destroy the well-oxygenated peripheral microextensions of the neoplasm, permitting complete excision of a previously nonresectable tumor or increasing the margin of resection of an initially resectable one, and that preoperative irradiation may reduce the viability of tumor cells, lessening the prospects of recurrence from local implantation or from lymphatic or hematogenous dissemination as a result of surgical manipulation.

Powers and Palmer (1968) reviewed the logic of preoperative irradiation and pointed out that benefit is possible only if (1) there are tumor cells capable of sustaining tumor growth, (2) the tumor cells are included in the radiation field, and (3) the radiation is administered in a manner that can favorably modify the tumor cells. It is evident that preoperative irradiation is not suitable for the patient whose tumor has already disseminated or whose tumor can be managed without such treatment.

What constitutes optimal preoperative irradiation remains to be determined, but clearly depends upon a variety of host and tumor factors. An analysis of the Memorial Sloan-Kettering Cancer Center (MSK) experience with preoperative irradiation and cystectomy forms the basis for this report.

MATERIALS AND METHODS

From 1949 to 1971, 451 patients with bladder cancer underwent radical cystectomy, usually with bilateral pelvic lymph node dissection, at MSK. Cystectomy has been indicated for superficially infiltrating tumors that are sufficiently multicentric in space, time, or both, to make conservative treatment impractical or impossible or that are of high grade, as well as for deeply infiltrating tumors unsuitable for segmental resection. The technique of radical cystectomy with bilateral pelvic lymph node dissection has been described (Whitmore 1975). In the usual surgical procedure, the bony and muscular walls of the pelvis and the major pelvic vessels were cleanly exposed, but the rectum was preserved.

The 451 patients included in this analysis may be divided into four groups: Group 1 (137 patients) underwent surgery alone in the interval 1949–1959.

Group 2 (109 patients) underwent surgery following a full course of radical megavoltage irradiation to the bladder in the interval 1949–1971. Such treatment was usually given elsewhere, rather than at MSK, and generally consisted of 6,000 rads to the bladder in 30 increments over six weeks by one of a variety of techniques. Patients were referred two months to eight years (average one year) following irradiation because of persistent, recurrent, or new lesions. These "radiation failures" are derived from an unquantitated total experience that must have included some successes and some failures who did not come for salvage cystectomy at MSK.

Group 3 (119 patients) received 4,000 rads in 20 increments of 200 rads over four weeks through fields encompassing the true pelvis, and underwent surgery four to 12 weeks (average 46 days) after irradiation in the interval 1959–1966.

Group 4 (86 patients) received 2,000 rads in five increments of 400 rads over one week to fields encompassing the bladder and true pelvis, followed by surgery within two weeks (average two days) in the interval 1966–1971.

All patients were subjected to a general evaluation that included complete history and physical examination, complete blood count, urinalysis, posteroanterior and lateral films of the chest, serum electrolyte and liver profiles, blood urea nitrogen and/or creatinine levels, and such other blood and/or radiographic studies as seemed indicated. Liver and bone scans and radiographic skeletal surveys were performed only for specific indications. Lymphangiographic examinations were not employed at all.

For purposes of clinical and pathologic staging, the classification system described by Marshall (1952) with modifications in the definition of pathologic stage D neoplasms (Whitmore et al. 1977b) has been used. The relationship of this classification to the TNM system has been set forth by Skinner (1977). Clinical staging was based upon the findings that resulted from cystoscopy, bimanual examination, and appropriate biopsies performed under anesthesia, and upon the adjunctive information derived from intravenous pyelograms. Pathologic staging was based upon the pathologist's evaluation of the surgical specimen from radical cystectomy and bilateral pelvic lymph node dissection. Discrepancies between the clinical and pathologic staging for each treatment group have been discussed elsewhere (Whitmore et al. 1977a,b).

Pelvic recurrences were defined as soft tissue recurrences within the pelvis with or without involvement of contiguous bone. Extrapelvic recurrences (or distant metastases) included all other categories of recurrent bladder neoplasm.

RESULTS

Table 1 demonstrates the similarity in distribution of clinical tumor stages, and Table 2 the similarity in distribution of pathologic tumor stages, among the treatment groups. Clinical staging error, tumor downstaging from irradiation, and selection bias are three factors that could affect the relationships between clinical (T) and pathologic (P) stage summarized in Table 3. In group 1 only

Table 1. *Comparison of Groups According to Clinical Stage*

Clinical Stage	Group 1 (137 cases)	Group 2 (109 cases)	Group 3 (119 cases)	Group 4 (86 cases)
Low O	7	1	9	1
A	17 (48%)	9 (43%)	13 (49%)	6 (34%)
B_1	42	37	36	22
High B_2	39	41	35	43
C	26 (52%)	17 (57%)	15 (51%)	9 (66%)
D_1	6	4	11	5

Table 2. *Comparison of Groups According to Pathological Stage*

Pathologic Stage	Group 1	Group 2	Group 3	Group 4
No tumor	—	15 (14%)	19 (16%)	3 (3%)
Low O	7	9	11	6
A	15 (38%)	20 (39%)	26 (39%)	7 (31%)
B_1	30	14	9	14
High B_2	31	13	18	17
C	20	12	8	12
D_1	16 (62%)	12 (47%)	9 (45%)	11 (65%)
D_2	18	14	16	16
D_3	—	—	3	—

Table 3. *Comparison of Pathologic Stage (P) Versus Clinical Stage (T)*

Group	$P < T$	$P = T$	$P > T$
1	6 (4%)	80 (58%)	51 (37%)
2	47 (43%)	31 (28%)	31 (28%)
3	48 (40%)	37 (31%)	34 (29%)
4	23 (27%)	27 (31%)	36 (42%)

Table 4. *Comparison of Groups According to Histologic Grade*

Histologic Grade	Group 1	Group 2	Group 3	Group 4
Low O	7	1	7	1
I	7 (49%)	5 (59%)	4 (45%)	6 (58%)
II	53	58	43	43
High III	66 (51%)	45 (41%)	61 (55%)	35 (44%)
IV	4	—	4	3

clinical staging error is operative; in group 2 all three factors are operative; in groups 3 and 4 clinical staging error and tumor downstaging from irradiation are operative. Furthermore, the $P < T$ error, largely attributable to tumor downstaging as a result of irradiation, is greater in group 3 than in group 4 because of the larger radiation dosage and longer interval between irradiation and cystectomy in group 3 patients.

Table 4 indicates the similarity in distribution of histologic grade among the treatment groups. Grade I and IV lesions were uncommon. Those lesions graded 0 represent cases of in situ carcinoma only.

Five-year results are summarized in Table 5. The overall impact of preoperative irradiation (groups 3 and 4) on five-year survival and deaths from recurrence is disappointingly small. A more optimistic view of the accomplishments of preoperative irradiation is provided by subsequent analyses, but these data clearly reflect the persisting magnitude of the bladder cancer problem. Approximately 20% of patients undergoing cystectomy for bladder cancer succumb from causes other than the cancer within five years.

An analysis of five-year survival rates relative to clinical stage and histologic grade for each of the treatment groups (Table 6) demonstrates that preoperative irradiation has not significantly altered survival rates in patients with low-stage tumors, regardless of tumor grade, although survival rates are appreciably better in patients with low-grade than high-grade tumors. Among patients with high-stage tumors, preoperative irradiation appears to improve survival rates for those with both low-grade and high-grade tumors, although survival rates are better in those with low-grade than high-grade lesions.

Table 5. *Five-Year Results*

Status at 5 Years	Group 1	Group 2	Group 3	Group 4
Alive N.E.D.*	45 (33%)	43 (39%)	50 (42%)	36 (42%)
Dead with recurrence	66 (48%)	35 (32%)	47 (39%)	35 (41%)
Without recurrence†	25 (18%)	26 (24%)	22 (18%)	15 (17%)
Lost to follow-up	1 (1%)	5 (5%)	—	—

* Later recurrence in one in group 1, three in group 2, five in group 3, and one in group 4.
† Treatment complications in 19 in group 1, 22 in group 2, 13 in group 3, and eight in group 4.

Table 6. *Five-Year Survival Rates According to Clinical Stage and Histologic Grade*

Group	Low Clinical Stage		High Clinical Stage	
	Low Grade	High Grade	Low Grade	High Grade
1	26/43 (60%)	9/23 (39%)	5/24 (21%)	4/46 (9%)
2	24/39 (62%)	2/8 (25%)	7/22 (32%)	10/35 (29%)
3	23/35 (66%)	11/23 (48%)	7/19 (37%)	10/42 (24%)
4	12/20 (60%)	3/9 (33%)	12/29 (41%)	9/28 (32%)

Table 7 lists all treatment failures due to bladder cancer according to clinical tumor stage and histologic grade for each treatment group. Except among patients with low-stage tumors, the incidence of pelvic and/or extrapelvic recurrence is generally lower in irradiated patients than in group 1 patients. The greatest decrease in pelvic and/or extrapelvic recurrence following irradiation was in patients with high-grade, high-stage lesions.

In Table 8 the incidence of pelvic recurrence alone is related to the clinical stage and histologic grade of the tumor in each treatment group. A clear decrease in the incidence of pelvic recurrence is noted in each group receiving radiation, regardless of the grade or stage of the tumor. The most conspicuous reduction in pelvic recurrence, however, is in patients with high-grade, high-stage tumors, in whom the greatest improvement in survival following preoperative irradiation was demonstrated (Table 6).

Table 7. *Pelvic and/or Extrapelvic Recurrence in Five or More Years According to Clinical Stage and Histologic Grade*

Group	Low Clinical Stage		High Clinical Stage	
	Low Grade	High Grade	Low Grade	High Grade
1	9/43 (21%)	12/23 (52%)	12/24 (50%)	34/46 (74%)
2	11/39 (28%)	5/8 (63%)	11/22 (50%)	11/35 (31%)
3	9/35 (26%)	12/23 (52%)	7/19 (37%)	25/42 (60%)
4	7/20 (35%)	4/9 (44%)	13/29 (45%)	12/28 (43%)

Table 8. *Pelvic Recurrence Alone in Five or More Years According to Clinical Stage and Histologic Grade*

Group	Low Clinical Stage		High Clinical Stage	
	Low Grade	High Grade	Low Grade	High Grade
1	7/43 (16%)	5/23 (22%)	6/24 (25%)	20/46 (43%)
2	3/39 (8%)	0/8 (0%)	5/22 (23%)	7/35 (20%)
3	4/35 (11%)	3/23 (13%)	3/19 (16%)	9/42 (21%)
4	2/20 (10%)	0/9 (0%)	4/29 (14%)	6/28 (21%)

Table 9 shows corresponding data for the incidence of pelvic and extrapelvic recurrences in each treatment group relative to tumor grade and clinical stage. Although a trend toward a reduced incidence of pelvic and extrapelvic recurrence is noted in the irradiated patients compared to the group 1 patients, regardless of grade and stage, the reductions are less impressive than those for pelvic recurrence only in the same patients (Table 8). This may be interpreted as signifying that pelvic recurrences are responsible for only some of the distant recurrences.

In Table 10 extrapelvic recurrence with or without pelvic recurrence is indicated for each treatment group relative to tumor grade and clinical stage. These data reveal no apparent advantage to prior irradiation in any treatment group and may mean that distant metastases are a dominant cause of treatment failure and are at least largely independent of preoperative irradiation and of the reduction in local recurrences following such irradiation.

In Table 11 the incidence of extrapelvic recurrence only for each of the treat-

Table 9. *Pelvic and Extrapelvic Recurrence in Five or More Years According to Clinical Stage and Histologic Grade*

Group	Low Clinical Stage		High Clinical Stage	
	Low Grade	High Grade	Low Grade	High Grade
1	2/43 (5%)	4/23 (17%)	4/24 (17%)	6/46 (13%)
2	4/39 (10%)	1/8 (13%)	1/22 (5%)	0/35 (0%)
3	2/35 (6%)	3/23 (13%)	0/19 (0%)	6/42 (14%)
4	0/20 (0%)	1/9 (11%)	3/29 (10%)	1/28 (4%)

Table 10. *Extrapelvic Recurrence With or Without Pelvic Recurrence in Five or More Years According to Clinical Stage and Histologic Grade*

Group	Low Clinical Stage		High Clinical Stage	
	Low Grade	High Grade	Low Grade	High Grade
1	2/43 (5%)	7/23 (30%)	6/24 (25%)	14/46 (30%)
2	8/39 (21%)	5/8 (63%)	6/22 (27%)	4/35 (11%)
3	5/35 (14%)	9/23 (39%)	4/19 (21%)	16/42 (38%)
4	5/20 (25%)	4/9 (44%)	9/29 (31%)	6/28 (21%)

Table 11. *Extrapelvic Recurrence Alone in Five or More Years According to Clinical Stage and Histologic Grade*

Group	Low Clinical Stage		High Clinical Stage	
	Low Grade	High Grade	Low Grade	High Grade
1	0/43 (0%)	3/23 (13%)	2/24 (8%)	8/46 (17%)
2	4/39 (10%)	4/8 (50%)	5/22 (23%)	4/35 (11%)
3	3/35 (9%)	6/23 (26%)	4/19 (21%)	10/42 (24%)
4	5/20 (25%)	3/9 (33%)	6/29 (21%)	5/28 (18%)

ment groups relative to tumor grade and clinical stage is indicated. These data support the interpretation expressed in the preceding paragraph. Because of evidence (van der Werf-Messing 1975, Wallace and Bloom 1976) that the favorable effects of preoperative irradiation on survival following cystectomy are limited largely to patients in whom tumor downstaging (P < T) occurs, we wished to examine the MSK experience in this regard.

Table 12 indicates five-year survival rates for treatment group relative to the presence (P < T) or absence (P ≥ T) of apparent downstaging. In the nonirradiated patients there is no difference; in groups 2 and 3 survival is better in the P < T patients than in the P ≥ T patients; in group 4 there is no difference between the P < T and P ≥ T patients, probably because the time-dosage factors did not allow for detectable tumor downstaging. Absence of therapeutic benefit from irradiation in group 4 seems an unlikely alternative explanation since the overall survival is better than in group 1.

Table 13 indicates the failures due to cancer within five years for each treatment group relative to P < T and P ≥ T status. Tumor downstaging, whether due to initial clinical overstaging or prior irradiation, diminishes the likelihood of death from bladder cancer. The data in Table 14 suggest, however, that the

Table 12. *Five-Year Survival According to P-T Relationship*

Group	P < T	P ≥ T
1	2/6 (33%)	43/130 (33%)
2	27/46 (59%)	16/58 (28%)
3	27/48 (56%)	24/71 (34%)
4	10/23 (43%)	26/63 (41%)

Table 13. *Recurrence in Five or More Years According to P-T Relationship*

Group	P < T	P ≥ T
1	2/6 (33%)	65/130 (50%)
2	9/46 (20%)	29/58 (50%)
3	13/48 (27%)	40/71 (56%)
4	6/23 (26%)	31/63 (49%)

Table 14. *Mortality Within Five Years From Causes Other Than Recurrence*

Group	P < T	P ≥ T
1	2/6 (33%)	23/130 (18%)
2	11/46 (24%)	15/58 (26%)
3	10/48 (21%)	11/71 (15%)
4	7/23 (30%)	8/63 (13%)

advantages demonstrated in Table 13 are at least partly offset by an increased mortality from other causes.

Table 15 indicates the incidence of pelvic recurrence alone in the various treatment groups relative to whether tumor downstaging was (P < T) or was not (P ≥ T) observed. The low incidence of pelvic recurrences in the downstaged compared to the nondownstaged patients in each of the irradiated groups is notable. Extrapelvic recurrence with or without pelvic recurrence (Table 16) was also less frequent in the P < T than in the P ≥ T category for each treatment group.

Analyses of the MSK material relative to whether the tumors were papillary or solid, greater or less than 4 cm in diameter, solitary or multifocal, and low or high grade provided no evidence that any of these factors significantly influenced the distribution into P < T and P ≥ T categories.

Table 17 indicates the five-year mortality rates from causes other than bladder cancer in each treatment group, and Table 18 some of the more conspicuous factors associated with such deaths. The similarities between the different treatment groups provide no basis for believing that prior radiation therapy contributed significantly to mortality.

Table 15. *Pelvic Recurrence Alone in Five or More Years According to P-T Relationship*

Group	P < T	P ≥ T
1	2/6 (33%)	36/130 (28%)
2	1/46 (2%)	13/58 (22%)
3	3/48 (6%)	16/71 (23%)
4	1/23 (4%)	11/63 (17%)

Table 16. *Extrapelvic Recurrence With or Without Pelvic Recurrence in Five or More Years According to P-T Relationship*

Group	P < T	P ≥ T
1	0/6 (0%)	29/130 (22%)
2	8/46 (17%)	16/58 (28%)
3	10/48 (21%)	26/71 (37%)
4	4/23 (17%)	20/63 (32%)

Table 17. *Mortality Under Five Years From Causes Other Than Recurrence*

Group	Hospital Mortality	Later Complication or Other Cause
1 (137)	19 (14%)	6 (4%)
2 (109)	17 (16%)	9 (8%)
3 (119)	13 (11%)	8 (7%)
4 (86)	8 (9%)	7 (8%)

Table 18. *Factors Associated With Deaths Within Five Years Without Recurrence**

Factor	Group 1 (25 cases)	Group 2 (26 cases)	Group 3 (21 cases)	Group 4 (15 cases)
Clinical				
Age 65 years or older	10	14	7	4
Cardiovascular disease and/or obesity	11 (72%)	18 (85%)	11 (81%)	11 (73%)
Obstructive uropathy on initial i.v. urogram	11	6	11	5
Surgical				
Pelvic surgery before radical cystectomy	11	12	6	7
Postoperative pelvic sepsis	6 (96%)	7 (54%)	11 (76%)	5 (67%)
Ureterosigmoidostomy or ureterocutaneous diversion	21	5	3	—
Oncologic				
Bladder cancer of high clinical pathologic stage	15	19	14	12
		(60%)	(73%)	(67%)	(80%)
Other primary cancer with or after bladder cancer	2	2	1	2

* Each patient usually had more than one factor.

Radiation therapy was usually well tolerated in groups 3 and 4, although transient cystitis and/or proctitis developed in 22 group 3 and two group 4 patients (Whitmore et al. 1977b). No technical difficulties with performance of cystectomy or urinary diversion were attributable to prior irradiation in groups 3 and 4. The sole postoperative complication attributable to prior irradiation was delay in healing of infected wounds. This was greatest in group 2 and was not noticeably different between groups 3 and 4, although a systematic analysis of this question remains to be carried out.

DISCUSSION

A valid criticism of the comparisons made in this study is that the various treatment groups were not randomized and that reliance was placed upon historical controls. Analysis with respect to age and sex, clinical presentations relative to type, number, size, histologic grade, and clinical stage of the tumor, clinical staging criteria, and technique of radical cystectomy with pelvic lymph node dissection revealed no significant differences among the four groups (Whitmore and Batata, unpublished data).

The data presented support the conclusion that planned preoperative irradiation with cystectomy has improved survival rates for patients with high-stage bladder cancers compared to patients with similar lesions treated by cystectomy alone. The absence of survival benefit from preoperative irradiation in patients with low-stage tumors is consistent with the logic behind preoperative irradiation.

This favorable effect of preoperative irradiation is achieved without significant effects on operative morbidity and mortality. The causes for this salutary effect on survival may be determined by examining the general causes of treatment failure (Powers and Palmer 1968):

1. New tumor formation. Cystectomy provides the best and only assured prophylaxis against new tumor formation in the bladder tumor patient.

2. Iatrogenic failure and incomplete resection of the primary tumor. The roles of incomplete resection, iatrogenic implantation, and iatrogenic lymphatic or hematogenous dissemination in fostering the development of local recurrence and of distant metastases remain uncertain. However, it is quite clear that preoperative irradiation reduces the incidence of local recurrence and is accompanied by improvement in survival.

3. Preexisting unrecognized metastasis, regional or distant. Whether or not preoperative irradiation materially alters the incidence of regional lymph node metastases and whether or not such alteration will affect survival has not been analyzed in this study. If 20–30% of patients with clinically stage B_2 or C tumors had limited (resectable) regional node metastases and if 10% of such patients were cured by cystectomy with pelvic lymph node dissection alone, the net gain in survival in the total experience would be only 2–3%. It will be difficult to demonstrate clinically an improved survival from preoperative irradiation mediated through an effect on regional metastases. Preexisting but unrecognized distant metastases are apparently the dominant cause of treatment failure in all groups and there is no logical reason to anticipate benefit from preoperative irradiation in such a setting.

4. Recognized metastases. Recognized distant metastases presently exclude patients from consideration for potentially curative preoperative irradiation with cystectomy, and since the clinical staging criteria used throughout the years encompassed by this experience remained the same, recognition of metastasis was not a variable in this study.

In evaluating the effects of preoperative irradiation, the experience with "radiation failures" after full-course irradiation (group 2) has been included in each table to provide a survey of total experience. However, it is appropriate to point out again the selective nature of this experience and the unquantifiable bias that results from the fact that the total irradiated bladder cancer population from which these patients were derived is not defined. Accordingly, although data from group 2 indicate that "salvage cystectomy" may be performed without prohibitive risks and with reasonable prospects of success, it is inappropriate to compare this experience further with that of group 3 and group 4 patients.

An inspection of the data in the various tables demonstrates no material differences in survival rates, local recurrence rates, or extrapelvic recurrence rates between otherwise comparable patients who received high-dose (4,000 rads in four weeks—group 3) and those who received low-dose (2,000 rads in one week—group 4) preoperative irradiation (Whitmore et al. 1977b).

Stage reduction $(P < T)$ is understandably greater in group 3 than in group 4, and since survival advantage accrues from (or is at least associated with) such reduction, a prognostic advantage is evident for group 3 patients that may become important when effective adjunct therapy is established.

Although the control of regional metastases remains a hypothetical advantage of high-dose over low-dose irradiation, precise definition of what constitutes a sufficiently high dose is lacking. Furthermore, the relative effectiveness of regional lymph node dissection and of optimal irradiation in achieving such control remains uncertain. Finally, circumstantial evidence already suggests that the vast majority of patients with recognized regional metastases have simultaneous unrecognized distant metastases that are destined to make the supplemental salvage from consistent control of regional metastases small at best (Whitmore and Marshall 1962, Dretler et al. 1972, Laplante and Brice 1973).

The complications attributable to preoperative irradiation, whether high-dose or low-dose, appear to be small and not appreciably different for group 3 and 4 patients. The principal advantage of low-dose preoperative irradiation over high-dose is the shortened treatment time, which has physical, psychologic, and economic advantages for the patient.

CONCLUSIONS

Analysis of the four MSK treatment groups leads to the following conclusions:

1. Planned preoperative irradiation improves the survival rates in patients with clinically high-stage tumors, probably by reducing the incidence of pelvic recurrences.

2. The favorable effects of preoperative irradiation are largely limited to those patients in whom tumor downstaging ($P < T$) may be demonstrable.

3. "Salvage cystectomy" is a practical therapeutic consideration in "radiation failures."

4. Administration of 4,000 rads in four weeks or 2,000 rads in one week followed by radical cystectomy with pelvic lymph node dissection gives equivalent results in terms of tumor control, operative mortality, and complications. However, practical advantages of the low-dose regimen make it the method of choice at MSK.

5. The optimal regimen of preoperative irradiation for the cystectomy candidate remains to be established.

6. The major cause of treatment failure in patients undergoing cystectomy for bladder cancer is distant metastasis, and the failure rate has not been materially altered by preoperative irradiation. Reduction of the problem of distant metastasis seems to depend on the development of selection criteria that will justify earlier cystectomy and/or upon the development of effective systemic adjunct therapy.

REFERENCES

Barnes, R. W., C. L. Turner, and R. T. Bergman. 1946. Treatment of bladder tumors. Calif. Med. 65:95–98.

Dretler, S. P., B. D. Ragsdale, and W. F. Leadbetter. 1972. The value of pelvic lymphadenectomy in the surgical treatment of bladder cancer. Trans. Am. Assoc. Genitourin. Surg. 64:79–81.

Emmett, J. L., and J. R. Winterringer. 1955. Experience with implantation of radon seeds for bladder tumors: Comparison of results with other forms of treatment. J. Urol. 73:502–515.

Laplante, M., and M. Brice, II. 1973. The upper limits of hopeful application of radical cystectomy for vesical carcinoma: Does nodal metastasis always indicate incurability? J. Urol. 109:261–264.

Magri, J. 1962. Partial cystectomy: A review of 104 cases. Br. J. Urol. 34:74–87.

Marshall, V. F. 1952. The relation of the preoperative estimate to the pathologic demonstration of the extent of vesical neoplasms. J. Urol. 68:714–723.

Powers, W. E., and L. A. Palmer. 1968. Biologic basis of preoperative radiation treatment. Am. J. Roentgenol. 102:176–192.

Riches, E. 1960. Choice of treatment in carcinoma of the bladder. J. Urol. 84:472–480.

Skinner, D. G. 1977. Current state of classification and staging of bladder cancer. Cancer Res. 37:2838–2842.

van der Werf-Messing, B. H. P. 1975. Carcinoma of the bladder $T_3N_xM_o$ treated by preoperative irradiation followed by cystectomy. Cancer 36:718–722.

Wallace, D. M., and H. J. G. Bloom. 1976. The management of deeply infiltrating (T_3) bladder carcinoma: Controlled trial of radical radiotherapy versus preoperative radiotherapy and radical cystectomy (first report). Br. J. Urol. 48:587–594.

Whitmore, W. F., Jr. 1975. Total cystectomy, *in* The Biology and Clinical Management of Bladder Cancer, E. H. Cooper and R. E. Williams, eds. Blackwell Scientific Publications, Oxford, pp. 193–227.

Whitmore, W. F., Jr., M. A. Batata, M. A. Ghoneim, H. Grabstald, and A. Unal. 1977a. Radical cystectomy with or without prior irradiation in the treatment of bladder cancer. J. Urol. 118:184–187.

Whitmore, W. F., Jr., M. A. Batata, B. S. Hilaris, G. N. Reddy, A. Unal, M. A. Ghoneim, H. Grabstald, and F. Chu. 1977b. A comparative study of two preoperative radiation regimens with cystectomy for bladder cancer. Cancer 40:1077–1086.

Whitmore, W. F., Jr., and V. F. Marshall. 1962. Radical total cystectomy for cancer of the bladder: 230 consecutive cases five years later. J. Urol. 87:853–868.

Cancer of the Genitourinary Tract, edited by
D. E. Johnson and M. L. Samuels.
Raven Press, New York © 1979.

CISCA Combination Chemotherapy for Metastatic Carcinoma of the Bladder

Melvin L. Samuels, M.D., Manuel E. Moran, M.D., Douglas E. Johnson, M.D.,* and R. Bruce Bracken, M.D.*

*Departments of Medicine and *Urology, The University of Texas System Cancer Center
M. D. Anderson Hospital and Tumor Institute, Houston, Texas*

The treatment of metastatic bladder cancer patients with chemotherapy has been a frustrating and depressing exercise. There has been no significant impact on survival and, indeed, worthwhile palliation has been only rarely seen. A review of our stage D patients for the years 1974 and 1975 shows a median survival of 13 weeks. Recently we reported on a new protocol for advanced bladder cancer patients (Sternberg et al. 1977) that produced a large number of partial responses, as well as significant palliation. This report, an extension of the initial preliminary findings, shows that complete response with a significant improvement in survival time can be achieved.

MATERIALS AND METHODS

Forty-one patients with stage D carcinoma of the bladder have been entered into the study during the past 18 months. Patients were required to have measurable lesions, except for two patients who had surgical removal of known metastatic disease (nodular mass in abdominal scar and multiple metastases in left axillary nodes). These two were considered to require adjuvant therapy and received the same treatment protocol.

Accessible lesions were carefully measured. In addition, pelvic and intraabdominal masses were studied by computerized transaxial tomography and sonography and evaluated independently by the Department of Diagnostic Radiology. Other radiographic studies included standard posteroanterior and lateral chest x-rays, bone surveys, pyelograms, and lymphangiograms. When indicated, liver-spleen scans and bone scans were done serially. An electrocardiogram and creatinine clearance were done before each treatment course, as were complete blood count tests for levels of blood urea nitrogen, serum creatinine, glucose, calcium, phosphorous, total protein, albumin, uric acid, bilirubin, alkaline phosphatase, and electrolytes, and urine analysis.

No patient was denied entry because of age. However, admission to the program was denied if the serum creatinine level was above 1.5 mg/100 ml or

Table 1. *CISCA Program*

---

1. Preliminary lab work on out-patient basis, including complete blood count, urinanalysis, SMA, and creatinine clearance.
2. Light supper evening of admission.
3. At 10:00 PM, Cytoxan 650 mg/m² i.v., followed by Adriamycin 50 mg/m² i.v. and then continuous infusion of 5% dextrose normal saline (D_5 N.S.) with added KCl at 100 ml per hour throughout night.
4. Hold breakfast and start second i.v. site at 8:00 AM with D_5 ¼ N.S. with 40 gm of mannitol per liter and run at 200 ml per hour for five liters.
5. At 8:00 AM give 12.5 gm mannitol i.v. in first site and follow with cis-platinum 100 mg/m² in 200 cc N.S. over two hours. Then keep open with D_5 N.S. with 20 mEq/l KCl at 50–75 ml per hour for 24 hours.
6. Watch for diarrhea.
7. Administer Thorazine liberally.

---

creatinine clearance was less than 55 ml per minute. Likewise, serious intrinsic heart disease requiring digitalis or a recent myocardial infarction was considered a high-risk complication prohibiting entry into the study.

The usual response criteria were employed. A complete response is the disappearance of all measurable lesions by both clinical and radiographic parameters. A partial response is a 50% decrease in the maximum diameter of a mass, and "plateau-stable" designates no change in tumor parameters for at least four months. Any detectable increase in mass implies progression, as does a mixed response.

The CISCA protocol employs cis-dichlorodiammineplatinum (DDP), cyclophosphamide, and Adriamycin administered over a two-day period (Table 1). Courses were repeated at 21-day intervals unless the serum creatinine rose above 1.5 mg/100 ml or the creatinine clearance dropped below 50 ml per minute. If heart disease supervened, Adriamycin was deleted from subsequent courses. In addition, nine patients received vincristine 2.0 mg i.v. on day 1 (Vin-CISCA).

PATIENT CHARACTERISTICS

Of the 41 patients, 12 were women. The mean age for the men was 60 years and for the women, 58 years. The nine patients above age 70 constituted 22% of the study population, while the four youngest patients, ages 32, 35, 39, and 41, constituted 10%. Thirty-four patients had high-grade transitional cell carcinoma, four had adenocarcinoma, two had squamous carcinoma, and one had an anaplastic spindle cell variant of transitional cell carcinoma. Twenty-six patients (63%) had received prior definitive radiotherapy consisting of 5,000 rads tumor dose. Sixteen had undergone a prior total cystectomy with "loop" and two had undergone a prior partial cystectomy.

Because tumor presentations have been found to be variable, they have been considered under four broad categories, including pulmonary, regional pelvic, skeletal, and visceral metastases producing an immediate increased hazard, such as liver metastases, brain metastases, or rectal invasion with large bowel obstruction. Hydronephorsis was considered a separate presentation.

RESULTS

Seven patients achieved a complete response and 10 achieved a partial response, for an overall response rate of 41%. In addition, three patients are "plateau-stable." The male patients tend to have pulmonary and skeletal metastases, while the female patients tend to fall into the regional pelvic tumor group. The pulmonary presentation showed the highest response rate, eight out of 13, or 61%, while the remaining categories showed a 30% response rate (Table 2). Thus, responses were seen among all the presentations, including bone metastases, pelvic mass, hydronephrosis, and even within the primary tumor site, where repeat cystoscopy was negative in three patients. Relief of bone pain and severe pelvic pain has been dramatic. Among the three patients with visceral presentations, one had widespread liver metastases. After four treatment courses, results of the liver function tests returned to normal and the technetium liver scan was much improved. This patient survived 56 weeks and received a total of eight courses. The responders and nonresponders are compared in Table 3. The nonresponders include a higher proportion of female patients, a higher mean age, and a larger proportion of patients receiving radiotherapy.

Figure 1 shows the survival curves of the responders and nonresponders. There is a highly significant difference between the survival curves of the two groups, with six deaths among the 20 responders and 10 among the 21 nonresponders. The survival curve for the entire group was compared with that for a historical control group consisting of 46 stage D_2 patients treated in M. D. Anderson Hospital in 1974–1975. There is a highly significant difference between these two curves, with a median survival for the study patients, all of whom died, of 13 weeks.

The nine Vin-CISCA patients are alive and still receiving therapy. Three are objective responders, two are plateau-stable, and four are nonresponders. There is one striking complete response in a 32-year-old woman, previously untreated, who presented with hypercalcemia (14 mg/100 ml), tumor-induced pyrexia with spikes to 39°C daily, a large pelvic mass, left hydronephrosis,

Table 2. *Presentations and Response in Patients With Advanced Bladder Cancer*

Category	Total No. Patients	Male/Female	Complete Response	Partial Response	Alive
Pulmonary	13	12/1	3	5	7
Regional pelvic	14	7/7	1	3	8
Hydronephrosis	9	6/3	2	1	8
Skeletal	7	7/0	1	1	3

Table 3. *Comparison of Responders With Nonresponders*

Patients	Total No. Patients	Male/Female	Mean Age (Yrs.)	No. Over 65 Yrs.	Prior XRT	Mean No. Courses
Responders	17	13/4	58	7 (41%)	7 (41%)	5.5
Nonresponders	21	14/7	62	12 (57%)	15 (71%)	3.0
Plateau-stable	3	2/1	59	1 (33%)	2 (67%)	4.0

and a left neck mass. She is in complete remission with a negative cystoscopy at 65 weeks.

TOXICITY

There were no deaths from CISCA chemotherapy. Immediate side effects were gastrointestinal and consisted of severe nausea and vomiting in 90% of the patients during the second day, and mild vomiting in the remaining 10%. The three instances of acute pneumonitis, noted during the early phase of this study (Sternberg et al. 1977), were probably secondary to aspiration. One episode of hypotension followed severe vomiting with diarrhea, but the patient responded

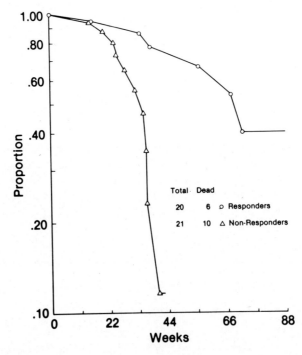

Figure 1. A comparison of the survival curves for responders and nonresponders reveals a statistically significant difference between the two curves ($p < 0.01$).

to fluid repletion and did not develop uremia. Diarrhea was seen to some degree in one third of the population. It was frequently severe, especially in those who had received prior radiotherapy to the bladder. Once established, it recurred with each course.

An acute severe anaphylactic reaction manifested by bronchospasm and cyanosis immediately followed the initiation of the first DDP treatment in a 50-year-old man. He responded to epinephrine, aminophylline, and corticosteroid therapy and was withdrawn from the study.

As previously noted, neutropenia was observed in 60% of patients during the first course, usually between days 10 and 16, and they rapidly recovered within four days (Sternberg et al. 1977). Thrombocytopenia was seen in 20% of patients during the first course, tended to worsen with successive courses, and was associated with hemorrhage in two patients, who required platelet transfusions.

Bacteriologically confirmed sepsis was seen in four patients. Three had a cystectomy and loop and one had only prior irradiation to the bladder. The organisms recovered were gram-negative rods (*Escherichia coli* in two and *Klebsiella* and *Pseudomonas* organisms in one each) and all patients responded promptly to antibiotic therapy with Keflin, Ticar, and tobramycin.

The major chronic toxicity with the CISCA program is renal damage induced by DDP. Five of the nine patients with unilateral hydronephrosis developed rapid elevations of serum creatinine to above 2.0 mg/100 ml so that further therapy could not be administered. This occurred during the first course of treatment.

Mild but transient elevation of the BUN and serum creatinine are universally seen after three to five courses of CISCA and usually peak between days 7 and 10, returning to pretreatment levels by day 21. However, we have seen persistent elevation of serum creatinine to levels at or near 2.0 mg/100 ml in five patients and we had to delete DDP from their courses of therapy. This elevation has occurred despite full hydration with mannitol diuresis and must be considered an unavoidable complication of repetitive DDP administration in some patients.

DISCUSSION

Yagoda and co-workers (Yagoda 1977, Yagoda et al. 1976, 1977) recently reviewed chemotherapy for bladder cancer patients and concluded that DDP is the single most active agent against metastatic bladder cancer, with a 50% response rate. These are partial responses, and while the addition of cyclophosphamide will slightly increase the number of responses, complete remissions are still not obtained. It is only when one adds Adriamycin, as in our protocol, that complete remissions are achieved. Adriamycin has unequivocal activity when administered systemically, as well as by direct bladder instillation, as Japanese workers have reported (Ozaki 1977).

We again emphasize that the major acute toxic manifestations with CISCA are vomiting, diarrhea, and gram-negative sepsis, bacteriologically proven in four patients. Acute transient elevations in serum creatinine are common, with the peak value of 1.8 mg/100 ml previously noted (Sternberg et al. 1977). However, chronic persistent elevations are seen in 12% of our current patients and this rate can be expected to worsen as we administer more than four courses of therapy (400 mg/m² of DDP). Thus, it seems quite clear that patients with only one functioning kidney and patients above age 60 should receive reduced doses of DDP, preferably after one or two full induction courses. Metastatic bladder cancer is rapidly fatal and the production of chronic uremia with plateau-stable serum creatinine values at or near 2.0 mg/100 ml may be the price we currently have to pay to achieve palliation with extended survival.

REFERENCES

Ozaki, Y. 1977. Bladder instillation of adriamycin in the treatment of bladder tumors. Jpn. J. Urol. 68:934–944.

Sternberg, J., R. Bracken, P. B. Handel, and D. E. Johnson. 1977. Combination chemotherapy (CISCA) for advanced urinary tract carcinoma. J.A.M.A. 238:2282–2287.

Yagoda, A. 1977. Future implications of Phase 2 chemotherapy trials in ninety-five patients with measurable advanced bladder cancer. Cancer Res. 37:2775–2780.

Yagoda, A., R. C. Watson, J. C. Gonzalez-Vitale, D. Grabstald, and W. F. Whitmore. 1976. Cis-dichlorodiammineplatinum (II) in advanced bladder cancer. Cancer Treat. Rep. 60:917–923.

Yagoda, A., R. C. Watson, W. F. Whitmore, H. Grabstald, M. P. Middleman, and I. H. Krakoff. 1977. Adriamycin in advanced urinary tract cancer: Experience in 42 patients and a review of the literature. Cancer 39:279–285.

Cancer of the Genitourinary Tract, edited by
D. E. Johnson and M. L. Samuels.
Raven Press, New York © 1979.

Phase II Trials in Bladder Cancer at Memorial Sloan-Kettering Cancer Center, 1975–1978

Alan Yagoda, M.D.

Solid Tumor Service, Department of Medicine, Memorial Sloan-Kettering Cancer Center, New York, New York

INTRODUCTION

In 1975 Memorial Sloan-Kettering Cancer Center (MSK) initiated a program to evaluate systemically the efficacy of chemotherapeutic agents in the treatment of patients with advanced urothelial tract cancers, i.e., carcinomas of the renal pelvis, ureter, bladder, and urethra. A survey of the literature at that time revealed few disease-oriented phase II studies; in fact, most reviews summarized data obtained from drug-oriented trials that included a small number of cases of bladder cancer. Frequently information concerning the kinds of patients treated, the measurable parameters evaluated, and the response criteria used was not adequately defined. However, these early studies established the potential efficacy of some antitumor agents in the treatment of patients with bladder cancer. During the past three years, 10 primary and 10 secondary drug-oriented phase II protocols in bladder cancer have been evaluated at MSK. This report will summarize and update the results of these trials in over 275 cases.

Measurable Parameters

A cardinal rule in phase II drug trials has been that patients with disease parameters that can be accurately measured should be selected to obtain a clear end point of response. Therefore, patients were selected at MSK for disease-oriented phase II trials in urothelial cancers who had objectively "measurable" parameters, such as pulmonary, hepatic, cutaneous, subcutaneous, or nodal metastases. In an attempt to enlarge the patient population for clinical studies, other metastatic lesions that could be defined bidimensionally were evaluated in patients with "measurable" disease. The accuracy of lymphangiograms and computerized transaxial tomograms (CT scans) was evaluated for "measurable" parameters, and lesions that can be precisely measured bidimensionally have now been accepted as a "measurable" parameter. Patients who had only "evaluable" lesions (i.e., intraabdominal, rectal, or pelvic masses poorly determinable by physical examination and the CT scan, lymphangitic spread of pulmonary metastases, or abnormal intravenous pyelograms, roentgenographic skeletal surveys, and/or radionuclide bone or liver scans) were excluded from primary disease-oriented trials. Generally, patients with "evaluable" disease received secondary protocols.

Potential inaccuracies in the assessment of objective changes in patients with "evaluable" lesions and in the subjective interpretation by both physicians and patients of favorable subjective benefit may result in aberrant response rates. In spite of careful patient selection for "measurable" parameters, reexamination of x-ray photographs and scans, observation of the subsequent course, and postmortem findings occasionally have resulted in some patients' being reassigned to the "evaluable" disease categories. Data from these patients are included in the overall results, but are also presented separately.

Response Categories

Another requirement of standard phase II drug trials has been a precise definition of the categories of response. In some clinical studies, major differences in remission rates may be related to aberrant definitions that have been used to evaluate response. The response criteria at MSK are outlined in Table 1.

All accessible lesions are measured by two or more perpendicular diameters and in over 95% of cases are reevaluated by the same observer (AY). Generally, pelvic and abdominal lesions are assessed by two observers, and all roentgenograms and CT scans are evaluated independently by Dr. Robin C. Watson, chief, MSK Department of Diagnostic Radiology.

Previously described methods employed to measure and define hepatomegaly by physical examination can be inaccurate. The anatomic landmarks used, i.e., the midline or the midclavicular or nipple lines, are sufficiently imprecise to raise doubts regarding findings on repeated examinations by the same or different observers. In addition, such imaginary anatomic lines limit investigators to the

Table 1. *Response Criteria*

CR	Complete disappearance of all measurable, radiologic, and biochemical abnormalities.
PR	Soft tissue lesions: >50% decrease in the *sum* of the products of two or more perpendicular diameters of all lesions for > one month. Abdominal or pelvic masses: >75% decrease by physical examination and/or >50% by CT in the *sum* of the products of two or more perpendicular diameters for > one month. Hepatomegaly: >50% decrease in the sum of all available measurements by physical examination and >50% decrease in all biochemical abnormalities and filling defects on scan for > one month. (In addition, if the pretreatment carcinoembryonic antigen (CEA) level is abnormal, a >50% decrease is required.)
MR	Minor remission: 25–49% decrease in tumor size, or biochemical abnormalities for > one month or >50% decrease for < one month.
STAB	Stable: 25% decrease or increase in tumor size or biochemical abnormalities for > three months.
PROG	Progression: >25% increase in tumor size or biochemical abnormalities or a mixed response.

use of only one to three measurements for evaluating liver size. The technique used at MSK (Yagoda and Kemeny 1978) represents an attempt to quantitate changes in liver size by using three to eight measurements at 5-cm intervals. While the patient lies in the supine position, breathing quietly, a ruler is placed on his chest wall on a horizontal plane at the level of the xiphoid. Marks are made on the rib cage at the xiphoid and 5, 10, 15, and 20 cm lateral to the xiphoid on each side. The extent of the liver below the costal margins at each of these points is recorded in centimeters and the sum of all measurements noted. In addition, the cephalad and caudad borders of the liver at its largest span (usually 5 or 10 cm to the right of the xiphoid) above and below the costal margin, measured by palpation, percussion, or the scratch technique, must be greater than 15 cm for a diagnosis of hepatomegaly. The MSK PR response criteria for malignant hepatomegaly are a >50% decrease in the sum of all available measurements by physical examination and a >50% decrease in all liver-related biochemical abnormalities. This method has been used at MSK for many years and seems to minimize errors and improve accuracy.

Patients who achieve MR, STAB, or mixed responses are not included in the overall objective (CR + PR) response rates. Most MR and mixed responses are brief and of little clinical benefit to patients, and patients in these categories are listed as nonresponders (PROG). However, MR and mixed responses do represent some evidence of potential drug activity and may indicate a need to modify dosages and schedules to induce complete or partial remissions. While stabilization may represent a response, it certainly does not represent an objective response. Any increase in survival in patients with "evaluable" or slow-growing disease who achieve stabilization is insufficient evidence of the efficacy of treatment, and statistical confirmation that patients with slow-growing tumors survive longer than those with fast-growing tumors is hardly proof of therapeutic benefit.

The durations of response for each phase II trial are measured from the initiation of protocol to progression. Generally, an adequate trial had been defined as two doses and one month survival (except for trials with Neocarzinostatin). The Karnofsky Performance Scale (PS) is used to evaluate subjective changes. Toxicity has been described as +1 (mild), +2 (moderate), +3 (severe, life-threatening, requiring hospitalization), and +4 (death directly or indirectly caused by complications of chemotherapy). Leukopenia is defined as a white blood count <4,500 mm³ and thrombocytopenia, <175,000 mm³.

Patient Characteristics

Another requirement is to define patient characteristics that may explain differences in response rates between clinical trials that use similar drugs and schedules. In the Karnofsky evaluation, these characteristics may lead to prognostic criteria favorable to the use of chemotherapy. All MSK studies include the following patient characteristics: median age; male-female ratio; percent grade III/IV lesions; PS; incidence of prior chemotherapy and types of agents given; incidence of prior irradiation and estimation of the extent of hematopoietic-producing bone marrow destroyed; incidence of radical surgery and presence of a urinary diversion; and intervals from diagnosis to metastasis, diagnosis or metastasis to protocol, and protocol to death or follow-up. In addition, the number of cases with a "measurable" disease parameter and the number of "measurable" and "evaluable" lesions are described in each study. Since the natural history of advanced bladder cancer is not well known and few prognostic factors have been identified, each of the above parameters could significantly alter response rates; therefore, each is a necessary component that should be included in all published reports of phase II trials in urothelial cancers.

MATERIALS AND METHODS

Initial Evaluation

Initial evaluation for each patient included a medical history and complete physical examination, and all accessible lesions were measured by two or more perpendicular diameters. Pelvic and intraabdominal lesions were generally measured by two physicians at MSK, one from the Solid Tumor Service, Department of Medicine, and one from the Urology Service, Department of Surgery. All pathologic material, such as urine and sputum cytology specimens, and biopsy specimens from bladder, lung, liver, lymph nodes, and skin, were reviewed in the Department of Pathology, MSK. Laboratory tests included a complete blood and platelet count, 12-channel screening profile, 24-hour urinary creatinine clearance, 5'-nucleotidase, and, during the past three years, CEA levels. Roentgenographic studies included bone surveys, standard posteroanterior, lateral, and stereoscopic chest x-ray photographs, intravenous pyelograms or loopograms, radionuclide bone and liver scans, lymphangiograms, and CT scans in patients found at laparotomy to have biopsy-proven lymph node involvement or nonresectable metastases. Appropriate measurements and diagnostic tests were always performed prior to administration of each dose or at three- to six-week intervals. Almost all subjective or symptomatic toxicities were recorded by one observer.

Protocols

The primary protocols, doses, and schedules are outlined in Table 2. In protocol I (Yagoda et al. 1977b), Adriamycin (ADR) was used as a single agent and, except in 18 cases, was administered as a single bolus in a dose of 45, 60, or 75 mg/m^2 every three weeks. Protocol II (Yagoda et al. 1977a) combined ADR and cyclophosphamide (CTX) in doses of 45 or 60 mg/m^2 and 450 or 600 mg/m^2, respectively, every three weeks. Subsequent doses were adjusted upward to ADR/CTX 60/450, 60/600, and 75/700 or downward to 35/350 mg/m^2.

Protocol III (Yagoda et al. 1976) used cis-diamminedichloride platinum II (DDP) administered intravenously every three or four weeks in a dose of 1.25

Table 2. *Primary MSK Protocols in Bladder Cancer: Drugs, Doses, and Schedules*

Protocol	Drugs	Doses (mg/m²)	Schedules (days)	Cycle (weeks)
I	ADR	15	1,2,3,4,5	1½–3
		8	1,2,3,7,8,9	—
		45–75	1	3–4
II	ADR	45–60	1	3
	CTX	450–600		
III	DDP	≅40–70	1	3–4
IV	DDP	70	1	3–4
	CTX	250–1,000		
V	DDP	70	1	3–4
	ADR	30–45		
VI	DDP	70	1	3–4
	CTX	250	2	
	ADR	30–45	3	
A	MTX	250	1	1½–2
		≅20–60	1	1
B	NCS	1,500–2,700 U	1,2,3,4,5	6–8
C	PALA	3,000–7,000	1	1

(two patients) or 1.6 mg/kg. All doses initially determined in mg/kg have been converted to mg/m² to permit comparison of results in protocols III–VI. Adequate hydration was given prior to and following DDP administration for two to six hours to maintain a urine diuresis of 100–125 ml/hr. Hospitalization was required to ensure adequate hydration in 85% of patients who received DDP. Patients with borderline renal function (creatinine clearance of 40–55 ml/min) received a dose of mannitol, 12.5 gm, at the time of DDP administration to increase urine output. Three patients received high-dose DDP (HD-DDP), 120 mg/m², with mannitol infusion by the method outlined by Hayes et al. (1977). Protocol IV (Yagoda et al. 1978a) used DDP, 70 mg/m², and CTX, 250, 500, 750, or 1,000 mg/m², administered intravenously every three to four weeks. Patients who had extensive prior irradiation started at 250 or 500 mg/m², while previously untreated patients received higher doses. Protocol V (Yagoda et al. 1978b) combined DDP, 70 mg/m², and ADR, 30, 45, or 60 mg/m², i.v., every three to four weeks. Protocol VI (Yagoda 1978) combined DDP, 70 mg/m², day 1, CTX, 250 mg/m², day 2, and ADR, 30 or 45 mg/m², day 3, every three to four weeks.

Patients who had progressive disease were given other agents. The schedule of methotrexate (MTX) administration was 250 mg/m², i.v., over a two-hour period, followed 24 hours later by citrovorum factor rescue, 15 mg p.o., every six hours for 12 doses or 50 mg i.v. followed by 5–10 mg p.o. every eight hours for 12 doses (Yagoda 1977). Sufficient intravenous hydration and intravenous and oral sodium bicarbonate were administered to induce a urine diuresis of 100–125 ml/hr and a urine pH of >8. Serum creatinine and blood urea nitrogen levels were monitored for two to three days after each dose. In addition, in some patients serum MTX levels were measured 24, 48, and 72 hours after infusion. Any increase above normal or expected values was treated vigorously with additional hydration, alkalinization, and additional doses of citrovorum factor. When response or stabilization occurred, patients were maintained on weekly i.v. MTX (without rescue) at doses of 0.5–1.5 mg/kg until progression was noted.

Neocarzinostatin (NCS), a new antitumor antibiotic, was administered in 20-minute infusions in doses of 1,500 2,000, 2,250, 2,500, or 2,750 units/m² for five consecutive days every six to eight weeks (Natale and Yagoda 1978). Since NCS is light sensitive, the bottle and tubing were covered with aluminum foil. Diphenhydramine was given routinely to prevent chills, fever, or allergic reactions.

Phase I–II trials with PALA, *N*-(phosphonoacetyl)-L-aspartic acid, a potent inhibitor of aspartate transcarbamylase activity, have been initiated at MSK and this agent is now included in the primary protocol group. Although PALA has been given by bolus in doses of 3,000–7,500 mg/m² weekly, most patients receive 3,750–4,500 mg/m² weekly.

Almost all patients in secondary protocols had received prior chemotherapy and many had a PS of less than 60. The following doses and schedules were used: CTX 20–40 mg/kg, i.v., every three to four weeks; vinblastine, 0.1–0.2 mg/kg, i.v., weekly; 5-fluorouracil, 300–400 mg/m² for five consecutive days, every four weeks; and bleomycin, 20 mg/m², in a continuous infusion for five to eight days.

RESULTS

There were 279 protocol cases. Twenty-five cases have not yet been evaluated and approximately 10% (25) have had inadequate trials. The results in 229 adequately treated patients, some of whom were treated after publication of the phase II trials, are summarized in Tables 3 and 4. Extensive toxicity data

Table 3. *Results of Primary MSK Protocols in Bladder Cancer*

Protocol	Drugs	No. Patients Entered	No. Not Yet Evaluated	No. Adequate Trials	No. CR	No. PR	CR + PR (%)	No. MR	No. PROG
I	ADR	52	2	42	1	6	17	4	31
II	ADR + CTX	20	0	18	0	3	17	0	15
III	DDP	33	2	30	0	11	37*	4	15
IV	DDP + CTX	40	1	34	0	15	44	2	17
V	DDP + ADR	30	1	29	2	12	48	1	14
VI	DDP + CTX + ADR	15	8	7	0	5	71	0	2
A	MTX	18	1	17	0	5	29	0	12
B	NCS	17	3	14	0	1	7	0	13
C	PALA	6	0	6	0	0	0	2	4
D	HD-DDP	3	1	2	0	0	0	1	1

* 50% in untreated patients.

Table 4. *Results of Secondary MSK Protocols in Bladder Cancer*

Drugs	No. Patients Entered	No. Not Yet Evaluated	No. Adequate Trials	No. Patients Responding			No. MR	No. PROG
				CR	PR	CR + PR (%)		
CTX	16	0	11	0	1	9	1	9
Bleomycin	6	0	4	0	0	0	0	4
Vincristine	5	1	3	0	0	0	0	3
Vinblastine	6	3	3	0	0	0	0	3
5-Fluorouracil	5	1	3	0	0	0	1	2
Alkeran	2	0	2	0	0	0	0	2
Hydroxyurea	2	0	2	0	0	0	0	2
6-Mercaptopurine	1	1	1	0	0	0	0	0
CTX + ADR + Vincristine	1	0	1	0	0	0	0	1
DDP + MTX	1	0	1	0	0	0	0	1

will not be presented, but can be obtained from published reports of each protocol.

Adriamycin Protocols

ADR used alone (protocol I) yielded clinically useful remissions (CR + PR) in only 17% of patients, but the response rate increased to 22% in patients who had no prior chemotherapy. Objective regression of disease, primarily in skin, lung, liver, and lymph nodes, was rapid and generally occurred within three to four weeks. Frequently the maximum extent of response was noted after two to four doses. The median duration of response was three months (range one to six months). Four patients achieved MR status, which persisted less than six weeks, and four more patients showed stabilization for four to nine months.

ADR was given in two schedules, a single dose and a loading dose. The response rate for single-dose therapy was 20%, versus 6% with the loading schedule. One patient who showed progression after two consecutive doses of 45 mg/m^2 responded to 75 mg/m^2. However, he refused additional therapy because of severe vomiting and persistent nausea, and exhibited rapid progression of disease six weeks later. Severe toxicity (+3, +4) occurred in 35% and was more frequent with high doses (60, 75, 90 mg/m^2).

ADR and CTX (protocol II) induced a similar response rate, 17%, to that achieved with ADR alone. Toxicity with this combination was more severe and 39% of patients required hospitalization.

Cis-platinum Protocols

DDP (protocol III) produced significant remissions in 37% of patients with advanced urinary tract cancers. However, the response rate increased to 50%

in patients who had no prior chemotherapy. Responses were extremely rapid, with subjective improvement noted in 12 to 48 hours and objective tumor regression in 24 to 72 hours. Except for one patient who required two doses, all patients responded after the first dose. The maximum response was generally obtained in one to two doses and additional tumor regression was not observed with subsequent DDP administration. The median duration of response was five months and, except for one patient who had an unmaintained remission for nine months, all patients relapsed within six to 10 weeks when DDP was not administered monthly. The major dose-limiting toxicity of protocol III was not deterioration of renal function or decreased auditory acuity, but unacceptable nausea and vomiting. In fact, most patients who responded to DDP eventually refused additional doses because of the latter toxicity, so many responses were unmaintained.

Although DDP seems to function in part as an alkylating agent, synergism has been described in experimental tumor models when DDP is combined with other alkylating agents, such as CTX. DDP and CTX were given to 40 patients, 35 of whom had adequate trials. The overall response rate was 44%, which was similar to that obtained with DDP used alone in previously untreated cases. The response rate in patients who had no prior chemotherapy was 46% (12/26), versus 33% (3/9) in previously treated cases. No difference in response rate occurred when CTX was given at doses of 250 to 750 mg/m². The median duration of response was seven months and the survival rate was identical to that of responders in protocol III. Toxicity resulted in cessation or temporary delay in therapy because of vomiting and nausea in 14 patients, myelosuppression in seven, hematuria in five, and mild nephrotoxicity in 19. Myelosuppression correlated with the dose of CTX and the extent of prior irradiation.

DDP and ADR (protocol V) were administered to 30 patients, 29 of whom have been evaluated. The overall response rate was 48%, with a median duration of 3+ months. The response rate in previously treated patients was 67% and in untreated patients, 50%. DDP and ADR produced more myelosuppression but less nausea and vomiting than DDP and CTX.

Protocol VI, which combines DDP, CTX, and ADR, administered sequentially, was started in May 1978. Thus far, 15 patients have been entered and seven have been evaluated. Preliminary results indicate a remission rate of 70%. Two patients are being reevaluated at this time and seem to have achieved complete regression of their indicator lesions. Although doses are well tolerated, one patient has had +3 toxicity. Patients in protocols IV and VI who obtained remission frequently had rapid tumor regression (probably due to DDP) and additional response (probably related to ADR) seven to 21 days later.

Other Primary Protocols

MTX (protocol A) induced remissions in five of 17 heavily pretreated patients. Responses have persisted from four to over six months. Two patients had almost complete clearing of adenopathy and skin metastasis. Generally toxicity has been mild, $+1$ to $+2$. Additional patient accrual will continue, and in future trials previously untreated patients will receive MTX.

The initial dose of NCS was 1,500 units/m^2 for five consecutive days. Cycles were to be repeated every four weeks, but myelosuppression required a schedule modification to every eight weeks. Forty-two of 51 courses were evaluable and myelosuppression occurred in 36% of courses at 1,500 units/m^2 and in 50–67% of courses at 2,000–2,750 units/m^2. Thrombocytopenia was more frequent than leukopenia and occurred earlier with high doses (28–34 versus 45–46 days, respectively, after the first dose). Most patients experienced fever and chills one-half to two hours postinfusion, which persisted for two to four hours and disappeared by the third or fourth dose. Two patients have had acute allergic reactions. Six patients described pain in known tumor-bearing sites one hour after each dose; discomfort persisted for four to six hours. One patient had histologic and biochemical evidence of acute hepatitis, probably attributable to NCS. There was no response in 14 previously treated patients. One of the three untreated patients achieved an objective response. The patient who obtained a PR after one cycle has remained without evidence of disease for over four months. Retreatment with NCS has been withheld because of persistent thrombocytopenia, $<100,000$ mm^3.

PALA has been administered in a phase I–II trial to five patients with advanced bladder cancer. All patients had extensive prior chemotherapy and a PS $<$ 70. Although the maximum extent of response was the achievement of MR status in two patients, further trials with different schedules or doses of PALA in previously untreated patients may produce better results.

Secondary Protocols

The results of secondary MSK protocols in bladder cancer (Table 3) are not surprising; only one of 32 patients has achieved partial remission. These backup protocols are used only after patients fail the primary MSK protocols. Most patients who receive secondary protocol therapy have low PS, poor marrow reserve, which necessitates decreased dosages, and a history of extensive prior chemotherapy. Methotrexate was originally a secondary protocol, but when responses were found in two heavily pretreated patients, the agent was moved to the primary protocol group.

DISCUSSION

Adriamycin is one of the most thoroughly studied drugs used against advanced urothelial tract cancers. Although earlier reports have described remissions in 35–55% (Yagoda et al. 1977b, Blum and Carter 1974), the overall response rates in recent studies are only 10–20%. In most trials, the durations of remissions are short, averaging three months. However, some patients respond for

28 to 52+ weeks. O'Bryan and co-workers (1977) have described an increased response rate when doses of 75+ mg/m^2 are employed, in contrast to that achieved with 30–45 mg/m^2, suggesting that the response rate is dose related. The major dose-limiting toxicity of ADR is cardiac toxicity. Since 60% of patients with bladder cancer are between the ages of 50 and 70 years and many already exhibit cardiac disease, ADR used alone for maintenance therapy may be of limited value. The combination of ADR and CTX was disappointing and there was no evidence of an additive or synergistic effect with this combination.

The most active agent in the treatment of transitional cell carcinoma of the urothelial tract has been DDP. Review of the literature (Yagoda 1978) has revealed 76 patients who received DDP, 67 of whom had adequate trials and 29 (43%) of whom obtained complete or partial remissions. The 95% confidence limit was 12–57%. The average duration of response with DDP was 4.5 months (range two to 48 months). Of particular interest is the report by Merrin (1978) of a complete remission of four years' duration in a patient who received only two 100 mg/m^2 doses of DDP.

Protocols IV, V, and VI included various DDP-combination regimens because of the findings by Soloway (1978) of increased antitumor activity with combination regimens in the FANFT (*N*-4-(5-nitro-2-furyl)-2 thiazolyl formamide)-induced bladder cancer model in mice. However, response rates in protocols IV and V are similar to those that could be achieved with DDP alone. Thus far, clinical evidence of an additive effect of ADR or CTX to DDP has not been found. The three-drug combination regimen, DDP, CTX, and ADR, was initiated because of the preliminary report by Sternberg and co-workers (1977). The sequential administration of ADR 48 hours after DDP had been suggested by the work of Soloway (1978). The results from protocol VI are still too preliminary and must await further patient accrual.

Comparison of patient characteristics (Table 5) and measurable parameters (Table 6) with the four DDP regimens reveals some differences in patient selection. The percent of males treated in protocol II is less than that in the other protocols. The percent of patients in protocols I and II with high-grade lesions is also low, 51% and 59%, versus 70% and 80% for protocols III and IV. In addition, more patients in protocols I and II have received prior chemotherapy. These differences may influence response rates. While the prognostic significance of various patient characteristics in bladder cancer is as yet undefined, further patient accrual from other studies may indicate that sex, tumor grade, and prior chemotherapy decrease the incidence of response to chemotherapeutic agents. Table 5 indicates that most patients entered into Phase II trials at MSK have "measurable" parameters.

Since remissions occur in approximately 45% (range 12–57%) of patients with transitional cell bladder cancer with DDP alone, additive or synergistic improvement with DDP-multidrug regimens will require either a higher CR rate or a statistically significant increase in the number of patients who achieve

Table 5. *DDP Phase II Trials in Adequately Treated Patients With Bladder Cancer*

Patient Characteristic	DDP (N = 30)	DDP CTX (N = 34)	DDP ADR (N = 29)	DDP CTX ADR (N = 7)
Age (yrs.)*	59 (39–73)	60 (30–79)	63 (35–77)	60 (47–71)
Males (%)	87	63	76	100
P.S.*	75 (30–90)	80 (30–90)	80 (50–100)	80 (50–90)
Tumor grade (%) III/IV	59	51	70	80
Prior urinary diversion (%)	50	54	24	43
Prior irradiation (%)	80	85	76	71
2+ ports	23	12	14	29
Prior chemotherapy (%)	33	26	21	14
Diagnosis to protocol (mos.)*	16 (0–72)	16 (3–135)	21 (2–149)	20 (6–140)
Protocol to follow-up (mos.)*	4 (1+–34)	6 (1.2–24+)	6+ (1.5–16+)	3+ (2.5–6+)

* Median, ( ) = range.

PR status. Preliminary results with DDP combination regimens in a small number of patients, particularly patients with "evaluable" disease parameters suggesting marked improvement in response rates above that expected with DDP used alone, demand cautious interpretation and confirmation by other investigators. Therefore, extended phase II and phase III trials in patients with so-called evaluable disease parameters will require prospective randomized studies that use DDP as the control arm.

Comparison of the results of the efficacy of MTX in published trials is extremely difficult because of differences in dosages, schedules, routes of administra-

Table 6. *Relationship Between Complete and Partial Response Rates and Measurable and Evaluable Parameters in DDP Phase II Trials*

Parameter	DDP (N = 30) All	DDP (N = 30) PR	DDP CTX (N = 34) All	DDP CTX (N = 34) PR	DDP ADR (N = 29) All	DDP ADR (N = 29) PR	DDP CTX ADR (N = 7) All	DDP CTX ADR (N = 7) PR
Measurable								
Lung, liver, skin, nodal, and subcutaneous lesions	23	9	25	11	27	13	6	4
Pelvic mass + CT	1	0	5	3	1	1	1	1
Lymphangiograms	2	0	2	1	1	0	0	0
Evaluable								
Abdominal mass	2	2	2	0	0	0	0	0
Osseous lesions	2	0	0	0	0	0	0	0

tion, case selection, patient characteristics, and response criteria. For example, some studies stress improvement in local or osseous metastases or simply a decrease in the amount of hematuria as indicative of a complete or partial remission (Altman et al. 1972, Turner et al. 1977). Although response rates as high as 56% (Turner et al. 1977) have been described, Gad-El-Mawla et al. (1978) have noted remissions in only 7% of patients with bilharzial bladder cancer. In the MSK study, MTX does appear to be an active agent and additional studies with high-dose MTX will continue.

Although Sakamoto and co-workers (1978) have described therapeutic activity with NCS, clinical studies at MSK indicate minimal benefit, particularly in previously treated patients. Presently, NCS is only being administered at MSK to patients who have had no prior chemotherapy.

Soloway (1978) has noted marked antitumor activity with the use of PALA alone and in combination with DDP in the FANFT model. Preliminary results in heavily pretreated patients suggest that PALA may be useful in the treatment of metastatic bladder cancer.

Cyclophosphamide is another agent that has been administered in a variety of schedules and dosages. While Merrin and co-workers (1975) noted responses in 50% of patients, the overall response rate in over 50 evaluable cases culled from various phase I and II trials (Yagoda et al. 1977a) is 10–25%.

New investigational agents as well as many older drugs, i.e., CTX, 5-fluoroura-cil, cytosine arabinoside, vinblastine, and vincristine, still require phase II disease-oriented studies in patients with urothelial tumors that use rigid response criteria and proper patient selection. At MSK, patients with advanced metastatic bladder cancer who have objectively measurable parameters will continue to be evaluated with single-agent therapy in an effort to define more precisely active chemotherapeutic drugs.

ACKNOWLEDGMENTS

The author gratefully acknowledges the technical and secretarial assistance of Mrs. Marjorie Freilich-Den and Mrs. Isa R. Irvin in the preparation of this manuscript. This investigation was supported in part by grant CA-05826 and contract N01-CM-57043, awarded by the National Cancer Institute, Department of Health, Education and Welfare.

REFERENCES

Altman, C. C., M. J. McCague, A. C. R. Pepi, and M. Cardozo. 1972. The use of methotrexate in advanced carcinoma of the bladder. J. Urol. 108:271–273.
Blum, R. H., and S. K. Carter. 1974. Adriamycin: A new anticancer drug with significant clinical activity. Ann. Intern. Med. 80:249–259.
Gad-El-Mawla, M. N., R. Hamsa, J. Cairns, T. Anderson, and J. L. Ziegler. 1978. Phase II trial of methotrexate in carcinoma of the bilharzial bladder. Cancer Treat. Rep. 62:1075–1076.
Hayes, D. M., E. Cvitkovic, R. B. Golbey, E. Scheiner, L. Helson, and I. H. Krakoff. 1977. High dose cis-platinum diammine dichloride. Cancer 39:1372–1381.

Merrin, C. 1978. Treatment of advanced bladder cancer with cis-diamminedichloroplatinum (II) (NSC 119875): A pilot study. J. Urol. 119:493–495.

Merrin, C., R. Cartagena, Z. Wajsman, G. Baumgartner, and G. P. Murphy. 1975. Chemotherapy of bladder carcinoma with cyclophosphamide and adriamycin. J. Urol. 114:884–887.

Natale, R. B., and A. Yagoda. 1978. Phase II trial of Neocarcinostatin (NCS 157365) in patients with bladder and prostate carcinoma, *in* Minutes of New Drug Liaison Meeting, National Cancer Institute, Sept. 20, 1978. Bethesda, Md.: National Cancer Institute, pp. 27–33.

O'Bryan, R. M., L. H. Baker, J. E. Gottlieb, S. E. Rivkin, S. P. Balcerzak, G. N. Grumet, S. E. Salmon, T. E. Moon, and B. Hoogstraten. 1977. Dose response evaluation of adriamycin in human neoplasia. Cancer 39:1940–1948.

Sakamoto, S., J. Ogata, K. I. Kegami, and H. Maeda. 1978. Effects of systemic administration of Neocarzinostatin, a new protein antibiotic on human bladder cancer. Cancer Treat. Rep. 62:453–454.

Soloway, M. S. 1978. Cisdiamminedichloroplatinum (II) (DDP) in advanced bladder cancer. (Abstract) Proc. Am. Assoc. Cancer Res. Am. Soc. Clin. Oncol. 19:366 (ASCO abstr. C-239).

Sternberg, J. J., R. B. Bracken, P. B. Handel, and D. E. Johnson. 1977. Combination chemotherapy (CISCA) for advanced urinary tract carcinoma: A preliminary report. J.A.M.A. 238:2282–2287.

Turner, A. G., W. F. Hendry, G. B. Williams, and H. J. G. Bloom. 1977. The treatment of advanced bladder cancer with methotrexate. Br. J. Urol. 49:673–678.

Yagoda, A. 1977. Future implications of phase 2 chemotherapy trials in ninety-five patients with measurable advanced bladder cancer. Cancer Res. 37:2775–2780.

Yagoda, A. 1978. Phase II trials with cis-diamminedichloride platinum II in the treatment of urothelial cancers. Cancer Treat. Rep. (in press).

Yagoda, A., and N. E. Kemeny. 1978. Chemotherapy of colorectal cancer: A critical analysis of response criteria and therapeutic efficacy, *in* Gastrointestinal Tract Cancer, M. Lipkin and R. A. Good, eds. Plenum Medical Book Company, New York, pp. 551–568.

Yagoda, A., R. C. Watson, J. C. Gonzalez-Vitale, H. Grabstald, and W. F. Whitmore. 1976. Cis-dichlorodiammineplatinum (II) in advanced bladder cancer. Cancer Treat. Rep. 60:917–923.

Yagoda, A., R. C. Watson, H. Grabstald, W. E. Barzell, and W. F. Whitmore. 1977a. Adriamycin and cyclophosphamide in advanced bladder cancer. Cancer Treat. Rep. 61:97–99.

Yagoda, A., R. C. Watson, N. Kemeny, W. E. Barzell, H. Grabstald, and W. F. Whitmore. 1978a. Diamminedichloride platinum II (DDP) and cyclophosphamide (CTX) in the treatment of advanced urothelial cancer. Cancer 41:2121–2130.

Yagoda, A., R. C. Watson, and W. F. Whitmore, Jr. 1978b. Diamminedichloride platinum II (DDP) and adriamycin in the treatment of advanced urothelial cancer. Paper presented at the National Bladder Cancer Project Symposium, Sarasota, Florida, Jan. 29–Feb. 1, 1978.

Yagoda, A., R. C. Watson, W. F. Whitmore, H. Grabstald, M. P. Middleman, and I. H. Krakoff. 1977b. Adriamycin in advanced urinary tract cancer: Experience in 42 patients, and a review of the literature. Cancer 39:279–285.

Cancer of the Genitourinary Tract, edited by
D. E. Johnson and M. L. Samuels.
Raven Press, New York © 1979.

Prophylaxis of Recurrent Bladder Cancer With Bacillus Calmette-Guérin

Alvaro Morales, M.D., and Anne Ersil, B.Sc.

Departments of Urology and Epidemiology, Queen's University, Kingston, Ontario, Canada

Because of the accessibility of the bladder, there is interest in the prophylaxis and treatment of superficial bladder cancer by intravesical instillation of antineoplastic agents. The early reports by Veenema et al. (1962, 1969) on the value of thio-TEPA in the prevention of tumor recurrence and ablation of superficial low-grade bladder cancer have been confirmed in other studies (Jones and Swinney 1961, Nieh et al. 1978). Intravesical instillations of other chemotherapeutic agents have been used to manage these lesions with variable success (Robinson et al. 1977, Banks et al. 1977, Bracken et al. 1977).

Little attention, however, has been paid to immunotherapy for superficial bladder tumors, which is surprising since such early neoplasms appear to be well suited to immunotherapeutic intervention. Animal experiments (Zbar and Rapp 1974) have shown that nonspecific active immunotherapy with *Mycobacterium bovis* (strain bacillus Calmette-Guérin, BCG) is most effective when the tumor burden is relatively small, a close contact between the vaccine and the tumor is achieved, and the dose and timing of the vaccine administration are adequate. In addition, experimental studies (Coe and Feldman 1966) have shown that, in contrast to the kidney, testis, and muscle, the bladder is an ideal organ for the extracutaneous production of delayed hypersensitivity reactions in the immunized host. Therefore, a protocol was designed in 1973 to evaluate the role of BCG as an adjuvant to surgery in the prevention of bladder tumor recurrence.

Preliminary results previously published (Morales et al. 1976) indicated that BCG treatment could alter the pattern of recurrence without inducing adverse long-lasting effects. In this report, the results of local and systemic BCG treatment in 20 patients are presented. The number of recurrences in this group of patients was significantly ($p < 10^{-3}$) reduced. Sixty percent remained tumor free for the duration of post-BCG follow-up.

MATERIALS AND METHODS

Twenty patients with histologically diagnosed transitional cell carcinoma of the bladder were treated. To enter the study, a patient had to have had at least two recurrences documented by separate endoscopic examinations within two years of the initiation of treatment. In every case the tumors were superficial (stages P1S to P1, UICC classification) and were completely resected, leaving no endoscopic evidence of residual tumor. There were 14 men and six women ranging in age from 43 to 88 years (mean 71).

Throughout the study, vaccine from the Institut Armand Frappier, Montreal, was used. One hundred twenty milligrams of the lyophilized vaccine were resuspended in 50 ml of sterile normal saline for use as a bladder instillation. Five milligrams of reconstituted BCG were employed for intradermal immunization.

The treatment protocol required that every patient receive weekly intradermal and intravesical immunizations with BCG. For the intradermal route, the anterior aspect of a thigh was cleaned with alcohol and allowed to dry. By means of a multiple-puncture apparatus (Heaf gun) with a six-prong head, 10 impacts were administered to an area approximately 5×5 cm. A small amount of the BCG suspension was spread over the area and allowed to dry. The vaccine was reapplied until it was all used. The area was dressed with a Telfa pad and the patient instructed to leave the area undisturbed for 24 hours. For intravesical administration, the patient was prepared for routine bladder catheterization under sterile conditions. A number 8F rubber catheter was inserted into the bladder, all urine removed, and a sample sent for routine culture. The BCG suspension was instilled into the bladder and the catheter removed immediately afterwards. The patient was instructed to retain the medication for no less than two hours, at which time he was allowed to void. Both the intradermal and intravesical administrations of the vaccine were repeated weekly for six weeks. For the intradermal applications, alternate thighs were used.

Cystoscopic examinations were performed at three- to six-month intervals from the onset of treatment. At endoscopy, biopsies were performed on any obvious tumor or area suggestive of recurrence with the aid of cold-cup forceps. In the absence of mucosal changes suggestive of recurrence, samples from preselected areas (usually four) were obtained. Urinary cytologic examinations were performed on fresh voided specimens and on samples obtained at the time of cystoscopy.

The response to therapy was classified as follows: (1) class A: no evidence of recurrence during the post-BCG follow-up period, (2) class B: a reduction of 50% or more in the number of recurrences and prolongation of 50% or more in the disease-free interval following therapy, and (3) class C: less than 50% reduction in the number of recurrences or less than 50% increase in the disease-free interval following treatment.

RESULTS

Figure 1 presents, for each of the 20 patients, the number of tumors as a function of time for the pre- and posttherapy terms. The durations of the follow-up periods differ among the subjects, the pre-BCG period ranging from seven to 43 months, the post-BCG from 12 to 40 months. The follow-up interval before treatment does not equal that after treatment for each subject. In the case of patient 1, for example, tumors were recorded for 23 months prior to the administration of BCG and for 29 months following therapy. For this comparison, an equal period before and after therapy was used. Thus, for patient 1, only tumors occurring within 23 months after treatment were counted. Data on the entire set of patients and the statistical analysis are summarized in Table 1.

The least squares method was used to estimate the slopes of the pre- and post-BCG linear regression lines. These convenient estimates are unbiased (Johnston 1972), despite the fact that serial correlations are probably present. Since the usual statistical test (t or F) of significance for the slopes may not be valid, we applied the Cochrane Q test (Sokal and Rohlf 1969) to determine trend. In this test, the patients were scored for the presence or absence of a tumor during four equal intervals before and after BCG therapy. Table 2 gives some details of the analysis. For the 20 patients in the trial, a statistically significant ($p < 10^{-3}$) positive (upward) trend in recurrence was detected for the pre-BCG period, while no trend ($p > 0.05$) is evident following BCG therapy. This analysis indicates that BCG administration reduces the number of recurrent tumors, disrupting the upward trend in the recurrence pattern.

Table 1. *Wilcoxon Signed-Rank Test*

Patient No.	No. Tumors Pre-BCG	No. Tumors Post-BCG	d_i	Rank of Absolute Value of d_i
1	9	0	9	18.5
2	6	0	6	13.5
3	8	1	7	16.0
4	6	0	6	13.5
5	4	2	2	2.5
6	9	0	9	18.5
7	6	2	4	9.5
8	5	2	3	5.5
9	16	2	14	20.0
10	4	0	4	9.5
11	6	0	6	13.5
12	6	3	3	5.5
13	3	0	3	5.5
14	7	4	3	5.5
15	4	0	4	9.5
16	6	0	6	13.5
17	8	0	8	17.0
18	2	0	2	2.5
19	4	0	4	9.5
20	1	0	1	1.0

$\Sigma(d_i > 0) = 210$, $\Sigma(d_i < 0) = 0$, $n = 20$ pairs; $\mu = n(n + 1)/4$; $\mu = 20(20 + 1)/4$; $\mu = 105$; $T = \min \{\Sigma(d_i > 0), \Sigma(d_i < 0)\}$; $T = 0$; $\sigma = (2n + 1)\mu/6$; $\sigma = (2 \times 20 + 1)105/6$; $\sigma = 26.8$; $Z = (T-\mu)/\sigma = 3.92$; $p < 10^{-3}$.

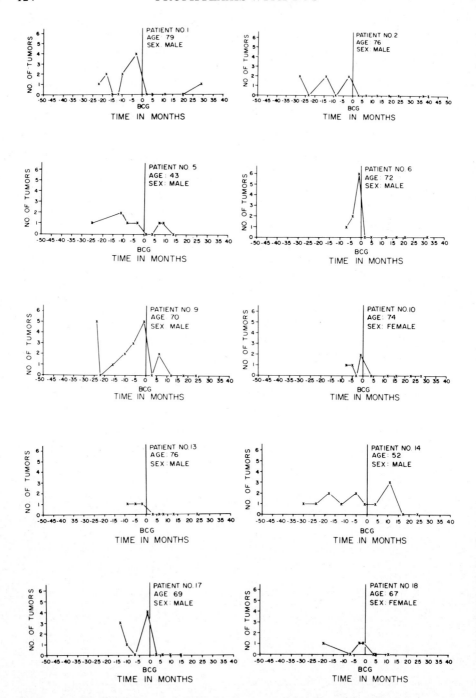

Figure 1. Number of tumors, in individual patients, as a function of time for the pre- and posttherapy periods.

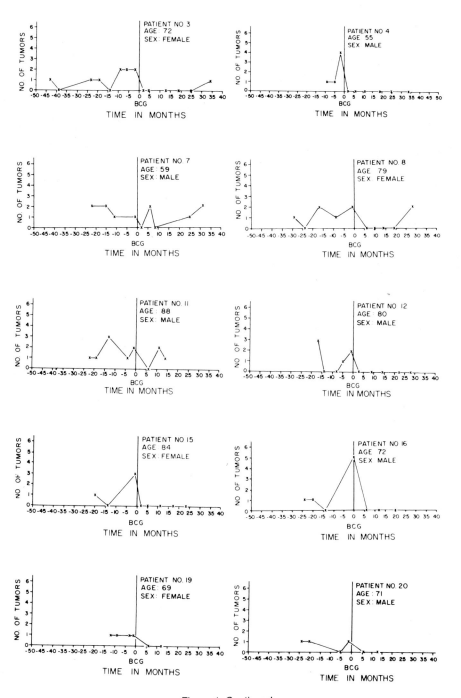

Figure 1 *Continued*

Table 2. *The Cochrane Q Test*

| | Number of Recurrences | | | | | | | | | |
| | Pre-BCG Interval | | | | | Post-BCG Interval | | | | |
Patient No.	1	2	3	4	Σ	1	2	3	4	Σ
1	0	1	0	1	2	0	0	0	0	0
2	0	1	0	1	2	0	0	0	0	0
3	0	1	1	1	3	0	0	0	0	0
4	1	0	1	1	3	0	0	0	0	0
5	0	1	0	1	2	0	0	1	0	1
6	1	1	0	1	3	0	0	0	0	0
7	1	1	1	1	4	0	1	0	0	1
8	0	1	1	1	3	0	0	0	0	0
9	0	1	1	1	3	0	1	0	0	1
10	0	1	0	1	2	0	0	0	0	0
11	0	0	1	1	2	0	0	0	0	0
12	1	0	1	1	3	0	0	1	1	2
13	1	0	1	1	3	0	0	0	0	0
14	1	1	1	1	4	1	1	0	0	2
15	0	0	0	1	1	0	0	0	0	0
16	0	0	0	1	1	0	0	0	0	0
17	0	0	0	1	1	0	0	0	0	0
18	0	0	0	1	2	0	0	0	0	0
19	1	1	0	1	3	0	0	0	0	0
20	0	0	0	1	0	0	0	0	0	0
Totals	7	11	10	20	48	1	3	2	1	7

$Q \sim \chi$ a b   ab   ab   b a

$Q = (a-1)[a\Sigma(\Sigma Y)^2 - (\Sigma\Sigma Y)^2]/a\Sigma\Sigma Y - \Sigma(\Sigma Y)^2$

$a = 4$

Pre-BCG

a b
$\Sigma\Sigma Y = 48$
b a
$\Sigma(\Sigma Y)^2 = 132$
a b
$\Sigma(\Sigma Y)^2 = 670$

$Q = (4-1)[4 \times 670-(48)^2]/(4 \times 48)-132$

$\chi^2{}_{.001.3} = 16.27$

$\therefore p < 10^{-3}$

Post-BCG

a b
$\Sigma\Sigma Y = 7$
b
$\Sigma(\Sigma Y)^2 = 11$
a b
$\Sigma(\Sigma Y)^2 = 15$

$Q = (4-1)[4 \times 15-(7)^2]/(4 \times 7)-11 = 1.94$

$\chi^2{}_{.05.3} = 7.82$

$\therefore p > 0.05$

Closer examination of the follow-up data reveals that it was feasible to divide the patients into three classes on the basis of response to treatment. Class A consists of those 12 out of 20 patients (60%) who remained entirely tumor free during the post-BCG follow-up. Class B, which accounts for 20% of the total group, is comprised of the four patients (1, 3, 8, and 9) in whom partial improvement was evident following BCG administration. In this class there was an average reduction of 84% in the number of tumors. Class C, the remaining

Table 3. *Number and Mean Ages (Years) of Patients According to Class*

Variable	Class A	Class B	Class C	Classes A & B	Classes B & C
Number of patients	12	4	4	16	8
Mean age at diagnosis	72.4	71.0	56.5	72.1	63.7
Mean age at treatment	73.8	75.5	58.5	74.2	67.0

20%, is made up of the four patients (5, 7, 11, and 14) whose pattern of recurrence was not apparently altered by the therapy under study.

The three classes were analyzed for factors that could account for the differences in response. A one-way analysis of variance (Ott 1977) showed that the differences in age among classes were significant both at diagnosis ($F = 4.13$; $df = 2,17$; $p < 0.05$) and at treatment ($F = 4.14$; $df = 2,17$; $p < 0.05$). Employing Fischer's test for multiple comparisons (Ott 1977), we concluded that mean ages at diagnosis and treatment in class C were significantly ($p < 0.05$) lower than those in class A or B. Mean age comparisons between classes are summarized in Table 3.

Untoward reactions to the vaccine were generally mild and brief. In most cases they consisted of general malaise, low-grade fever, and bladder irritability (dysuria and urinary frequency) lasting a few days and not requiring specific treatment. In four subjects, however (8, 12, 15, and 20), symptoms of bladder irritability were severe enough to require the use of urinary analgesics (phenazopyridine) and anticholinergic medication. Patients 15 and 20 responded promptly to the medication, but BCG therapy had to be stopped after five or six treatment sessions for patients 8 and 12. Patient 12 developed a severe inflammation of the bladder mucosa and secondary partial bilateral ureteric obstruction. The most severe reaction was observed in patient 8, in whom migratory polyarthritis and cutaneous erythema of the palms occurred, in addition to urinary symptoms. In three other patients a lower urinary tract infection with *Escherichia coli* was documented during treatment. In all three patients a rapid response to antibiotics was obtained.

DISCUSSION

In this trial, the simultaneous intradermal and intravesical administration of BCG favorably altered the pattern of recurrence of superficial bladder cancer in most patients. Sixty percent of patients with a previous history of multiple recurrences have remained tumor free for 12 to 40 months. In agreement with results found with other solid tumors (Eilber et al. 1975), the response to therapy with BCG was not an all-or-nothing phenomenon. In 20% of the patients recurrence was detected in the post-treatment period, but its frequency was reduced by 84%, which corresponded to an increase in mean disease-free interval from

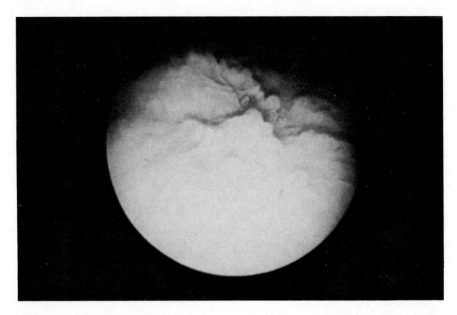

Figure 2. Endoscopic aspect of bladder three months after onset of treatment showing raised mucosal lesions suggestive of recurrence.

four months before treatment to 20 months after treatment. It is conceivable that a longer period of immunization could have improved the outcome in these patients, but such a possibility remains to be proven.

Undesirable side effects directly attributable to the regimen of immunizations were tolerable. For most patients they were minor and self-limiting, and, except for the lower urinary tract manifestations, have been common findings during BCG therapy (Sparks et al. 1973). The more severe side effects encountered in two of our patients were not treated with specific medication; in retrospect, antituberculous therapy should have been used in these two cases. Severe systemic effects have been reported in two of six patients treated with intravesical instillations of BCG in the presence of tumor, but both patients responded rapidly to isoniazid administration (Douville et al. 1978). McKneally et al. (1978) have used postoperative intrapleural BCG adjuvant therapy in lung cancer patients who receive isoniazid routinely. The use of this drug appeared to prevent the more severe systemic manifestations without having a detrimental effect on the effectiveness of the vaccine. Our present experience with intravesical administration of BCG suggests that the routine use of prophylactic isoniazid or an alternative antituberculous medication is not necessary, but such treatment is mandatory in the presence of severe reactions.

The endoscopic appearance of the bladder epithelium may be deceptive following BCG therapy. A reddened, velvety mucosa may represent a severe inflammatory reaction or, alternatively, carcinoma in situ. On the other hand, we have observed raised mucosal lesions highly suggestive of tumor recurrence (Figure 2) that on histologic examination proved to be granulomatous inflammation (Figure 3).

Adequate biopsy specimens during follow-up cystoscopic examinations are particularly important, since they provide objective evidence of response to treatment. Tissue samples obtained with cold-cup forceps were superior for this purpose.

The histologic picture of biopsy specimens from patients treated with BCG frequently disclosed marked inflammatory infiltrates and granulomatous reaction, as shown in Figures 3 and 4. Similar findings have been observed in experimental animal tumors treated with BCG (Hanna et al. 1973, Bloomberg et al. 1975), although the intracavitary instillation of the vaccine has failed to produce inflammatory reactions in the intact bladder.

The experimental studies of Coe and Feldman (1966) showed that delayed hypersensitivity reactions can be induced in the bladders of immunized hosts. These reactions can be produced clinically by the intravesical and intradermal administration of a vaccine in the presence of a disrupted vesical epithelium; therefore, instillations of the vaccine should be started within a few days of the endoscopic procedure and the resulting mucosal disruption. This presumably would facilitate localization of the bacterial antigens in the bladder and promote the inflammatory reaction detrimental to the tumor. Similar results may be obtained, in the presence of an intact urothelium, by the direct intratumoral

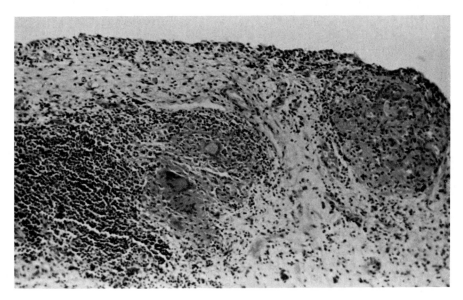

Figure 3. Histologic appearance of biopsy specimen from bladder seen in Figure 2. Note the marked inflammatory reaction with formation of granulomas.

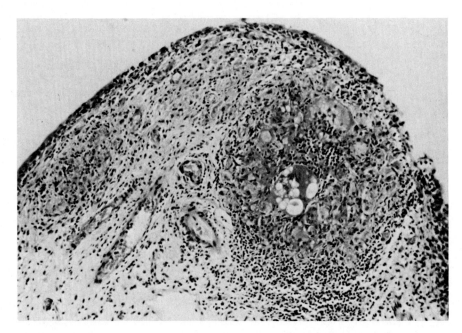

Figure 4. Characteristic granulomatous reaction in bladder following BCG treatment.

injection of BCG. DeKernion et al. (1975) reported the successful destruction of a vesical melanoma after a single intratumoral injection of BCG induced an active inflammatory granulomatous reaction; the patient had been previously immunized with BCG.

In this trial, age appeared to be a possible determinant of treatment success. The 16 subjects who showed complete or partial response to treatment were significantly older, on the average ($p < 0.05$), than the four for whom the vaccine proved ineffective. Definitive answers on the role of age as a prognostic variable will require a larger patient population. No other factor emerged as a predictor of therapeutic success. Intradermal response to tuberculin was positive in three patients prior to treatment, two of whom have remained tumor free, while the third showed an early recurrence. Systemic and local reaction to the vaccine appeared to have no bearing on the therapeutic response; the four patients who experienced more severe effects varied considerably in their treatment outcomes. Two patients remained tumor free, while the other two did not complete the regimen as their reactions warranted cessation of treatment. One of the latter two showed some improvement nonetheless, while in the other the pattern of recurrences was unchanged. This lack of therapeutic response may have been a consequence of incomplete treatment.

In vitro evaluation and monitoring of immune responsiveness in cancer patients, particularly those receiving immunotherapy, is of undeniable relevance (Weese et al. 1977), but the value of currently available techniques is the subject of increasing controversy (Bean 1977, Catalona et al. 1977, Morales and Eidinger 1976). We are investigating the effect of BCG on natural cytotoxic reactivity to monitor and predict clinical response to treatment. Experimental studies indicate that this may be a relevant mechanism of action for some forms of immunotherapy (Wolfe et al. 1976, Herberman et al. 1977), and recent human studies support this possibility (Saal et al. 1977, Morales et al. 1977).

This study was designed to investigate the role of BCG as an adjuvant to surgery in the prevention of tumor recurrences; the effect of the vaccine alone on the destruction of superficial tumors is presently under study. In the report of Douville et al. (1978), who employed a protocol similar to ours, evidence of tumor remission was found. The significance of this observation is evident because immunotherapy may provide an avenue for treatment of extensive superficial lesions not amenable to endoscopic resection and of "flat" carcinoma in situ of the bladder.

Although several trials are now in progress to determine the role of BCG in early and advanced bladder cancer, excluding our own (Morales et al. 1976), we are aware only of the published results of Fraley et al. (1976), who have documented response to therapy in at least one patient with metastatic disease. We have used BCG to treat a small number of patients with metastatic transitional cell carcinoma (unpublished observations), with the primary object of defining the parameters of toxicity and establishing whether toxicity was predictable, reversible, or both (phase I trial). Notwithstanding the lack of objective response in this group of seven patients, the vaccine was considered safe for further use in the prevention of recurrence and in the treatment of existing superficial bladder neoplasms. The results presented here, essentially a phase II investigation, permit a reasonable judgement on the degree of efficacy and nature of adverse effects of BCG in a particular dose and form of administration. Definitive answers on the ultimate value of BCG in both the prevention and treatment of bladder cancer require a larger-scale phase III trial.

ACKNOWLEDGMENT

This project was supported in part by the Ontario Cancer Foundation, grant 292.

REFERENCES

Banks, N. D., J. E. Pontes, R. M. Izbicki, and J. M. Pierce, Jr. 1977. Topical instillation of doxorubicin hydrochloride in the treatment of recurrent superficial transitional cell carcinoma of the bladder. J. Urol. 118:757–760.

Bean, M. A. 1977. Some immunological considerations relevant to the study of human bladder cancer. Cancer Res. 37:2879–2884.

Bloomberg, S. D., S. A. Brossman, M. S. Haussman, A. Cohen, and J. D. Battenberg. 1975. The effects of BCG on dog bladder. Invest. Urol. 12:423–427.

Bracken, R. B., D. E. Johnson, L. Rodriguez, M. L. Samuels, and A. Ayala. 1977. Treatment of multiple superficial tumors of bladder with intravesical bleomycin. Urology 9:161–163.

Catalona, W. J., R. K. Oldham, R. B. Herberman, J. Djeu, and G. B. Cannon. 1977. Lack of specificity of lymphocyte-mediated cytotoxicity against the bladder cancer cell line T-24. J. Urol. 118:254–257.

Coe, J. E., and J. D. Feldman. 1966. Extracutaneous delayed hypersensitivity particularly in the guinea pig bladder. Immunology 10:127–135.

DeKernion, J. B., S. H. Golub, R. K. Gupta, M. Silverstein, and D. L. Morton. 1975. Successful transurethral intralesional BCG therapy of bladder melanoma. Cancer 36:1662–1667.

Douville, Y., R. Roy, R. Charrois, A. Kibrite, M. Martin, L. Dionne, L. Coulonval, and J. Robinson. 1978. Recurrent bladder papillomata treated with bacillus Calmette-Guerin: A preliminary report (Phase I trial). Cancer Treat. Rep. 62:551–552.

Eilber, F. R., D. F. Morton, E. C. Holmes, F. C. Sparks, and K. P. Ramming. 1975. Adjuvant immunotherapy with BCG in the treatment of regional lymph node metastases from malignant melanoma. N. Engl. J. Med. 294:237–240.

Fraley, E. E., P. H. Lange, and T. R. Hakala. 1976. Recent studies on the immunobiology and virology of human urothelial tumors. Urol. Clin. North Am. 3:31–49.

Hanna, M. G., M. J. Snodgrass, B. Zbar, and H. J. Rapp. 1973. Histological and ultrastructural studies of tumor regression in inbred guinea pigs after intralesional injection of *Mycobacterium bovis* (BCG). Natl. Cancer Inst. Mongr. 39:71–85.

Herberman, R. B., M. E. Nunn, H. T. Holden, S. Staal, and J. Y. Djeu. 1977. Augmentation of natural cytotoxic reactivity of mouse lymphoid cells against syngeneic and allogeneic target cells. Int. J. Cancer 19:555–563.

Johnston, J. 1972. Econometric Methods. 2nd ed. McGraw-Hill Book Co., New York.

Jones, H. D., and J. Swinney. 1961. Thiotepa in the treatment of tumors of the bladder. Lancet 2:615–617.

McKneally, M. F., C. M. Maver, and H. W. Kausel. 1978. Regional immunotherapy of lung cancer using post-operative intrapleural BCG, *in* Immunotherapy of Cancer: Present Status of Trials in Man. W. D. Terry and D. Windhorst, eds. Raven Press, New York, pp. 161–171.

Morales, A., G. D. Bonnard, J. H. Dean, and R. B. Herberman. 1977. In vitro augmentation of the NK and K cell activities by co-cultivation with mumps virus. Fed. Proc. 36:1325.

Morales, A., and D. Eidinger. 1976. Immune reactivity in renal cancer: A sequential study. J. Urol. 115:510–513.

Morales, A., D. Eidinger, and A. W. Bruce. 1976. Intracavitary bacillus Calmette-Guerin in the treatment of superficial bladder tumors. J. Urol. 116:180–183.

Nieh, P. T., J. J. Daly, N. M. Heaney, and G. R. Prout. 1978. The effect of intravesical thio-tepa on normal and tumor urothelium. J. Urol. 119:59–61.

Ott, L. 1977. An Introduction to Statistical Methods and Data Analysis. Duxbury Press, Boston, 654 pp. See especially pp. 384–388.

Robinson, M. R. G., M. B. Shetty, B. Richards, J. Bastable, R. W. Glashan, and P. H. Smith. 1977. Intravesical epodyl in the management of bladder tumors. J. Urol. 118:972–973.

Saal, J. G., G. Riethmuller, E. P. Eiber, M. Hadam, H. Ehinger, and W. Schneider. 1977. Regional BCG therapy of malignant melanoma: In vitro monitoring of spontaneous cytolytic activity of circulating lymphocytes. Cancer Immunol. Immunother. 3:27–33.

Sokal, R. R., and F. J. Rohlf. 1969. Biometry—The Principles and Practice of Statistics in Biological Research. W. H. Freeman & Co., San Francisco, pp. 613–616.

Sparks, F. C., M. J. Silverstein, J. S. Hunt, C. M. Haskell, Y. H. Pilch, and D. L. Morton. 1973. Complications of BCG immunotherapy in patients with cancer. N. Engl. J. Med. 289:827–830.

Veenema, R. J., A. L. Dean, Jr., M. Roberts, B. Fingerhut, B. K. Chewry, and H. Tarasally. 1962. Bladder carcinoma treated by direct instillation of thio-tepa. J. Urol. 88:60–63.

Veenema, R. J., A. L. Dean, Jr., A. C. Uson, M. Roberts, and F. Longo. 1969. Thiotepa bladder instillations: Therapy and prophylaxis for superficial bladder tumors. J. Urol. 101:711–715.

Weese, J. L., R. K. Oldham, D. C. Tormey, A. Morales, M. H. Cohen, T. C. Alford, P. E. Shorb, N. T. Tsangaris, W. H. West, G. B. Cannon, J. H. Dean, H. Djeu, J. L. McCoy, and R. B. Herberman. 1977. Immunological monitoring in carcinoma of the breast. Surg. Gynecol. Obstet. 145:209–218.

Wolfe, S. A., D. E. Tracey, and C. S. Henney. 1976. Induction of "natural killer cells" by BCG. Nature 262:584.

Zbar, B., and H. J. Rapp. 1974. Immunotherapy of guinea pig cancer with BCG. Cancer 34:1532–1540.

TESTICULAR CARCINOMA

Cancer of the Genitourinary Tract, edited by
D. E. Johnson and M. L. Samuels.
Raven Press, New York © 1979.

Surgical Treatment of Nonseminomatous Germinal Testis Tumors

William J. Staubitz, M.D.

Department of Urology, Veterans Administration Hospital and State University of New York at Buffalo School of Medicine, Buffalo, New York

In 1958, in an effort to evaluate the efficacy of lymphadenectomy and to improve survival in patients with nonseminomatous testis tumors, a prospective study was established (Staubitz et al., 1959). All patients with stage I or II tumors were to be treated, following radical orchiectomy, by transabdominal bilateral retroperitoneal lymphadenectomy. None was to receive pre- or postoperative irradiation. The guidelines established for this study did not vary until its completion in 1970. Preoperative evaluation included history and physical examination, chest tomograms, intravenous pyelograms, venacavagrams, and bilateral pedal lymphangiograms. If clinical or radiographic evidence of disease outside the retroperitoneum existed (stage III), lymphadenectomy was not attempted.

MATERIALS AND METHODS

Surgical Technique

Our surgical approach is based on the fundamental knowledge of testicular lymphatic drainage acquired by Jamiesen and Dobson (1910). Their work, recently confirmed by Sayegh et al. (1966) and Chiappa et al. (1966), shows the primary node receptacles are near L-2 on the left and are usually located between L-1 and L-3 on the right. They have further shown that crossover drainage does occur, usually from right to left. Furthermore, retrograde filling of para-aortic nodes has been documented. In view of this complex and sometimes unpredictable lymphatic network, our aim is to remove all accessible lymph node-bearing tissue en bloc in the retroperitoneum.

A vertical xyphoid-to-pubis midline incision is made. Upon entering the abdominal cavity, we undertake a thorough search for metastatic disease. If distant organs are involved, no dissection is attempted, as is the case if suspicious lymph nodes above the renal hilum are shown to contain metastatic tumor by frozen section examination.

If no metastatic disease is evident cephalad to the renal pedicles, mobilization of the right colon and small bowel is begun. The right lateral peritoneal reflection is incised and the ascending colon and cecum are mobilized. Subsequently, the parietal peritoneum of the small bowel mesentery is incised to Treitz's ligament. The entire small intestine and right colon then can be eviscerated, exposing the retroperitoneum and major vessels. Dissection is begun at the level of the renal pedicles. Care is taken to remove all lymphatic and areolar tissue in the lateral pockets, which are bounded by the vena cava or aorta, the renal pelvis, and the posterior abdominal wall.

The major vessels are circumferentially dissected clean. The spermatic arteries and veins are bilaterally included in the dissection. Both ureters are identified, tagged, and closely observed throughout the procedure; they mark the lateral boundaries of dissection. The en bloc removal is then continued inferiorly, with all nodal tissue behind and between the great vessels removed, allowing the aorta and vena cava to be lifted from their beds anchored only by the major lumbar tributaries. The inferior mesenteric artery is routinely sacrificed, with no adverse effects noted to date. Dissection is carried distally to the bifurcation of the iliac vessels on the uninvolved side and to the internal ring on the ipsilateral side. If any segment of spermatic cord was left behind during the previous orchiectomy, it is removed.

At the end of the procedure, all lymphatic and areolar tissue has been removed from the area bordered proximally by and including the renal pedicles, laterally by the course of the ureters, and distally by the bifurcation of the iliac vessels and/or the internal ring on the involved side. An x-ray photograph of the operative field is then taken. If, according to the previously obtained lymphangiogram, opacified nodes remain at the site of dissection, they are searched for and removed.

After the dissection is completed, the mobilized duodenum, small bowel, and colon are replaced in their original positions and sutured to the parietal peritoneum, and a routine appendectomy is performed. The wound is closed in layers by means of retention sutures.

Complications

In the 65 patients treated, complications occurred in eight, or 12%. There was one case each of severe wound infection, postoperative hemorrhage (reexplored and controlled), ureteropelvic junction obstruction due to periureteral fibrosis (relieved by lysis one year later), wound dehiscence, ventral hernia (repaired successfully one year later), renal pedicle accident (requiring intraoperative nephrectomy), and massive gastrointestinal bleeding on the fifth operative day. The last patient died, and an autopsy revealed multiple gastrointestinal ulcerations.

Absence of ejaculation occurred in most patients, although incomplete recording of preoperative and postoperative sexual histories precluded accurate documentation of the precise incidence. In those patients who experienced failure

Table 1. *Results With Stage I Nonseminomatous Testis Tumors*

Histology of Tumor	No. of Patients	3-Year Survival		5-Year Survival	
		No.	(%)	No.	(%)
Embryonal cell carcinoma	28	26/28	(93%)	20/23	(87%)
Teratocarcinoma	11	11/11	(100%)	7/8	(87%)
Teratocarcinoma + embryonal cell carcinoma	4	4/4	(100%)	3/3	(100%)
Embryonal cell carcinoma + choriocarcinoma	2	1/2	(50%)	1/2	(50%)
Total	45	42/45	(93%)	31/36	(86%)

to ejaculate, no adverse social or psychological reactions have become manifest to date.

RESULTS

The results with 72 patients explored during the period from 1958 to 1970 are presented. In seven of these disease extended above the renal pedicle and was unresectable. Each received chemotherapy consisting of actinomycin D alone or in combination with Cytoxan and methotrexate; three received irradiation as well. Six died within one year and the last died of disease within five years.

The results obtained in the 65 patients whose tumors were resectable are shown in Tables 1 and 2. As shown in the tables, 30% of these patients had metastatic tumors in the retroperitoneal nodes and thus had stage II disease; 75% have survived three years, while 71% have survived five years or more. In stage I patients, 93% have lived three years and 86% have lived five or more years.

Table 2. *Results With Stage II Nonseminomatous Testis Tumors*

Histology of Tumor	No. of Patients	3-Year Survival		5-Year Survival	
		No.	(%)	No.	(%)
Embryonal cell carcinoma	14	12/14	(86%)	10/12	(83%)
Teratocarcinoma + embryonal cell carcinoma	1	0/1	(0%)	0/1	(0%)
Teratocarcinoma + choriocarcinoma	2	1/2	(50%)	1/2	(50%)
Embryonal cell carcinoma + choriocarcinoma	3	2/3	(67%)	1/2	(50%)
Total	20	15/20	(75%)	12/17	(71%)

DISCUSSION

An area of concern in treating patients with nonseminomatous germinal testis tumors is which surgical approach to use. Should one employ a unilateral dissection, using the thoracoabdominal approach, or a bilateral dissection, using the transabdominal route? Recent reports (Maier et al. 1969, Skinner and Leadbetter 1971, Walsh et al. 1971) favor a unilateral approach, arguing that bilateral metastatic node involvement is rare. Our experience does not support this. In the present series of 65 patients undergoing a bilateral retroperitoneal lymphadenectomy, 9% had bilateral involvement, but more important, over 30% of the stage II patients had bilateral extension of metastatic disease. This supports the work of Jamiesen and Dobson (1910), who demonstrated the crossover of the lymphatic system draining the testes. Since one third of stage II patients have this degree of node involvement, unilateral dissection seems inadequate, regardless of the route used.

Those favoring the unilateral route point out that it results in a much lower incidence of failure to ejaculate, whereas after bilateral dissection, in which the surgery is much more extensive, absence of ejaculation is common because the sympathetic nerve chain is more frequently disturbed. However, when dealing with a highly malignant disease in a young individual, we believe that all efforts must be directed toward achieving a cure and that disturbances of nonfatal physiologic functions may be necessary to attain the best survival rate. A more thorough dissection increases the likelihood of removing all tumor, as our survival figures indicate.

CONCLUSION

This experience with patients with stage II nonseminomatous testis tumors clearly demonstrates that surgery can be used as a primary treatment to control 70% of patients with retroperitoneal lymph node metastases. This surgical technique is, therefore, recommended as primary therapy in patients with stage I and II disease.

REFERENCES

Chiappa, S., C. Uslenghi, G. Bonadonna, P. Marano, and G. Ravasi. 1966. Combined testicular and foot lymphangiography in testicular carcinomas. Surg. Gynecol. Obstet. 123:10–14.

Jamiesen, J. K., and J. F. Dobson. 1910. The lymphatics of the testicle. Lancet 1:493–495.

Maier, J. G., K. E. van Buskirk, M. H. Sulak, R. H. Perry, and D. T. Schamber. 1969. An evaluation of lymphadenectomy in the treatment of malignant testicular germ cell neoplasms. J. Urol. 101:356–359.

Sayegh, E., T. Brooks, E. Sacher, and F. Busch. 1966. Lymphangiography of retroperitoneal lymph nodes. J. Urol. 95:102–107.

Skinner, D. G., and W. F. Leadbetter. 1971. The surgical management of testis tumors. J. Urol. 106:84–93.

Staubitz, W. J., I. V. Magoss, M. H. Lent, E. M. Sigman, and J. T. Grace. 1959. Surgical management of testicular tumors. N.Y. State J. Med. 59:3959–3963.

Walsh, P. C., J. J. Kaufman, W. F. Coulson, and W. E. Goodwin. 1971. Retroperitoneal lymphadenectomy for testicular tumors. J.A.M.A. 217:309–312.

Cancer of the Genitourinary Tract, edited by
D. E. Johnson and M. L. Samuels.
Raven Press, New York © 1979.

Testis Carcinoma: What Role Radiotherapy?

John G. Maier, M.D., Ph.D.

*Department of Radiation Oncology, Fairfax Hospital, Falls Church, Virginia, and
Department of Radiology, George Washington University School of Medicine,
Washington, D.C.*

In the U.S. today, a patient presenting with clinical stage I or II carcinoma of the testis will most likely be treated by an ipsilateral inguinal orchiectomy, a bilateral retroperitoneal lymphadenectomy, and chemotherapy if the resected lymph nodes contain metastatic disease. This presentation will analyze the appropriateness of such treatment and suggest an alternative for stage I disease.

PATHOLOGY

A histologic classification of germ cell tumors of the testis has evolved from that established by Dixon and Moore (1952, 1953). The emphasis today is on listing the actual tumor types seen in the primary orchiectomy specimen. The World Health Organization and the Armed Forces Institute of Pathology (AFIP) (Mostofi and Price 1973) have agreed upon the following classification:

1. Seminoma—classical, anaplastic, spermatocytic;
2. Embryonal carcinoma—adult, infantile (yolk sac), polyembryoma;
3. Teratoma—mature, immature;
4. Teratocarcinoma—teratoma and embryonal carcinoma; and
5. Choriocarcinoma.

While each of the above histologic varieties may occur as a single cell line (in 60% of cases in AFIP series), they also may occur in combination with other varieties. When a pure seminoma is found in the primary lesion, it invariably remains a single cell line if metastases occur. This is not true of the other four types, which may metastasize as the same or another variety or several in combination. Unfortunately, most reported series include all categories, exclusive of seminoma, within the broad single category of carcinoma. This is done partly for convenience, but primarily because of a lack of adequate numbers of patients with this rather rare tumor. There simply are not enough patients in the various subtypes for valid comparisons of treatment modalities. Therein lies a major dilemma that is often overlooked. In a small series, an unusual weighting of a particular cell type could bias results radically.

CLINICAL DIAGNOSTIC STUDIES

Accuracy of staging of testis tumor patients has improved in recent years, and the significant impact this has had on selection of treatment must be considered. Recommended diagnostic studies include chest x-ray exam, whole lung tomogram, excretory urogram, lymphangiogram, computerized tomographic body scan, serum beta human chorionic gonadotropin (HCG), urine HCG, serum alpha-fetoprotein, complete blood count, routine urinalysis, liver chemistries, and blood urea nitrogen.

Assessment of paraaortic lymph node metastases by lymphangiography became possible in most institutions approximately 15 years ago. Several reports have demonstrated an accuracy rate of approximately 75% (Maier and Schamber 1972). The highest error rate occurs in patients in whom no metastatic disease can be identified radiographically in the paraaortic region, but who do have occult microscopic disease. This may include as many as 30% of patients, but the error rate may be reduced by using abdominal tomography in conjunction with lymphangiography. More recently, abdominal computerized tomography has offered further improvement in accuracy of diagnosis.

With the development of radioimmunoassay techniques, two tests for tumor markers in testis tumor patients have been exceedingly helpful. These are the serum beta human chorionic gonadotropin (β-HCG) and serum alpha-fetoprotein. These tumor markers may be elevated from the primary testis tumor alone. It is advisable to have both preorchiectomy and postorchiectomy studies. If a positive titer persists after orchiectomy, metastatic disease is invariably present. On the other hand, a negative titer is no guarantee that metastatic disease is not present. Much more information is needed to know how often metastatic disease is present in the face of negative markers. Although radioimmunoassays of serum levels are about 200 times more sensitive than previous urinary assays, the false-negative incidence is not known.

STAGING

Following histologic classification and clinical diagnostic studies, it is essential to *clinically* stage each patient if treatment modalities are to be compared. Too often a pathologic staging is based on the findings at lymphadenectomy. If primary irradiation is employed following orchiectomy, a comparison with surgical series staged by histologic examination of the nodes is impossible. A comparison of the Walter Reed Hospital staging system (Maier and Sulak 1973) and the UICC system (1968) is shown in Table 1. The 1977 American Joint Committee system (Manual for Staging of Cancer 1977) is yet another system. None of these systems allows for positive tumor markers or use of computerized tomographic body scans as yet.

The staging system used at Walter Reed Hospital combines clinical, radiologic, and surgicopathologic findings. Clinical stage I indicates tumor confined to the

Table 1. *Staging Systems of Walter Reed General Hospital and the UICC*

Walter Reed System	UICC System
Stage IA—Tumor confined to one testis; no clinical or roentgenographic evidence of spread beyond; testing may include excretory or retrograde urogram, lymphangiogram, inferior venacavogram, and chest roentgenogram.	T_0—No evidence of primary tumor.
	T_1—Tumor occupying less than half of the testis and surrounded by palpably normal gland.
	T_2—Tumor occupying half or more of the testis, but not producing enlargement or deformity of the testis.
Stage IB—Same as in stage IA, but with histologic evidence of metastases to iliac or paraaortic lymph nodes at time of retroperitoneal lymph node dissection.	T_3—Tumor confined to the testis, but producing enlargement or deformity of the testis.
Stage II—Clinical or roentgenographic evidence of metastases to femoral, inguinal, iliac, or paraaortic lymph nodes; no demonstrable metastases above the diaphragm or to visceral organs.	NO—No deformity of regional nodes on lymphogram.
	NX^+—When it is impossible to assess the regional nodes, the symbol NX is used, permitting eventual addition of histologic information; thus, NX^+ or NX^-.
Stage III—Clinical or roentgenographic evidence of metastases above the diaphragm or other distant metastases to body organs.	T_4—Tumor extending to the epididymis or beyond the testis, to epididymis only, or to other structures.
	N_1—Regional nodes deformed on lymphogram.
	N_2—Fixed, palpable abdominal nodes.
	M_1—Distant metastases present including lymph nodes outside the abdomen.

From Maier, Sulak, and Mittemeyer (1968) and UICC (1968).

testis. It is subdivided into IA and IB when the patient undergoes retroperitoneal lymphadenectomy. In this system, IA indicates the absence of microscopic metastases in the lymph nodes below the diaphragm and IB indicates the presence of microscopic metastases. This system was the first attempt to correlate clinical and surgicopathologic staging and to allow some comparison between the results of radiation and surgical treatment.

TREATMENT

Until the advent of effective multiagent chemotherapy for testis carcinoma, patients with clinical stage I or II disease had been treated by one of three methods over the last 25 years. All three methods are preceded by an inguinal orchiectomy. The three include:

1. Primary irradiation to drainage lymphatics of testis;
2. Retroperitoneal lymphadenectomy, followed by postoperative irradiation when nodes contain metastatic disease;
3. So-called sandwich technique, with preoperative irradiation to drainage lymphatics of testis below the diaphragm, followed by retroperitoneal lymphadenectomy and postoperative irradiation.

A summary of contemporary reports of these three treatment methods in the last 10 years has been reported previously (Maier and Lee 1977) and is shown in Tables 2–4. These reports were selected because they represented the largest series available during this period and because lymphangiography had been performed for clinical staging in patients undergoing primary irradiation or "sandwich therapy." In the surgical series, paraaortic nodal evaluation

Table 2. *Results of Primary Treatment With Radiotherapy Following Orchiectomy**

Report	Stage I Disease Patients NED at 3–5 Years (%)	Stage II Disease Patients NED at 3–5 Years (%)
Van der Werf-Messing (1976)	26/29 (90%)	16/35 (46%)
Peckham and McElwain (1974, 1975)	66/78 (85%)	17/29 (59%)
Batterman et al. (1973)	21/30 (70%)	5/19 (26%)
Maier and Mittemeyer (1977)	25/29 (86%)	9/11 (82%)
Total	138/166 (83%)	47/94 (50%)

* Stages I and II combined: 185/260 (71%).

Table 3. *Results of Primary Treatment With Lymphadenectomy and Postoperative Radiotherapy**

Report	Stage I Disease Patients NED at 3–5 Years (%)	Stage II Disease Patients NED at 3–5 Years (%)
Whitmore (1970)	184/204 (90%)	78/159 (49%)
Walsh et al. (1971)	41/44 (93%)	12/20 (60%)
Bradfield et al. (1973)	28/40 (70%)	11/34 (32%)
Skinner and Leadbetter (1971)	27/30 (90%)	15/27 (56%)
Maier and Sulak (1973)	80/109 (73%)	44/97 (45%)
Staubitz et al. (1969)	15/17 (88%)	7/8 (88%)
Hussey et al. (1977)	97/124 (78%)	24/62 (39%)
Total	472/568 (83%)	191/407 (47%)

* Stages I and II combined: 663/975 (68%).

Table 4. *Results of "Sandwich Techniques"; Preoperative and Postoperative Irradiation**

Report	Stage I Disease Patients NED at 3–5 Years (%)	Stage II Disease Patients NED at 3–5 Years (%)
Nicholson et al. (1974)	23/27 (85%)	6/9 (67%)
Earle et al. (1973)	12/12 (100%)	9/20 (45%)
Hussey et al. (1977)	4/5 (80%)	17/25 (68%)
Quivey et al. (1977)	7/7 (100%)	3/4 (75%)
Maier and Mittemeyer (1977)	29/30 (97%)	17/21 (81%)
Total	75/81 (93%)	52/79 (66%)

* Stages I and II combined: 127/160 (79%).

Table 5. *Walter Reed Hospital Testis Carcinoma Trial: Three-Years NED Rate*

Regimen	Stage I Patients (%)	Stage II Patients (%)	Total (%)
Orchiectomy + radiation	25/29 (86%)	9/11 (82%)	34/40 (85%)
Orchiectomy, lymphadenectomy, and radiation	29/30 (97%)	17/21 (81%)	46/51 (90%)
Total	54/59 (92%)	26/32 (81%)	80/91 (88%)

was available from the resected nodes examined histologically, but lymphangiograms were not available prior to surgery in most cases.

It is interesting that the results obtained by methods 1 and 2 are quite similar. Unfortunately, there have been very few randomized prospective studies comparing different treatment methods. In one study, summarized in Table 5 (Maier and Mittemeyer 1977), results with orchiectomy and irradiation were compared to those with orchiectomy, lymphadenectomy, and irradiation. A later paper in this symposium (pp. 149–158) will analyze such treatment in more detail.

DISCUSSION

When an inguinal orchiectomy followed by primary irradiation to the drainage lymphatics is performed for stage I carcinoma of the testis, a cure rate of 85–90% is obtained. Unfortunately, the results for stage II have been only about 50%. There seems to be little question that primary irradiation alone for stage II disease is not satisfactory. Considerable variation exists in the size of lymph node metastases in stage II disease, and while a small mass of tumor metastases in the paraaortic lymph nodes should respond to radiotherapy better than a large one, there are few published data on this point.

Tyrrell and Peckham (Peckham and McElwain 1974, 1975, Tyrrell and Peckham 1976) have examined the relationship between radiation response of carcinomas in the retroperitoneal lymph nodes and tumor volume. These authors found good local control of tumor deposits less than 2 cm in diameter. Twelve of 14 patients with such deposits were alive from 2½ to more than 11 years after irradiation, although one patient had needed chemotherapy for pulmonary metastases and another had undergone a retroperitoneal lymphadenectomy. However, of the 15 patients who had bulky metastases (more than 2 cm in diameter), only five were living without evidence of disease 3½ years or longer after irradiation, and three of these five had had lymphadenectomies. Tyrrell and Peckham suggest that small tumor deposits are well vascularized and thus fully oxygenated, which could make them relatively radiosensitive. Bulky deposits, on the other hand, are likely to contain necrotic areas associated with hypoxic cells and thus would be less radiosensitive.

The next logical question is, how effective is radiotherapy in controlling micrometastases? Obviously, such information is available only indirectly. Of patients with apparent stage I disease, 15–25% can be expected to have occult retroperitoneal metastases. In the Walter Reed Hospital series (Maier and Mittemeyer 1977), 24 patients had adequate preoperative lymphangiograms that were interpreted as normal. However, metastatic disease in the lymph nodes was found in six patients (25%) undergoing bilateral retroperitoneal lymphadenectomy.

Tyrrell and Peckham treated 85 patients with apparent stage I disease by primary irradiation. Only four patients (4.7%) had a recurrence in the irradiated tissue. Of the 29 patients treated in the Walter Reed series (Maier and Mittemeyer 1977) by primary irradiation for stage I disease, four failed treatment. All four failures were due to lung metastases without evidence of retroperitoneal recurrence. Lung metastases may have been present at the time of initial diagnosis but unrecognized. Urinary β-HCG studies on these four patients were initially negative, but serum radioimmunoassay studies were not performed.

It would appear from the data available that the results in stage I testis carcinoma patients treated primarily by irradiation are comparable to those in patients treated by retroperitoneal lymphadenectomy. If this is true, then the next logical question is, what are the incidence and nature of complications from each of these modalities of treatment?

Data on the incidence and types of injury from various doses of radiotherapy became available as early as 1950. As is well known, the higher the tissue dose, the greater the incidence and severity of injury. The small intestine appears to be at greatest risk in primary irradiation to the drainage lymph nodes below the diaphragm. Ulceration, perforation, and obstruction may occur if the dose exceeds 5,000 to 5,500 rads in five to six weeks. The series described above employed 4,500 to 5,000 rads and small intestinal complications were at a minimum.

When long segments of the spinal cord are irradiated, the limit of tolerance is about 4,000 rads in four weeks, while short segments may tolerate as much as 5,000 rads in five weeks. The spinal cord appears to be most sensitive to irradiation at about the level of the 10th thoracic vertebra, where its blood supply is weakest. For stage I disease, elective irradiations to the mediastinum and left supraclavicular regions is not presently recommended. The top of the radiation portal is located at the level of the diaphragm, at about the 11th thoracic vertebra.

Hematopoietic depression with such radiotherapy is mild and includes transient leukopenia and thrombocytopenia. It is seldom a limiting factor. According to Golbey (1976), prior irradiation is not a limiting factor in the Velban-actinomycin-bleomycin (VAB) IV chemotherapy program at Memorial Sloan-Kettering Cancer Center. Also, the response of tumor to subsequent chemotherapy is the same regardless of whether or not radiotherapy has been administered previously.

The complications following retroperitoneal lymphadenectomy are not well documented. The most distressing morbidity associated with a bilateral retroperitoneal lymphadenectomy is aspermia. This does not appear to be a result of retrograde ejaculation, but of the lack of ductus deferens peristalsis and of seminal vesicle contractions secondary to sympathectomy. Sexual function is otherwise intact, with patients able to have the sensation of orgasm but with a dry ejaculate.

Some authors have advocated less than a bilateral lymphadenectomy. However, the lymph nodes that are the primary retroperitoneal landing sites for these tumors are those located between the aorta and inferior vena cava, just distal to the renal vessels. These nodes are in a direct line of lymphatic flow from the spermatic cord and therefore are the primary lymphatic drainage fields for these cancers. If a satisfactory surgical margin around these nodes is to be obtained, a bilateral dissection is necessary. Thus, the surgery normally is carried out from the level of the renal vessels to the bifurcation of the aorta.

In an effort to prevent aspermia, Ray and co-workers (1974) limited the resection on the contralateral side to above the level of the inferior mesenteric artery. However, this did not prevent aspermia in most instances. Preservation of preoperative semen specimens may be one solution to this problem. However, storage techniques now available cannot guarantee long-term survival of viable sperm. Furthermore, the genetic consequences of storing sperm in this manner are uncertain.

In these days of cost-consciousness, another factor to be considered is the relative costs of primary irradiation and lymphadenectomy. Primary irradiation can be given on an outpatient basis and in almost all instances the patient can continue to be employed in his usual occupation. Patients undergoing lymphadenectomy are usually hospitalized seven to 10 days and then undergo a period of convalescence before returning to work. When the surgical fee, hospitalization expenses, and anesthesiology fee are taken into consideration, the overall cost of lymphadenectomy is approximately three times that of radiotherapy.

One main reason promulgated by lymphadenectomy enthusiasts for lymphadenectomy is the definite determination of the presence of lymph node metastases, their number and size. The presence of positive metastases is considered an indication for sequential elective chemotherapy. However, very little survival data are available thus far for such treatment. Perhaps the largest series was that reported recently by Vugrin et al. (1978), in which 60 pathologic stage II testis carcinoma patients underwent retroperitoneal lymphadenectomy and elective chemotherapy with the reduced VAB IV regimen. There were 11 failures, for an 82% NED rate. The group was broken down into subgroups on the basis of size of tumor and number of involved nodes, with median follow-up times of 10 and 17 months. Some of those with more advanced disease received postoperative irradiation. While combined modality treatment is described elsewhere in this monograph (pp. 149–158), the early results with lymphadenectomy and postoperative chemotherapy have not proven superior to the "sandwich technique" of pre- and postoperative irradiation combined with lymphadenectomy.

SUMMARY

A review of the three treatment methods formerly used for stage I and II testis carcinoma revealed that primary radiotherapy following inguinal orchiectomy remains a viable alternative for stage I testis carcinoma patients. Its cure rates are comparable to those for retroperitoneal lymphadenectomy. No hospitalization is required for patients treated by radiotherapy, and patients remain fertile. The present cost for radiotherapy is approximately one-third that for lymphadenectomy. Less than 5% of treatment failures occur in the paraaortic lymph node areas following primary irradiation. Multiagent chemotherapy, including the VAB IV program, is not precluded by primary radiotherapy and can be quite successful should disease recur.

REFERENCES

Batterman, J. J., J. F. M. Delemarre, A. A. M. Hart, E. A. van Slooten, and A. H. Tierie. 1973. Testicular tumors: A retrospective study. Arch. Chir. Neerl. 25:457–469.

Bradfield, J. S., R. U. Hagen, and D. O. Ytredal. 1973. Carcinoma of the testis: An analysis of 104 patients with germinal tumors of the testis other than seminoma. Cancer 31:633–640.

Dixon, F. J., and R. A. Moore. 1952. Atlas of Tumor Pathology. Sec. VIII, Fasc. 31b and 32. Tumors of the Male Sex Organs. Armed Forces Institute of Pathology, Washington, D.C.

Dixon, F. J., and R. A. Moore. 1953. Testicular tumors: A clinicopathological study. Cancer 6:427–454.

Earle, J. D., M. A. Bagshaw, and H. S. Kaplan. 1973. Supervoltage radiation therapy of the testicular tumors. Am. J. Roentgenol. Rad. Ther. Nucl. Med. 117:653–661.

Golbey, R. 1976. Testicular Tumor Conference: Cooperative Studies Discussion Groups. National Cancer Institute, Washington, D.C.

Hussey, D. H., K. H. Luk, and D. E. Johnson. 1977. The role of radiation therapy in the treatment of germinal cell tumors of the testes other than pure seminomas. Radiology 123:175–180.

Maier, J. G., and S. N. Lee. 1977. Radiation therapy for nonseminomatous germ cell testicular cancer in adults. Urol. Clin. North Am. 4:477–493.

Maier, J. G., and B. T. Mittemeyer. 1977. Carcinoma of the testis. Cancer 39:981–986.

Maier, J. G., and D. T. Schamber. 1972. The role of lymphangiography in the diagnosis and treatment of malignant testicular tumors. Am. J. Roentgenol. Rad. Ther. Nucl. Med. 114:482–491.

Maier, J. G., and M. H. Sulak. 1973. Radiation therapy in malignant testis tumors. Part II. Carcinoma. Cancer 32:1217–1226.

Manual for Staging of Cancer. 1977. American Joint Committee for Cancer Staging and End Results Reporting, Chicago.

Mostofi, F. K., and E. B. Price, Jr. 1973. Atlas of Tumor Pathology. 2nd series, Fasc. 8. Tumors of the Male Genital System. Armed Forces Institute of Pathology, Washington, D.C.

Nicholson, T. C., P. C. Walsh, and M. B. Rotner. 1974. Lymphadenectomy combined with preoperative and postoperative cobalt 60 teletherapy in the management of embryonal carcinoma and teratocarcinoma of the testes. J. Urol. 112:109–110.

Peckham, M. J., and T. J. McElwain. 1974. Radiotherapy of testicular tumors. Proc. R. Soc. Med. 67:300–303.

Peckham, M. J., and T. J. McElwain. 1975. Testicular tumors. Clin. Endocrinol. Metab. 4:665–692.

Quivey, J. M., K. K. Fu, K. A. Herzog, J. W. Weiss, and T. L. Phillips. Malignant tumors of the testes: Analysis of treatment results and sites and causes of failure. Cancer 39:1247–1253.

Ray, B., S. I. Hajdu, and W. F. Whitmore, Jr. 1974. Distribution of retroperitoneal lymph node metastases in testicular germinal tumors. Cancer 33:340–348.

Skinner, D. G., and W. F. Leadbetter. 1971. The surgical management of testis tumors. J. Urol. 106:84–93.

Staubitz, W. J., I. V. Magoss, T. J. Grace, and W. G. Shenk, III. 1969. Surgical management of testis tumors. J. Urol. 101:350–355.

Tyrrell, C. J., and M. J. Peckham. 1976. The response of lymph node metastases of testicular teratoma to radiation therapy. Br. J. Urol. 48:363–370.

Union Internationale Contre le Cancer. 1968. T.N.M. Classification for Malignant Tumours. U.I.C.C., Geneva.

van der Werf-Messing, B. 1976. Radiotherapeutic treatment of testicular tumors. Int. J. Rad. Oncol. Biol. Phys. 1:235.

Vugrin, D., E. Cvitkovic, W. F. Whitmore, Jr., and R. B. Golbey. 1978. Prophylactic chemotherapy of testicular germ cell carcinomas (nonseminomas) Stage II following orchiectomy and retroperitoneal dissection. Clin. Bul. 8:81.

Walsh, P. C., J. J. Kaufman, W. F. Coulson, and W. E. Goodwin. 1971. Retroperitoneal lymphadenectomy for testicular tumors. J.A.M.A. 217:309.

Whitmore, W. F., Jr. 1970. Germinal tumors of the testis, *in* Proceedings of the Sixth National Cancer Conference. J. B. Lippincott Co., Philadelphia, pp. 219–245.

Cancer of the Genitourinary Tract, edited by
D. E. Johnson and M. L. Samuels.
Raven Press, New York © 1979.

Experience With Preoperative Radiotherapy and Lymphadenectomy for Germinal Cell Tumors of the Testis Other Than Pure Seminoma

David H. Hussey, M.D.

Department of Radiotherapy, The University of Texas System Cancer Center M. D. Anderson Hospital and Tumor Institute, Houston, Texas

The treatment for stages I and II malignant tumors of the testis other than pure seminoma remains a subject of controversy. It is generally agreed that the primary tumor should be treated with an inguinal orchiectomy. However, the best way to manage the regional lymph nodes is still debated. In the United States, the regional lymphatics have usually been treated with a periaortic lymphadenectomy, and if the specimen is positive, postoperative radiotherapy or chemotherapy has usually been delivered. However, lymphadenectomy alone, radiotherapy alone, and lymphadenectomy with pre- and postoperative radiotherapy or with chemotherapy have all been advocated for treating early nonseminomatous tumors.

This paper is an analysis of the results of treatment for nonseminomatous testicular tumors at The University of Texas System Cancer Center M. D. Anderson Hospital and Tumor Institute. In that institution, most patients with testicular tumors other than pure seminoma have been treated by orchiectomy and lymphadenectomy, with or without postoperative radiotherapy. However, a selected group of patients with clinical evidence of regional node metastasis have been treated with preoperative radiotherapy and lymphadenectomy, with or without postoperative irradiation. The principle objective of this paper is to compare the results obtained with preoperative irradiation and lymphadenectomy with those achieved with lymphadenectomy alone or with lymphadenectomy and postoperative radiation therapy.

CLINICAL MATERIAL

Between March 1944 and September 1973, 279 patients with nonseminomatous germinal cell tumors of the testis received all or a significant part of their treatment at M. D. Anderson Hospital. Of these, 186 patients presented with tumors limited to the primary site or to the regional lymphatics below the diaphragm (stages I and II).

This report is based on an analysis of 165 patients with stages I and II nonseminomatous tumors treated with orchiectomy and lymphadenectomy with or without radiation therapy. Twenty-one patients who were treated with orchiectomy alone (nine patients) or orchiectomy plus radiation therapy (12 patients) have been excluded.

The clinical material has been classified by the Dixon and Moore system (1952), which is of prognostic importance: group I—seminoma, pure; group II—embryonal carcinoma, pure or with seminoma; group III—teratoma, pure or with seminoma; group IV—teratoma with embryonal carcinoma and/or choriocarcinoma, with or without seminoma; and group V—choriocarcinoma, pure or with embryonal carcinoma and/or seminoma.

Most patients were treated with an orchiectomy elsewhere before referral to M. D. Anderson Hospital. However, in every case the diagnosis was confirmed by the Department of Pathology at M. D. Anderson Hospital. Patients with an initial diagnosis of pure seminoma who were later found to have nonseminomatous metastases have been excluded from the analysis.

The following clinical staging system* has been employed for this analysis:

Stage I   Tumor clinically limited to the testis and spermatic cord.
Stage II   Clinical or radiographic evidence of tumor spread beyond the testis, but limited to the regional lymphatics below the diaphragm.
Stage IIA   Moderate-sized retroperitoneal metastasis.
Stage IIB   Massive retroperitoneal metastasis.
Stage III   Metastasis beyond the diaphragm.
Stage IIIA   Extension above the diaphragm, but still confined to the mediastinal and/or supraclavicular lymphatics.
Stage IIIB   Extranodal metastasis.

The patients were staged on the basis of the initial clinical evaluation, including lymphangiography. The surgical findings at lymphadenectomy did not alter the clinical staging. The clinical evaluation included a complete history and physical examination, complete blood count, liver function tests, blood-urea nitrogen, urinalysis, and chorionic gonadotropin titer. The radiographic studies included a chest x-ray, excretory urogram, and, more recently, a pedal lymphangiogram.

TREATMENT METHODS

The primary tumor was usually treated by a radical orchiectomy through an inguinal incision with high ligation of the spermatic cord. If the patient

---

* This differs from the current M. D. Anderson Hospital staging system, which classifies patients with extension through the capsule and/or to the spermatic cord with negative lymphangiograms as stage IIA. There were eight patients in this category, with a three-year NED rate of 50%.

was referred after an incisional biopsy or a scrotal orchiectomy, an inguinal orchiectomy or resection of the spermatic cord was usually carried out before proceeding with treatment of the regional lymphatics.

The treatment of the regional lymphatics has undergone several modifications throughout the years as the causes of treatment failure have been defined (Castro 1969, Hussey, Luk, and Johnson 1977). Most patients were treated by periaortic lymphadenectomy. When the surgical specimen was positive, postoperative radiotherapy was usually delivered to the periaortic and ipsilateral iliac areas. In most instances, the postoperative dose was 4,000 to 5,000 rads in 4½ to 5 weeks.

Beginning in the early 1960s, a selected group of patients were treated with preoperative irradiation and lymphadenectomy, with or without postoperative radiotherapy. In the early years, preoperative radiotherapy was used only for patients with massive retroperitoneal disease (stage IIB). The aim was to improve resectability and diminish the chance of tumor dissemination by the surgical procedure. Since 1969, preoperative radiotherapy has been used for all patients with stage II tumors.

The patients selected for preoperative radiotherapy received 2,500 rads in three weeks to the periaortic and ipsilateral iliac areas, followed one to two weeks later by a bilateral periaortic lymphadenectomy. If the surgical specimen was positive, an additional 2,000 to 3,000 rads was usually delivered to the area of involvement marked by surgical clips. If the specimen was negative, the patient usually received no further treatment, although in some patients a dose of 2,000 to 3,000 rads was delivered postoperatively.

The mediastinal and supraclavicular areas were not routinely irradiated prophylactically because the next manifestation of disease with nonseminomatous tumors is usually extranodal spread. Elective chemotherapy was usually not employed for patients with stage I or II disease, although it has been used for some patients with positive nodes in recent years.

RESULTS

The results are outlined by clinical stage and treatment method in Table 1. Ninety-six patients were treated with lymphadenectomy alone, 35 with lymphadenectomy and postoperative radiotherapy, and 34 with preoperative radiotherapy and lymphadenectomy, with or without postoperative radiotherapy. The analysis includes six patients in the lymphadenectomy plus postoperative radiotherapy group and four patients in the preoperative radiotherapy plus lymphadenectomy group who were found to have unresectable tumors at laparotomy. Thirty-six months with no evidence of disease (three-year NED rate) was used as an indicator of cure, since 98% of treatment failures occurred within 36 months.

The results for patients with stage I nonseminomatous testicular tumors are quite good, with 81% alive with no evidence of disease at three years. The

Table 1. Results for Nonseminomatous Testicular Tumors by Treatment Method After Orchiectomy: Patients NED at 36 Months and Sites of Failure

Stage	Node Dissection Only		Node Dissection + Postop XRT		Preop XRT + Node Dissection ± Postop XRT		Total Patients NED
	Negative Nodes	Positive Nodes	Negative Nodes	Positive Nodes	Negative Nodes	Positive Nodes	
I	71/85 2 Scrotal 1 PA 1 PA+MED+ENM 2 MED+ENM 1 SC+ENM 6 ENM 1 LFU	3/4 1 LFU	3/3	9/14 1 PA+ENM 1 MED+SC+ENM 3 ENM	4/5 1 ID		90/111 (81%)
IIA	2/2	0/4 1 PA 1 PA+MED+SC 2 PA+ENM		4/15* 1 Pelvis 1 Pelvis+ENM 2 PA+ENM 1 SC 4 ENM 1 ID 1 Uncertain	12/13 1 ENM	2/6† 2 MED+ENM 2 ENM	20/40 (50%)
IIB		0/1 1 PA+MED+ENM		0/3* 2 PA+ENM 1 PA+MED+SC+ENM	1/2 1 SC+ENM	2/8* 2 PA+ENM 1 PA+MED+ENM 3 ENM	3/14 (21%)

* Includes three patients with unresectable tumors.
† Includes one patient with unresectable tumor.
Abbreviations: ENM = extranodal metastasis; ID = intercurrent disease; LFU = lost to follow-up; MED = mediastinum; PA = periaortic; and SC = supraclavicular.

three-year NED rate for patients with stage IIA tumors was only 50%, although the results were better for those treated with preoperative irradiation (74%). The results for patients with massive abdominal disease (stage IIB) are poorer, with only three of 14 patients (21%) alive with no evidence of disease at three years. However, all three of the survivors with stage IIB disease were treated with preoperative radiotherapy.

Hematogenous metastasis was the most frequent cause of treatment failure. Elective irradiation of the mediastinum and left supraclavicular area is not indicated for these tumors since only one patient developed mediastinal or supraclavicular metastasis without evidence of extranodal spread.

Correlation of Staging With Lymphadenectomy Findings

The pathology findings at lymphadenectomy were correlated with the clinical staging in 131 patients with stage I or II tumors treated initially with orchiectomy and lymphadenectomy (Table 2). These correlations represent conservative figures since the lymphadenectomy specimens were not routinely serially sectioned.

Of 106 patients with stage I tumors, 18 had positive nodes at lymphadenectomy. This 17% incidence of occult disease in periaortic nodes justifies elective treatment of the periaortic nodes. Even teratomas, pure or with seminoma (group III), which show a more benign course than other histopathological types, had a 9% incidence of occult disease in the periaortic area.

With stage II tumors, 23 of 25 patients treated initially with orchiectomy

Table 2. *Incidence of Positive Nodes at Laparotomy by Clinical Stage* and Histopathology (131 Patients Treated Initially by Orchiectomy and Lymphadenectomy)†*

	Histology‡	Stage I	Stage II
II	Embryonal carcinoma, pure or with seminoma	24% (8/33)	94% (15/16)
III	Teratoma, pure or with seminoma	9% (2/23)	50% (1/2)
IV	Teratoma, with embryonal carcinoma or choriocarcinoma, with or without seminoma	13% (6/45)	100% (4/4)
V	Choriocarcinoma, pure or with embryonal carcinoma, and/or seminoma	40% (2/5)	100% (3/3)
Total		17% (18/106)	92% (23/25)

* The 87 patients staged by lymphangiography had a similar incidence of positive nodes at lymphadenectomy: stage I, 18% (13/73); stage II, 93% (13/14).

† Includes six patients with stage II disease who were found to have unresectable tumors at laparotomy.

‡ Dixon and Moore classification (1952).

and lymphadenectomy were found to have positive nodes at surgery, for a false-positive staging rate of only 8%.

Correlation of Laparotomy Findings With Frequency of Extranodal Metastasis

Patients with positive nodes at laparotomy have a high risk of developing distant metastasis (Table 3). In this series, 28 of 55 patients (51%) with positive nodes developed extranodal spread. The incidence of extranodal metastasis for patients with negative nodes was only 11%. Although the incidence of extranodal metastasis for patients with negative nodes following preoperative radiotherapy (10%, 2/20) was similar to that observed for patients not receiving preoperative irradiation (11%, 10/90), patients treated with preoperative radiotherapy presented with more advanced disease initially.

Dose Relationships

The relationship between local control in the periaortic lymph nodes and the radiation dose delivered is shown in Table 4. The fact that there were only two periaortic failures in 87 patients (2%) with negative nodes who did not receive radiotherapy indicates that postoperative radiotherapy is not necessary for patients with negative nodes at lymphadenectomy.

When positive nodes were found at lymphadenectomy, radiotherapy reduced the incidence of failure in the periaortic area significantly. There were five periaortic failures in nine patients (56%) who had positive nodes resected at lymphadenectomy and did not receive radiation therapy. In contrast, there were only two periaortic failures in 35 patients (6%) who had positive nodes resected and were irradiated.

Table 3. *Incidence of Extranodal Metastasis by Clinical Stage and Nodal Status at Lymphadenectomy**

	Laparotomy Findings	
Clinical Stage	Negative Nodes	Positive Nodes
I	11%	28%
	(10/93)	(5/18)
IIA	7%	52%
	(1/15)	(13/25)
IIB	50%	83%
	(1/2)	(10/12)
Total	11%	51%
	(12/110)	(28/55)

* Includes four patients with stage IIA disease and six with stage IIB who were found to have unresectable tumors at laparotomy.

Table 4. *Incidence of Failure in the Periaortic Area by Radiation Dose and Tumor Burden (Stages I, IIA, and IIB)*

Status of Periaortic Lymph Nodes	No XRT	Tumor Dose (rads)		
		2,000–3,000	3,000–4,500	4,500–5,500
No tumor at lymphadenectomy	2/87	0/11	0/7	0/5
Tumor resected*	5/9	1/2	0/5	1/28
Gross tumor remaining†	—	2/2	4/4	2/5

* Lymphadenectomy specimen positive, but gross tumor completely resected.
† Includes one patient with gross tumor remaining after lymphadenectomy and 10 patients with unresectable tumor at laparotomy.

The minimum dose required for local control when all evident disease is resected cannot be determined from this series, since only seven patients in this category were treated with doses of fewer than 4,500 rads. If there was gross disease in the periaortic area, a dose of 4,500 to 5,500 rads was required to achieve any salvage.

Complications occur if doses in the range of 4,500 to 5,500 rads are combined with lymphadenectomy. Three of 69 patients (4%) treated with a combination of radiotherapy and lymphadenectomy or radiotherapy and laparotomy developed complications. These included two patients with intestinal obstructions and one with extensive retroperitoneal fibrosis. All three patients had been treated with a bilateral lymphadenectomy, followed by postoperative radiotherapy to a dose of 5,000 rads in 5 weeks.

Preoperative Radiotherapy

The results achieved with preoperative radiotherapy and lymphadenectomy are compared with those obtained with lymphadenectomy alone or with lymphadenectomy and postoperative radiotherapy in Table 5. In general, patients treated with preoperative irradiation presented with more advanced disease than those in the other treatment categories.

With stage I patients, the results with preoperative radiotherapy were similar to those achieved with patients not receiving preoperative irradiation. Four of five patients treated with preoperative radiotherapy had no evidence of disease at three years. The only treatment failure was due to intercurrent disease (an auto accident).

With stage IIA patients, the results with preoperative radiotherapy were superior to those achieved in the other treatment groups. The three-year NED rate for patients receiving preoperative irradiation was 74%, as compared to only 29% for patients not receiving preoperative radiotherapy ($\chi^2 = 8.12$; $p < .005$). A dose of 2,500 rads preoperatively significantly influenced the lymphadenectomy findings in these patients. Although 90% of patients treated initially with an orchiectomy and lymphadenectomy, without preoperative irradiation,

Table 5. *Influence of Preoperative Radiotherapy on Surgical Findings at Laparotomy and Results of Treatment*

Stage	Surgical Findings		Results		
	% With Nonresectable Tumors	% With Positive Nodes	% With Failure in Periaortic Area	% With Extranodal Metastasis	3-Year NED Rate
I					
Preop XRT	0%	0%	0%	0%	80%*
	(0/5)	(0/5)	(0/5)	(0/5)	(4/5)
No preop XRT	0%	17%	3%	14%	81%
	(0/106)	(18/106)	(3/106)	(15/106)	(86/106)
IIA					
Preop XRT	5%	32%	0%	26%	74%
	(1/19)	(6/19)	(0/19)	(5/19)	(14/19)
No preop XRT	14%	90%	29%	43%	29%
	(3/21)	(19/21)	(6/21)	(9/21)	(6/21)
IIB					
Preop XRT	30%	80%	30%	70%	30%
	(3/10)	(8/10)	(3/10)	(7/10)	(3/10)
No preop XRT	75%	100%	100%	100%	0%
	(3/4)	(4/4)	(4/4)	(4/4)	(0/4)

* One patient who died of intercurrent disease (an auto accident) is listed as failure.

were found to have positive nodes at surgery, only 32% of patients treated with preoperative radiation therapy had positive nodes at lymphadenectomy. This difference is statistically significant ($\chi^2 = 14.76$; $p < .001$). Although the incidence of subsequent distant metastasis was lower in the group receiving preoperative radiotherapy, the difference is not statistically significant.

In the present series, the only survivors among patients with bulky abdominal disease (stage IIB) were three patients who had been treated with preoperative radiotherapy. The prognosis for patients with stage IIB disease is poor because most have unresectable tumors on initial presentation and there is a high incidence of extranodal metastasis. Three of four patients who had laparotomies initially without preoperative radiotherapy were found to have unresectable tumors at surgery (Table 5). However, only three of 10 patients who had preoperative radiotherapy to a dose of 2,500 rads had unresectable tumors at laparotomy. The incidence of extranodal metastasis in patients with stage IIB disease is very high (79%, 11/14). Consequently, the treatment approach should include all three modalities (surgery, radiotherapy, and chemotherapy).

DISCUSSION

The results with preoperative radiotherapy and lymphadenectomy at M. D. Anderson Hospital are similar to those achieved with a similar treatment regimen at the Walter Reed General Hospital (Table 6) (Maier and Mittemeyer 1977). In the Walter Reed study, 97% of patients with stage I nonseminomatous tumors

Table 6. *Influence of Preoperative Radiotherapy on the Surgical Findings at Lymphadenectomy and the Three-Year NED Rate: A Comparison of M. D. Anderson and Walter Reed Results*

	% With Positive Nodes		3-Year NED Rate	
Stage	MDAH	Walter Reed	MDAH	Walter Reed
I				
Preop XRT	0%	3%*	80%†	97%*
	(0/5)	(1/30)	(4/5)	(29/30)
No preop XRT	17%	25%‡	81%	73%§
	(18/106)	(6/24)	(86/106)	(80/109)
II				
Preop XRT	48%	52%*	59%	81%*
	(14/29)	(11/21)	(17/29)	(17/21)
No preop XRT	92%	91%‡	24%	45%‖
	(23/25)	(32/35)	(6/25)	(44/97)

* 3,000 rads preoperatively to the periaortic and ipsilateral iliac areas, followed by bilateral lymphadenectomy and 1,500 rads postoperatively, and 4,000 rads to the mediastinum and supraclavicular area. From Maier and Mittemeyer (1977).
† One patient who died of intercurrent disease (an auto accident) is listed as failure.
‡ From Maier and Schamber (1972).
§ Clinical stage I and negative nodes at lymphadenectomy (prelymphangiogram era); five-year survival; treated with lymphadenectomy only. From Maier et al. (1969).
‖ Clinical stage I and positive nodes at lymphadenectomy (prelymphangiogram era) (unresectable cases excluded); five-year survival; treated with lymphadenectomy and postoperative radiotherapy. From Maier et al. (1969).

treated with preoperative radiotherapy, bilateral lymphadenectomy, and postoperative radiotherapy were alive with no evidence of disease at three years. By comparison, the five-year survival rate for a historical control group (clinical stage I and negative nodes at surgery) treated with lymphadenectomy alone was only 73% (Maier et al. 1969). In stage II patients, a three-year NED rate with preoperative radiotherapy was 81%, whereas the five-year survival rate for those who did not receive preoperative irradiation (clinical stage I and positive nodes at lymphadenectomy) was only 45%. (Three- and five-year rates are compared because three-year NED rates are not available for lymphangiogram-staged patients at Walter Reed. Experience at M. D. Anderson Hospital has shown that over 98% of treatment failures occur within three years.)

Both the M. D. Anderson and Walter Reed studies have shown that preoperative radiotherapy significantly reduces the incidence of positive nodes at lymphadenectomy. In the Walter Reed study, the frequency of positive lymphadenectomy specimens was 3% with stage I disease and 52% with stage II disease when preoperative radiotherapy was given. By comparison, 25% of patients with stage I disease and 91% of patients with stage II had positive lymphadenectomy specimens when the lymphadenectomy was performed immediately, without preoperative irradiation (Maier and Schamber 1972). These results are similar to those reported from M. D. Anderson Hospital, where 48% of patients with stage II disease treated with preoperative radiation therapy had positive nodes at lymphadenectomy, as compared to 92% of those treated with orchiectomy and immediate lymphadenectomy.

The most likely explanation for the superior results with preoperative radiotherapy is that moderate doses of irradiation (2,500 to 3,000 rads) reduce the number of clonogenic cells in the periaortic area, diminishing the frequency of tumor dissemination by the surgical procedure. This explanation is supported by the lower incidence of positive lymphadenectomy specimens observed in patients treated with preoperative irradiation.

The high incidence of subsequent extranodal metastases in patients with positive nodes at lymphadenectomy and the increasing effectiveness of chemotherapeutic agents have prompted some institutions to replace radiotherapy with chemotherapy as a component of the initial therapeutic effort. The assumption is that if surgery cannot cure the patient, elective chemotherapy is necessary. However, the experience at M. D. Anderson Hospital and Walter Reed General Hospital has shown that high cure rates can be achieved with preoperative radiotherapy and lymphadenectomy, with or without postoperative irradiation. Before radiotherapy is discarded as part of the initial treatment regimen, the advocates of adjunctive chemotherapy should show that their treatment modality can achieve similar cure rates without prohibitive toxicity.

ACKNOWLEDGMENT

This investigation was supported in part by Grant CA 06294, awarded by the National Cancer Institute, Department of Health, Education and Welfare.

REFERENCES

Castro, J. R. 1969. Lymphadenectomy and radiation therapy in malignant tumors of the testicle other than pure seminoma. Cancer 1:87–91.

Dixon, F. J., and R. A. Moore. 1952. Atlas of Tumor Pathology. Sec. VIII, fasc. 31b and 32. Tumors of the Male Sex Organ. Armed Forces Institute of Pathology, Washington, D.C.

Hussey, D. H., K. H. Luk, and D. E. Johnson. 1977. The role of radiation therapy in the treatment of germinal cell tumors of the testis other than pure seminoma. Radiology 123:175–180.

Maier, J. G., and B. T. Mittemeyer. 1977. Carcinoma of the testis. Cancer 39:981–986.

Maier, J. G., K. E. Van Buskirk, M. H. Sulak, R. H. Perry, and D. T. Schamber. 1969. An evaluation of lymphadenectomy in the treatment of malignant testicular germ cell neoplasms. J. Urol. 101:356–359.

Maier, J. G., and D. T. Schamber. 1972. The role of lymphangiography in the diagnosis and treatment of malignant testicular tumors. Am. J. Roentgenol. 114:482–491.

Cancer of the Genitourinary Tract, edited by
D. E. Johnson and M. L. Samuels.
Raven Press, New York © 1979.

Velban Plus Continuous Infusion Bleomycin (VB-3) in Stage III Advanced Testicular Cancer: Results in 99 Patients With a Note on High-Dose Velban and Sequential Cis-platinum

Melvin L. Samuels, M.D., Douglas E. Johnson, M.D.,* Barry Brown, Ph.D.,† R. Bruce Bracken, M.D.,* Manuel E. Moran, M.D., and Andrew von Eschenbach, M.D.*

*Departments of Medicine, *Urology, and † Biomathematics, The University of Texas System Cancer Center M. D. Anderson Hospital and Tumor Institute, Houston, Texas*

Our last review of the Velban-bleomycin programs (Samuels et al. 1976) focused primarily on earlier experience. The initial program, Velban plus biweekly intramuscular bleomycin (VB-1), demonstrated a sharp increase in response and survival, and Table 1 summarizes these data for nonseminomatous germinal malignant lesions. The important point is the 28% cure rate, with the longest survival beyond eight years. The poor response in patients with embryonal carcinoma to VB-1, below, prompted VB-3 with or without cis-platinum.

1. VB-1
   Velban 0.4 mg/kg total dose days 1 and 2. Bleomycin 30 units i.m. twice weekly × 10 weeks. Additional courses of Velban unchanged. Bleomycin 30 units i.m. twice weekly × 5 weeks; repeat at 4-week intervals.
2. Bleomycin-COMF (14-day program)
   Bleomycin 30 units i.m. twice weekly × 4 weeks; Cytoxan 200 mg/m^2 i.v. daily × 14 days; Oncovin 2.0 mg i.v. days 1 and 7; methotrexate 15 mg/m^2 twice weekly × 4 weeks; 5-fluorouracil 400 mg/m^2 i.v. daily days 1–5.
   a. Initial therapy for seminoma, stage III-B.
   b. Failures of VB-1 program.
   c. Consolidation for teratocarcinoma.
3. VB-2 and VB-3 (continuous-infusion bleomycin)
   a. Bleomycin 30 units per liter normal saline over 24 hours × 5 days; Velban 0.4 mg/kg days 5 and 6 (VB-2).
   b. Velban 0.4–0.6 mg/kg days 1 and 2; bleomycin 30 units per liter normal saline over 24 hours × 5 days (days 2 through 6) (VB-3).
4. VB-3 plus sequential cis-platinum, 100 mg/m^2 upon recovery from myelosuppression, × 2 at 7-day intervals, course 1; single dose of cis-platinum,

Table 1. *Results With Velban-Intermittent Bleomycin (VB-1) (1970–1973)*

Histologic Group	Total No. of Patients	Response Complete	Partial	No. Failed	No. Alive NED
Embryonal carcinoma	26	7 (26%)	13	3	4
Teratocarcinoma	24	11 (46%)	5	1	10
Total	50	18 (36%)	18	4	14

course 2; then VB-3 alone, $\times$ 2, courses 3 and 4. Total dose of cis-platinum 300 mg/m^2.

The most significant change was the adoption of the new technique for the administration of bleomycin (VB-3). Data from Drewinko's laboratory (Drewinko et al. 1972) suggested that continuous exposure of cancer cells to bleomycin over one cell cycle markedly improved cell kill. Recent data in the Lewis lung tumor have tended to confirm the superiority of continuous-infusion over intermittent bleomycin administration (Sikic et al. 1978). Patient entry into the VB-3 program began July 1973, and initial results demonstrated its superiority over earlier programs (Samuels et al. 1975, 1977). Enough time has now elapsed to report the impact of this program on survival.

The newest major advance appears to be the introduction of cis-diamminedichloroplatinum (cis-platinum) (DDP) into current programs, and we will add a note on our results with VB-3 plus sequential cis-platinum.

PATIENT POPULATION

The study population consists of 99 stage III testis cancer patients entered between July 1, 1973, and January 31, 1977. Entry was stopped for this study at this point to allow for at least 18 months of follow-up of all patients. Our studies have shown that patients in complete remission at 18 months after inception of therapy rarely fail (we have had only one such patient in this study, who failed at 100 weeks).

We have demonstrated that complete response with potential cure is directly related to net tumor burden (Samuels et al. 1976) and, thus, it has become necessary to stratify stage III presentation into six groups as follows:

III-A   Disease confined to supraclavicular nodes.

III-B-1   Gynecomastia, either unilateral or bilateral with or without elevation of biomarkers. Estrogen levels may be elevated. No gross tumor detectable.

III-B-2   Minimal pulmonary disease. Up to five metastatic masses in each lung, with the largest diameter of any single lesion no larger than 2.0 cm.

III-B-3   Advanced pulmonary disease. Any mediastinal or hilar mass, neo-plastic pleural effusion, or intrapulmonary mass greater than 2.0 cm in diameter.

III-B-4   Advanced abdominal disease. Any palpable abdominal mass, ureteral displacement, or obstructive uropathy.

III-B-5   Visceral disease (excluding lung). The liver is the most common organ involved. Also included are the gastrointestinal tract (second and third portions of the duodenum) and brain. Inferior vena caval invasion is considered in this category.

The III-A presentation is restricted to failed stage II patients and is rare. Gynecomastia as an isolated new finding (III-B-1) is also unusual and found as an early manifestation of a failed stage II or failed stage III (complete responder) presentation. Only 5% of the VB-3 study patients were III-A or III-B-1. Note that minimal abdominal disease does not appear in this classification. All stage III pulmonary presentations must be presumed to include positive para-aortic nodes independent of lymphangiogram findings, which are false-negative in 16–24% of patients (Hermanek 1977). Likewise, we do not include elevation of biomarkers in this classification. Levels of biomarkers have frequently been seen to fall rapidly to normal with gross tumor still abundantly demonstrable. Hence, these laboratory values must not be used as isolated findings on which to judge complete response. In our experience, patients showing isolated elevation of biomarkers are rare and almost invariably will show tumor, usually retroperitoneal, if the search is diligently and, if necessary, invasively pursued.

Table 2 summarizes the clinical and histologic data for the VB-3 study patients. Special note should be made of the fact that 75% of these patients have advanced disease (III-B-3, B-4, B-5). While most reported series show a predominance of patients with embryonal cell carcinoma, our study population shows the following distribution: 45% embryonal carcinoma, 45% teratocarcinoma, and

Table 2. *Clinical and Histologic Data for 99 Vinblastine-Continuous Infusion Bleomycin (VB-3) Patients*

Clinical Presentation	Total No. of Patients	No. Evaluable	Histologic Group		
			Embryonal Carcinoma	Terato-carcinoma	Chorio-carcinoma
Minimal disease (III-A, B-1, B-2)	26	26	13	10	3
Advanced disease					
B-3	31	27	12	13	1
B-4	25	23	11	12	1
B-5	17	15	5	6	4
Total	99	91	41	41	9

Table 3. *Time to Stage III Conversion for 43 Stage II Patients*

Histologic Group	Total No. of Patients	Mean Age	Mean Time to Metastases (wks.)	No. of Metastases Beyond 6 Months
Embryonal carcinoma	23	30	20	6
Teratocarcinoma	17	25	31	6
Choriocarcinoma	3	29	17	1

10% choriocarcinoma (one case of pure choriocarcinoma, one choriocarcinoma plus seminoma, and seven choriocarcinoma plus embryonal carcinoma). Cases of pure seminoma are excluded from this report. Eight patients had unrelated medical complications (one each with myocardial infarction and malignant hypertension, two with bleeding peptic ulcers, and four with radiation enteritis) that were responsible for inadequate chemotherapy and early death. However, all 99 patients were included in survival studies.

Table 3 summarizes the data on the 43 failed stage II patients in our study group who had undergone prior retroperitoneal node dissection and radiotherapy. These represent almost half of our study population.

RESPONSE AND SURVIVAL

Of the 91 evaluable patients, 59, or 65%, responded completely. In addition, there were 27 partial responses, for an overall response rate of 95%. Table 4 breaks down response by histologic group. Thus, patients with embryonal carcinoma show a 68% complete response rate, those with teratocarcinoma a 63% response rate, and those with choriocarcinoma a 56% response rate.

The effects of disease presentation and prior radiotherapy were studied for each of the three major histologic categories. Table 5 demonstrates that patients with minimal disease and embryonal carcinoma had a 100% complete response rate, with only one failure for a 92% salvage rate. Prior radiotherapy does

Table 4. *Response of Evaluable VB-3 Patients by Histologic Group*

Histologic Group	Total No. of Patients	No. CR*	Mean Survival CR (wks.)	No. PR†	Mean Survival PR (wks.)
Embryonal carcinoma	41	28	142	11	63
Teratocarcinoma	41	26	117	12	56
Choriocarcinoma	9	5	116	4	44
Total	91	59		27	

* Complete responders.
† Partial responders.

Table 5. *Effect of Prior Radiotherapy and Clinical Presentation on Response of Patients With Embryonal Carcinoma*

Clinical Presentation	Prior Radiotherapy*			No Prior Radiotherapy		
	Total No.	No. CR	No. Dead	Total No.	No. CR	No. Dead
Minimal disease	10	10	1	3	3	0
Advanced disease	10	5	8	18	10	9
Total	20	15	9 (45%)	21	13	9 (43%)

* Indicates failed stage II presentation, in contrast to stage III at presentation.

not exert a deleterious effect. However, prior radiotherapy with advanced disease presentations is associated with a fall in the complete response rate to 50%; furthermore, three complete responders failed, giving a stable complete response rate of only 20%. For patients with advanced disease and no prior radiotherapy, the complete response rate is 56% with only one failure.

Table 6 summarizes the effects of the same variables on patients with teratocarcinoma. The complete response rate for those with minimal disease is now 80% but three subsequently failed, for a salvage rate of only 50%. The numbers are too small to reflect a radiotherapy effect. For patients with advanced disease, the complete response rates are about 60% for both the radiotherapy and nonradiotherapy groups, with no significant difference in the failure rate.

Results with Dixon and Moore (1952) group 5 patients are summarized in Table 7. Note that the two patients who received prior radiotherapy at the time of stage II presentation responded completely after converting to stage III, but later relapsed and died. Three of seven patients who were stage III at presentation responded completely to chemotherapy and have not failed. Thus, the overall salvage for this group is only 33%.

The effect of increasing Velban dosage on complete response is indicated in Table 8. Four dosage programs were studied, with the dose of bleomycin remain-

Table 6. *Effect of Prior Radiotherapy and Clinical Presentation on Response of Patients With Teratocarcinoma*

Clinical Presentation	Prior Radiotherapy			No Prior Radiotherapy		
	Total No.	No. CR	No. Dead	Total No.	No. CR	No. Dead
Minimal disease	6	5	2	4	3	3
Advanced disease	9	6	5	22	12	11
Total	15	11 (73%)	7 (47%)	26	15 (58%)	14 (54%)

Table 7. *Effect of Prior Radiotherapy and Clinical Presentation on Response of Patients With Choriocarcinoma*

Clinical Presentation	Prior Radiotherapy			No Prior Radiotherapy		
	Total No.	No. CR	No. Dead	Total No.	No. CR	No. Dead
Minimal disease	1	1	1	2	2	0
Advanced disease	1	1	1	5	1	4
Total	2	2	2 (100%)	7	3	4 (56%)

ing fixed at 30 units per day by continuous infusion for five successive days. At the lowest Velban dose, less than 0.4 mg/kg, there was only a 38% complete response rate, with 33% of these patients relapsing. At the next level, 0.4 to 0.45 mg/kg, the complete response rate was 57%, but the failure rate was still high at 29%. Only three patients in this group received 0.45 mg/kg; the remainder received 0.4 mg/kg. Increasing the Velban dose to 0.5 mg/kg or greater resulted in a striking increase in the complete response rate to 85% with only one failure. The survival time study proves these data to be mature, with all complete responders living and well beyond 18 months.

Cis-platinum was used as primary induction therapy in nine patients and as secondary therapy for VB-3 failures in 16 (Table 9). Three patients who received initial VB-3 therapy were placed on cis-platinum, 100 mg/m^2 every seven days for three doses. Mannitol diuresis was used during each dose. The reasons for this change of therapy included an erythema multiforme skin reaction in one patient, a rapidly progressive choriocarcinoma with retinal metastasis in a second, and a large mediastinal teratoma in a third. All three received the three initial doses of cis-platinum, followed by a four-week rest period and then one or two additional doses. They are in complete remission and doing well. (Radiotherapy was added for the patient with eye metastases.) The remaining six patients in the primary therapy group received VB-3 followed by sequential cis-platinum, 100 mg/m^2, after recovery from myelosuppression. This was usually about day 18 to 20. A second pulse of cis-platinum followed in seven days. However,

Table 8. *Response and Survival Rates According to Velban Dose*

Velban Dose (mg/kg)	No. of Patients	No. Receiving Prior XRT	No. CR	No. CR Surviving	Mean Survival (wks.)
<0.4	24	18	9 (38%)	6	80
0.4–0.45	49	18	28 (57%)	20	103
0.5	14	6	12 (86%)	12	95
≥0.6	12	1	10 (83%)	9	87
Total	99	43	59 (60%)	47	

Table 9. *Results With Cis-Platinum in 25 Stage III Testis Cancer Patients*

Therapy	No. of Patients	No. With Advanced Presentations	Histologic Grade			No.* NED
			2	4	5	
Primary†	9	8	2	5	2	8
Secondary‡	16	14	4	10	2	6

* All living beyond 18 months.

† Includes three patients receiving pulse-dose DDP every seven days as solitary therapy and six receiving DDP as sequential therapy with VB-3.

‡ Includes nine complete response failures on VB-3, four partial responders, and three non-responders.

the second course of VB-3 was followed with only one dose of cis-platinum at 100 mg/m² and a third and fourth course were given without cis-platinum. Five of the six patients are in complete remission. Figure 1 shows an example of a complete response in a teratocarcinoma patient with an advanced pulmonary presentation.

Of the 16 VB-3 failures, nine had achieved prior complete response, and complete stable responses were reinduced in two, whereas four achieved further partial responses. The latter four patients then underwent thoracotomies and all are in stable complete remission beyond 18 months. The remaining seven patients showed no further response. These results demonstrate that cis-platinum as a single agent can induce complete response when used sequentially with VB-3 and, further, that there is apparently no cross-resistance in many patients who have failed VB-3. Figure 2 compares the survival curves of the complete responders and the partial and nonresponders.

TOXICITY

Bacteriologically unproven febrile reactions occurring during the period of maximum leukopenia are very common and are treated empirically with a prophylactic antibiotic program consisting of Keflin, Ticar, and full-dose tobramycin or amikacin on day 6. There is an increased risk of acute tubular necrosis when aminoglycoside therapy follows within days of cis-platinum administration (Gonzales-Vitale et al. 1978). However, by giving cis-platinum sequentially *after* hematologic recovery, we have never encountered any difficulty. Aminoglycoside therapy follows the completion of VB-3 and is discontinued several days prior to administration of cis-platinum. Bacteriologically proven septicemia occurred in 17 courses among 14 patients. Six cases were caused by *Staphylococcus aureus* or *epidermdiis,* while the remainder were caused by gram-negative bacilli, with *Klebsiella* organisms and *Escherichia coli* predominating. Table 10 shows the relation between different Velban doses and septicemia. With low-dose Velban, the incidence of proven septicemia is 2.3% per course, and this increases fourfold when the Velban dosage is raised to 0.5 mg/kg or more. This increase is primarily

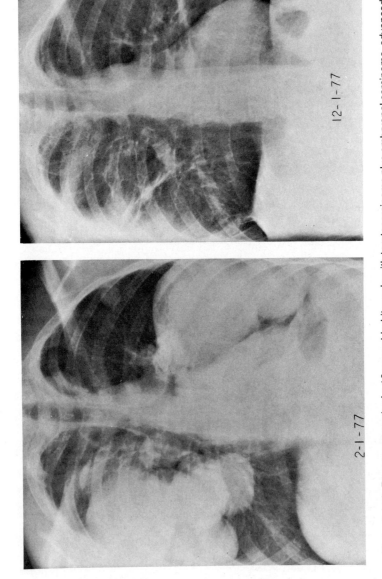

Figure 1. Left, Roentgenograph of a 16-year-old white male with teratocarcinoma plus embryonal carcinoma, advanced pulmonary presentations. Right, Same patient after four courses of VB-3. The Velban dose was 0.6 mg/kg for each course. Pulse-dose cis-platinum was used sequentially during the first and second courses. Patient remains in stable complete remission beyond 18 months.

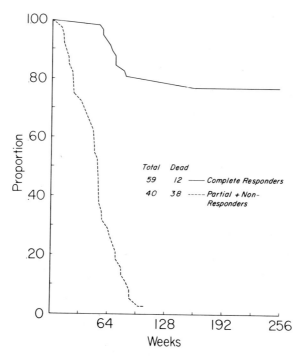

Figure 2. There is a highly significant difference ($p < 0.001$) between the survival curves of the complete responders and the partial and nonresponders.

due to the increased severity of the stomatitis, aciniform skin reactions, and paralytic ileus. Thus, meticulous attention to oral hygiene, skin care, fluid balance, and antibiotic administration is mandatory.

Our mean dose of bleomycin exceeds 700 mg. There were only two cases of bleomycin-induced interstitial pneumonitis and both involved only minimal clinical and radiographic findings, without hypoxemia. The patients' recovery was uneventful. In addition, three patients presented with hypersensitivity pneumoni-

Table 10. *Relation of Velban Dose to Sepsis*

Dose	No. of Patients	No. of Courses	No. of Proven Infections*	No. of Deaths from Infection
Low (≤0.45 mg/kg)	73	351	8 (2.3%)	0
High (≥0.5 mg/kg)	26	98	9 (9.2%)	1†

* Culture positive.
† Death due to *Serratia* organisms.

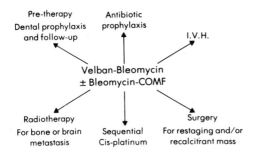

Figure 3. Supplementary measures for VB-3. I.V.H. = intravenous hyperalimentation.

tis induced by bleomycin (Holoye et al. 1978) and all responded dramatically to corticosteroid therapy. Monitoring procedures for bleomycin-induced lung disease must be meticulously performed and include careful historical data on exertional dyspnea, serial spirometry, careful auscultation of the lungs for dry "cellophane" rales, and serial gallium scans. We now do a gallium scan following every two courses of therapy and find that it may produce the earliest abnormal finding. The forced vital capacity is a very useful test to perform serially, and we regard a fall of greater than 10% from base value as significant.

Figure 3 summarizes the various supplementary measures that are necessary if the chemotherapy protocol is to be successful. Thus, dental prophylaxis with repair of all major oral disease is necessary prior to initiation of chemotherapy, as the program uniformly produces stomatitis. Intravenous hyperalimentation is necessary in malnourished patients and is especially useful for those with advanced disease, who require multiple courses as rapidly as possible. The antibiotic program previously discussed is introduced on treatment day 6, when granulocytopenia is at its nadir, and is continued for six to eight days until recovery is evident. Leukocyte transfusions are not necessary, as the period of leukopenia is brief. Fluid balance is critical, and at least four liters daily should be administered. Acne is frequently a severe problem and we have found 1% Cleocin in 70% alcohol applied locally twice daily following pHisohex scrubs to be useful.

DISCUSSION

It is clear that testicular cancer is not a homogeneous entity, but a collection of many different clinical presentations and histologic types. Therefore, a single chemotherapy program will not suffice, as there must be provisions within a given protocol for this great variability. Embryonal carcinoma is the histologic type most responsive to Velban-bleomycin. Thus, cases involving minimal disease and embryonal presentations respond very well to 0.4 mg/kg of Velban with continuous-infusion bleomycin, and one can expect a 90% salvage rate, with or without prior radiotherapy. The situation is clearly different with advanced embryonal presentations, for which the salvage rate varies from 20% (prior radiotherapy) to 50% (no prior radiotherapy). Escalation of the Velban dose is indicated in the non-radiotherapy population if the physician has experience with the program and can closely monitor the patient. Sequential cis-platinum appears to be of value. Substitution of less myelosuppressive drugs for Velban in the prior-radiotherapy, advanced-disease group may be the best initial approach for these patients. They present a very special problem, being at greater risk from high-dose Velban and responding poorly to the conventional dose.

Teratocarcinoma presents yet another and more complex problem. Cases with minimal disease presentation show only a 50% salvage rate, as do those with advanced disease presentation, irrespective of prior radiotherapy, so high-dose Velban becomes necessary. Among the 26 patients previously described who were treated with 0.5 mg/kg or higher of Velban, 18 had teratocarcinoma. The complete response rate was above 80%, indicating that an increase in dose will probably improve the salvage rate. The place of cis-platinum in the teratocarcinoma protocols is not certain, judging from other reports. Einhorn and Donohue noted six complete responses among 12 teratocarcinoma patients, but one responder died, giving only a 40% potential salvage rate (Einhorn and Donohue 1977). This is not better than our original VB-1 data (Samuels et al. 1976). If cis-platinum is to be added, pulse-dose administration would seem most appropriate. Animal data suggest that administration every seven days is superior to daily administration (Presnov et al. 1978), as does the report of Higby and co-workers (1974) of their human data, although the risk of nephrotoxicity is increased.

Choriocarcinoma most frequently presents as advanced disease with "white" lungs and hemoptysis or large abdominal masses with liver metastasis. While response to Velban-bleomycin is the rule (Samuels et al. 1976), stable complete remissions beyond 18 months are attainable in only one third of patients. Does cis-platinum have anything to add to existing programs? Among five of 50 choriocarcinoma patients reported by Einhorn and Donohue (1977), three responded completely, but only two complete responders are alive (40%). Further, the data are not mature, so the survival rate will probably deteriorate further. This is a depressing revelation, since the report of Higby and co-workers (1974) demonstrated striking activity of cis-platinum as a solitary agent. Thus, it is apparent that new cis-platinum programs are needed for treating patients with choriocarcinoma.

Unsettled is the problem of maintenance chemotherapy. Bacillus Calmette-Guérin and Velban are being used, but still produce a 20% failure rate among complete responders (Einhorn and Donohue 1977). The administration of bleomycin-COMF consolidation following VB-1 resulted in a 44% cure rate for patients with stage III teratocarcinoma (Samuels et al. 1976), suggesting that consolidation therapy should be studied. This has not been done to date, but clearly the subject should be addressed, as all programs today have at least a 20% relapse rate among complete responders and it would seem that this could be sharply reduced.

The final verification of the efficacy of a program must come from statistical analysis of survival data. Comparisons of the number of complete responses

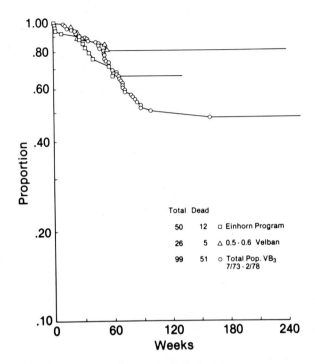

Figure 4. Comparison of the survival curves of 99 VB-3 patients, 50 patients treated with cis-platinum plus Velban and bleomycin, and 26 high-dose Velban patients.

among various programs are not valid, since the treatment populations are different and response criteria variable. We emphasize that our population consists of 75% advanced presentations, heavily irradiated (45%), with a high percentage of teratocarcinoma and choriocarcinoma patients, while Einhorn and Donohue's population (1977) consists of 50% advanced presentations, 60% embryonal carcinoma patients, and less than 10% who received prior irradiation, if seminoma patients are excluded. Figure 4 compares the survival curves of our 99 VB-3 patients with Einhorn and Donohue's 50 patients who received high-dose Velban. There is no significant difference between the two curves (Wilcoxon two-tailed test = 0.91, one-tailed test = 0.45). We have also included the survival curve of our 26 patients who have received high-dose Velban. While this curve looks better, analysis again shows no significant difference. However, the mean survival time, ignoring censoring, is 2.6 times as long in our high-dose Velban group as in the entire population of 99 patients, suggesting a true difference may exist and larger numbers might demonstrate this difference.

CONCLUSIONS

The current Velban-continuous infusion bleomycin program (VB-3) has achieved a 50% salvage rate, a clear improvement over our initial VB-1 program, which produced a 28% salvage rate. Embryonal carcinoma is exquisitely sensitive to VB-3, with the minimal disease presentations showing better than a 90% salvage rate. Administration of cis-platinum to this population is unwarranted. Teratocarcinoma and choriocarcinoma are more resistant to VB-3. The administration of 0.5 mg/kg of Velban further improves complete response and survival, but acute toxicity becomes formidable and this dose should not be used by the inexperienced generalist or internist. The more aggressive VB-3 programs should be restricted to experienced oncology services in well-endowed hospitals. The addition of sequential large-dose cis-platinum to this program further improves response and is indicated in patients with advanced presentations. Administration of cis-platinum follows sequentially after hematological recovery from VB-3 and does not add to the toxicity of the program. It is given in pulse doses at seven-day intervals.

When special attention is paid to dental prophylaxis, skin care, prophylactic antibiotics, and fluid balance, the death rate from infection can be expected to be 1–2% or less. Careful monitoring of chest x-rays, spirometry, and gallium scans will allow the diagnosis of bleomycin-induced interstitial pneumonitis to be made at an early, completely reversible stage, as was the case in two of our patients (2% incidence).

There is no question that antibiotic prophylaxis in the granulocytopenic patient and the early detection of bleomycin-induced interstitial pneumonitis with the gallium scan have made VB-3 a much safer program. We remain impressed with the total lack of chronic side effects. All of our complete responders have returned to full-time employment without disability. The task is now to achieve a 100% salvage rate.

REFERENCES

Dixon, F. J., and R. A. Moore. 1952. Atlas of Tumor Pathology. Sec. 8, fasc. 316 and 332. Tumors of the Male Sex Organs. Armed Forces Institute of Pathology, Washington, D.C.

Drewinko, B., J. Novak, and S. C. Barranco. 1972. The response of human lymphoma cells in vitro to bleomycin and 1,3-cis-(chloroethyl)-nitrosourea. Cancer Res. 32:1206–1208.

Einhorn, L. H., and J. P. Donohue. 1977. Chemotherapy for disseminated testicular cancer. Urol. Clin. North Am. 4:407–426.

Gonzales-Vitale, J. C., D. M. Hayes, E. Cvitkovic, and S. S. Sternberg. 1978. Acute renal failure after cis-dichlorodiammine-platinum (II) and gentamicin cephalothin therapy. Cancer Treat. Rep. 62:683–697.

Hermanek, P. 1977. Testicular cancer, histologic classification and staging, topography of lymph node metastases. Recent Results Cancer Res. 60:202–211.

Higby, D. J., D. J. Wallace, D. Albert, and J. F. Holland. 1974. Diamminodichloroplatinum in the chemotherapy of testicular tumors. J. Urol. 102:100–105.

Holoye, P. Y., M. A. Luna, B. Mackay, and C. W. M. Bedrossian. 1978. Bleomycin hypersensitivity pneumonitis. Ann. Intern. Med. 88:47–49.

Presnov, M. A., A. L. Konovalova, L. F. Romanova, Z. P. Sofina, and A. I. Stetsenko. 1978. Chemotherapy of transplantable mouse tumors with cis-dichlorodiamminoplatinum (II) alone and in combination with sarcolysin. Cancer Treat. Rep. 62:705–715.

Samuels, M. L., P. Y. Holoye, and D. E. Johnson. 1975. Bleomycin combination chemotherapy in the management of testicular neoplasia. Cancer 36:318–326.

Samuels, M. L., D. E. Johnson, and P. Y. Holoye. 1977. Continuous intravenous bleomycin (NSC-125065) therapy with vinblastine (NSC-49842) in stage III testicular neoplasia. Cancer Chemother. Rep. 59:563–570.

Samuels, M. L., V. J. Lanzotti, P. Y. Holoye, L. E. Boyle, T. E. Smith, and D. E. Johnson. 1976. Combination chemotherapy in germinal tumors. Cancer Treat. Rev. 3:185–204.

Sikic, B. I., E. G. Mimnaugh, and T. E. Gram. 1979. Improved therapeutic index of bleomycin order administered by continuous infusion in mice. Cancer Treat. Rep. (in press).

Cancer of the Genitourinary Tract, edited by
D. E. Johnson and M. L. Samuels.
Raven Press, New York © 1979.

Adjuvant Chemotherapy in Metastatic Testicular Neoplasia: Results With Vinblastine-Bleomycin

Melvin L. Samuels, M.D., Douglas E. Johnson, M.D.,* and
R. Bruce Bracken, M.D.*

*Departments of Medicine and *Urology, The University of Texas System Cancer Center
M. D. Anderson Hospital and Tumor Institute, Houston, Texas*

The therapy for patients with metastatic nonseminomatous germinal neoplasia to the retroperitoneal lymph nodes, termed stage II disease, has been classically surgery and radiotherapy. The five-year survival rate with such therapy is generally about 50%. This figure is much better than the poor results with other primary tumors with regional node metastases, such as malignant melanoma, bladder cancer, and breast cancer.

The chemotherapeutic control of widely disseminated testicular cancer (stage III disease) has improved strikingly, with significant long-term survivals and probable cures (Einhorn and Donohue 1977, Samuels et al. 1975, 1976). Thus, even though the 50% survival rate with local modalities of therapy in stage II appears remarkable, it would seem that this could be improved upon by adjuvant chemotherapy, using protocols effective in stage III disease. Adjuvant chemotherapy may also be useful for patients with stage II disease, but would be unsuitable for patients with stage I disease (limited to the testis), for whom there is now a better than 90% five-year survival rate with radical orchiectomy alone (Johnson 1977).

This report summarizes our experience with the administration of adjuvant vinblastine-bleomycin chemotherapy programs since 1971, when bleomycin first became generally available for clinical trials in the United States.

PATIENTS AND METHODS

The study population consists of 32 patients who had all undergone orchiectomy followed by surgery for metastatic disease. Patients seen after December 1977 are not included. The patients have been stratified into a larger group of 27 young male subjects, mean age 25.8 years, who had recently undergone partial or complete retroperitoneal node dissection for stage II disease, and a smaller group of five male subjects with stage III disease, mean age 25 years, who had undergone thoracotomy for pulmonary metastases (four patients) or laparotomy with nephrectomy and node dissection for extensive retroperitoneal disease (one patient). The youngest patient was 16, the oldest 50, and all except one were caucasian. In addition to surgery, six stage II patients had received radiotherapy to the para-aortic nodal region and ipsilateral iliac and inguinal nodes.

The stage II patients were further stratified by examination of the operative records describing the para-aortic node dissection. If the surgeon was able to identify tumor at the time of operation, we classified the presentation as gross disease. There are 21 patients in this subgroup. The remaining six patients demonstrated microscopic disease only.

The chemotherapy programs using vinblastine, intermittent biweekly bleomycin and vinblastine, and continuous infusion bleomycin have been described in the literature (Samuels et al. 1975, 1976) and will not be detailed here. One point concerning vinblastine dosage needs emphasis. The stated range of vinblastine dosage is 0.4 to 0.6 mg/kg in two divided fractions, days 1 and 2. Those patients presenting with residual tumor following retroperitoneal node dissection received the larger dosage of 0.6 mg/kg. Also, five of seven patients presenting with a choriocarcinoma component in their primary tumor received 0.5 or 0.6 mg/kg, while the others received 0.4 mg/kg. The highest single dose of vinblastine given was 53 mg in two fractions. Severe toxic manifestations (myalgia, myelosuppression) can be expected with higher dosage. Further, patients who received prior radiotherapy should not receive more than 0.4 mg/kg or 30 mg, whichever is lower. One patient presenting with persistent paralytic ileus following node dissection in another hospital received only half-dose vinblastine plus intermittent bleomycin, and a second patient presenting in 1969 with stage III disease after thoracotomy received only vinblastine.

Since July 1973, we have used the vinblastine-continuous infusion bleomycin program rather than the intermittent biweekly bleomycin program, as it gives superior results in patients with stage III disease. Recent experimental evidence suggests continuous infusion bleomycin is also superior in the Lewis lung tumor model (Sikic et al., in press). A third program, bleomycin plus COMF (cyclophosphamide, vincristine, methotrexate, and 5-fluorouracil), has been used in teratocarcinoma patients for consolidation and rarely as initial therapy (Samuels et al. 1975). This protocol can be administered to outpatients, whereas vinblastine-continuous infusion bleomycin must be monitored in the hospital, primarily because of severe myelosuppression.

Each patient was scheduled to receive four courses of chemotherapy following completion of surgery, radiotherapy, or both. However, one patient received only two courses because of peripheral neuropathy, one received three courses because of bleomycin-induced interstitial pneumonitis, and four received five or more courses because of bulky retroperitoneal disease at surgery. Follow-up examinations were routine every three months and included chest x-ray exams, complete blood count, and analysis for the presence of alpha-fetoprotein, lactic dehydrogenase isoenzymes, and, recently, human chorionic gonadotropin (HCG) measured by the HCG-beta subunit radioimmunoassay.

A contemporary group of stage II patients treated at M. D. Anderson Hospital with classical radiation and surgery but no chemotherapy served as a historical control population. The five-year period commencing January 1, 1973, and ending December 31, 1977, was chosen for review. Forty-four patients were treated during this time, and they were stratified according to gross or microscopic para-aortic nodal disease, as were the adjuvant patients. An additional 17 patients referred to M. D. Anderson Hospital during this period had received radiotherapy and surgery at other institutions and now presented with stage III disease.

RESULTS

The 32 patients who received adjuvant chemotherapy show a mean survival time of 163 weeks. There have been four deaths, with the remaining patients living and well. (The longest survivor, at 442 weeks, is a postthoracotomy patient who received five courses of vinblastine alone, the only nonbleomycin patient in the group.) Twenty-two of the 32 patients have been followed for two years or more and the estimated proportion surviving at two years is 89% (standard error 6%).

The 27 stage II adjuvant patients show a mean survival of 144 weeks, with three dead and 24 free of gross disease. One death resulted from radiation enteritis with small bowel obstruction at 32 weeks, with the remaining two deaths from tumor. These three deaths were among the 21 patients who presented with gross retroperitoneal disease at the time of surgery. The six stage II patients with microscopic retroperitoneal disease are all alive and well.

Among the five stage III adjuvant patients, one died of sepsis during the third course of chemotherapy (vinblastine-intermittent bleomycin) and *Candida* organisms were cultured from his blood but not found at postmortem. The remaining four patients, all postthoracotomy, are alive and well with a mean survival of 295 weeks.

Table 1 summarizes the data and gives the distribution of patients by Dixon

Table 1. *Survival by Presentation of Patients Receiving Adjuvant Chemotherapy*

Presentation	Total No. Patients	Mean Age	Dixon-Moore Classification			No. NED*	No. Dead	Mean Survival (wks.)
			2	4	5			
Gross disease	21	24	5	12†	4	18	3‡	125
Microscopic disease	6	28	3	3	0	6	0	228
Stage III, adjuvant	6	25	1	4	0	4	1§	240
Total	32		9	19	4	28	4	

* No evident disease.
† Three with choriocarcinoma.
‡ Two tumor deaths at 116 and 172 weeks. The remaining death was from radiation enteritis at 32 weeks.
§ Chemotherapy death, third course.

and Moore (1952) histopathologic classification. In this classification, group 2 is pure embryonal carcinoma, group 4 is teratocarcinoma mixed with embryonal carcinoma, choriocarcinoma, or both, and group 5 is pure choriocarcinoma or, more commonly, choriocarcinoma plus embryonal carcinoma. Seven chorio-carcinoma patients in the gross disease group (Dixon and Moore groups 4 and 5) are alive and well, although a previous study suggested that choriocarcinoma worsens the prognosis of patients with stage III disease in vinblastine-bleomycin programs (Samuels et al. 1976).

Of the 21 patients with gross disease, only three had abnormal levels of bio-markers before surgery and all values returned to normal after the retroperitoneal node dissection was completed. Tumor was found in extranodal connective tissue in eight patients, which is ordinarily considered a poor prognostic sign. In five patients only a partial nodal tumor dissection could be accomplished. After completion of chemotherapy, a second laparotomy was performed and no viable tumor was found in these patients.

The results of the three treatment programs for patients with stage II disease are summarized in Table 2. Note that the two tumor deaths occurred with the intermittent bleomycin program, while the one therapy death occurred in the continuous infusion bleomycin group. Table 3 summarizes the data on the 44 stage II patients treated with surgery and radiotherapy. Twelve patients in this group remain free of disease, while 32 patients have progressed to stage III disease. This gives a disappointing control rate of 27%. Reasons for the apparent failures are the high percentage of gross nodal presentations and the presence of choriocarcinoma. Further, it appears that invasion of the spermatic cord together with nodal disease is associated with aggressive disease and early failure. A comparison of the survival curves for the adjuvant and nonadjuvant chemotherapy populations (Figure 1) shows a highly significant difference ($p < 0.01$).

The major toxicity associated with the vinblastine-bleomycin programs is leukopenia. Virtually all patients develop a severe but short-lived depression

Table 2. *Survival According to Treatment Program in Patients With Stage II Disease*

Adjuvant Treatment	Total No. Patients	Nodal Disease		No. Patients Dead	No. Patients NED
		Gross	Microscopic		
Vinblastine with intermittent bleomycin (VB-1)	6	4	2	2*	4
Vinblastine with continuous infusion bleomycin (VB-3)	19	17	2	1†	18
Bleomycin-COMF	2	0	2	0	2

* Both deaths in the gross tumor group.
† Death from radiation enteritis.

Table 3. *Summary of Data on 44 Stage III Patients Treated With Radiotherapy and Surgery Alone, 1973–1977*

Outcome	Total No. Patients	Gross Nodal Disease	Cord Invasion	Vascular Invasion Primary	Chorio-carcinoma Present	No. Patients NED
Disease controlled	12	2 (16%)	1 (8%)	2 (16%)	0 (0%)	12 (100%)
Disease not controlled (converts to stage III)	32	16 (50%)	6 (19%)	4 (11%)	6 (19%)	15 (47%)

in leukocytes to less than 1,000/mm^3, usually seen between days 6 and 8, and recovery is evident by days 12 to 14. Stomatitis is also a universal finding. Two patients developed sepsis, with one death from *Candida* septicemia, as previously noted. We have observed only one case of bleomycin interstitial pneumonia, which occurred at a total dosage of 450 mg of bleomycin. The patient was treated with prednisone and fully recovered. His pulmonary function is normal three years later.

Also of note were single instances of severe peripheral neuritis secondary to vinblastine administration, activation of a duodenal ulcer, and retroperitoneal fibrosis with obstructive uropathy in a patient who previously received radiotherapy.

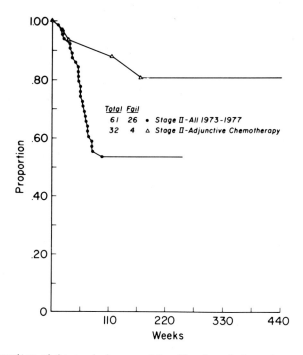

Figure 1. Comparison of the survival curve of the 32 adjuvant chemotherapy patients with that for a control population of 61 patients.

There were three patients with double primaries, two of the opposite testis and one of the colon. All three received adjuvant therapy for stage II disease and are in complete clinical remission.

COMMENTS

An acceptable adjuvant chemotherapy program must be able to induce complete clinical remissions in patients with advanced, widely disseminated cancer and have both acceptable acute toxicity and minimal or no long-term deleterious effects. We believe that vinblastine-continuous infusion bleomycin fulfills these requirements.

Tyrrell and Peckham (1976) divide stage II disease into small volume disease, in which the nodes are 2.0 cm or less in maximum diameter (II-A), and bulky disease, in which the metastatic deposits are greater than 2.0 cm in maximum diameter (II-B). Although they achieved a control rate of 52% overall using radiotherapy alone, stage II-A patients showed an 85% rate of long-term control, which fell to 33% with stage II-B patients. The authors suggest that chemotherapy be used to reduce II-B nodal disease prior to radiotherapy and that surgery be used to remove residual disease. Earle et al. (1973) report 85% of stage II seminoma patients achieve disease-free survival with radiotherapy, but "approximately one half of stage II carcinoma patients [nonseminomatous germinal neoplasia] succumb to their disease." They further note that one year of disease-free survival in the carcinoma patient following standard radiation therapy "means that a patient has a very low risk of recurrence." The results with surgery alone do not appear significantly different from those with radiotherapy. Staubitz (1977) attempted to operate on 72 presumed stage II patients, but found seven inoperable. Twenty of the remaining 65 patients were truly operable stage II, and 12 of these (60%) survived five years. The remaining 45 patients were considered stage I, and 31 (68%) survived five years. In this study inoperable patients succumbed rapidly, usually within one year, and serious postoperation complications, including one death, occurred in 9.7%.

The observed failure rate of 11% in our stage II adjuvant population, which included 78% with advanced presentations and extensive retroperitoneal disease, supports the concept of adjuvant chemotherapy. We would emphasize that our program primarily involves surgery and chemotherapy, with radiation therapy assuming a minor role. We view radiotherapy as chiefly useful for bulky retroperitoneal disease. However, valuable time must not be wasted with elaborate high-dose radiation therapy protocols, for there is the added risk of reduced marrow tolerance to chemotherapy, loss of time in a rapidly evolving tumor, and, uncommonly, production of leukopenia, forcing a delay of several months or more before chemotherapy can be administered.

In our view, all presumed stage I patients (low levels of biomarkers, negative lymphangiogram results) should undergo node dissection, as false-negative lymphangiogram results are noted in 15% of our series and up to 24% in other reports (Hermanek 1977). Biomarker levels are low in patients with stage I disease and seldom higher in those with stage II (11% of our study group). In 152 successive lymphadenectomies, Johnson (1977) noted a 6.5% complication rate with no deaths. He observed that true stage I patients with teratoma, seminoma, or both, have a 100% five-year survival rate, whereas those with teratocarcinoma plus embryonal carcinoma, choriocarcinoma, or both, have a 93% five-year survival rate and those with pure embryonal carcinoma have a 74% five-year survival rate. Thus, stage I disease remains primarily a surgical problem, with the possible exception of that involving embryonal carcinoma. Nodal dissection is required for staging, even though ejaculatory incompetence with sterility will result in most patients. Sperm banking is offered in our institution prior to surgery.

Our present programs appear capable of managing patients with retroperitoneal cancer, so we would discourage the use of cis-diamminedichloroplatinum in patients with stage II disease. This drug is now an integral part of many stage III programs (Einhorn and Donohue 1977), but we do not endorse its use with stage II disease. The major drawbacks are acute renal toxicity, ototoxicity, and the increased risk of aminoglycoside renal toxicity (Samuels et al. 1977, Dentino et al. 1977). The vinblastine-bleomycin program produces acute, reversible, short-lived toxicity with minimal or no significant long-term complications.

REFERENCES

Dentino, M. E., M. N. Yum, R. J. Rohn, L. H. Einhorn, and F. C. Luft. 1977. The long-term effect of cis-platinum diamminedichloride (CPDD) on renal function in man. Proc. Am. Assoc. Cancer Res. 18:116.

Dixon, F. J., and R. A. Moore. 1952. Atlas of Tumor Pathology. Sec. 8, fasc. 316 and 332. Tumors of the Male Sex Organs. Armed Forces Institute of Pathology, Washington, D.C.

Earle, J. D., M. A. Bagshaw, and H. S. Kaplan. 1973. Supervoltage radiation therapy of the testicular tumors. Am. J. Roentgenol. Rad. Ther. Nucl. Med. 117:653–661.

Einhorn, L. H., and J. Donohue. 1977. Cis-diamminedichloroplatinum, vinblastine, and bleomycin combination in disseminated testicular cancer. Ann. Intern. Med. 87:293–297.

Hermanek, P. 1977. Testicular cancer, histologic classification and staging, topography of lymph node metastases. Recent Results Cancer Res. 60:202–211.

Johnson, D. E. 1977. Retroperitoneal lymphadenectomy: Indications, complications, and expectations. Recent Results Cancer Res. 60:221–230.

Samuels, M. L., P. Y. Holoye, and D. E. Johnson. 1975. Bleomycin combination chemotherapy in the management of testicular neoplasia. Cancer 36:318–326.

Samuels, M. L., V. J. Lanzotti, P. Y. Holoye, L. E. Boyle, T. E. Smith, and D. E. Johnson. 1976. Combination chemotherapy in germinal tumors. Cancer Treat. Rev. 3:185–204.

Sikic, B. I., E. G. Mimnaugh, and T. E. Gram. 1979. Improved therapeutic index of bleomycin when administered by continuous infusion in mice. Cancer Treat. Rep. (in press).

Staubitz, W. J. 1977. Surgical treatment of non-seminomatous germinal testes tumors. Recent Results Cancer Res. 60:215–226.

Tyrrell, C. J., and M. J. Peckham. 1976. The response of lymph node metastases of testicular teratoma to radiation therapy. Br. J. Urol. 48:363–370.

Cancer of the Genitourinary Tract, edited by
D. E. Johnson and M. L. Samuels.
Raven Press, New York © 1979.

Platinum Combination Chemotherapy in Disseminated Testicular Cancer

Lawrence H. Einhorn, M.D.

Department of Medicine, Indiana University Medical Center, Veterans Administration Hospital, Indianapolis, Indiana

Although testicular cancer accounts for only 1% of all malignant tumors in males, it ranks first in incidence of cancer deaths in the 25–34-year age group (MacKay and Sellers 1966). Thus, cancer of the testis has a significant impact on the social, economic, and emotional status of this young population.

In 1960, Li and associates introduced the first major chemotherapeutic regimen for advanced testicular cancer with a combination of actinomycin-D, chlorambucil, and methotrexate (Li et al. 1960). Subsequent studies confirmed a 50–70% response rate, which included 10–20% complete remissions (Ansfield et al. 1969, MacKenzie 1966). The past 15 years have also seen the development of many new agents with substantial activity, notably vinblastine (Samuels and Howe 1970), bleomycin (Blum et al. 1973), and mithramycin (Kennedy 1970). A major significant achievement of these single-agent studies was the demonstration not only that complete remissions could be obtained in disseminated testicular cancer, but that approximately half of these complete remissions were permanent (Ansfield et al. 1969, MacKenzie 1966, Samuels and Howe 1970, and Kennedy 1970). Most relapses occurred within two years of initiation of chemotherapy.

Combination chemotherapy has produced excellent long-term complete remissions in other chemosensitive diseases, such as Hodgkin's disease (DeVita et al. 1970). Likewise, most recent attempts at improved chemotherapy in testicular cancer have been with combination chemotherapy. One of the most widely used combinations has been vinblastine and bleomycin (Samuels et al. 1975).

Cis-diamminedichloroplatinum is one of a group of coordination compounds of platinum identified by Rosenberg and co-workers (1965) that strongly inhibit bacterial replication. This agent has significant activity in refractory advanced testicular cancer and, furthermore, is ideal for combination chemotherapy because of its relative lack of myelosuppression (Higby et al. 1974). We believe that platinum is the most effective agent in the treatment of disseminated testicular cancer.

MATERIALS AND METHODS

One hundred twenty-nine patients with disseminated testicular cancer were the subjects of these studies. Fifty patients were treated from August 1974 to September 1976 as follows:

1. Platinum, 20 mg/m^2 i.v. (over 15 minutes) daily for five days, once every three weeks for three courses. A fourth course was given if complete remission not achieved with three courses. Saline hydration was started at least 12 hours prior to platinum administration and continued throughout the five-day course at rate of 100 cc/hour of normal saline.

2. Bleomycin, 30 units i.v. weekly for 12 weeks.

3. Vinblastine, 0.2 mg/kg i.v. daily for two days every three weeks. Vinblastine was given six hours before bleomycin, and maintenance vinblastine (0.3 mg/kg every four weeks) was initiated after completion of bleomycin and continued for two years.

Three patients were inevaluable because of early death (due to massive carcinoma) prior to completion of two weeks of therapy.

Initially, bacillus Calmette-Guérin (BCG) immunotherapy was given if complete remission was achieved in an attempt to augment host cell-mediated immunity and prolong complete remission. More recently we have questioned the value of administering BCG to such patients, and in the past two years we have not employed any immunotherapy. Since the relapse rate remains at a very low level despite cessation of BCG, it appears unlikely that BCG contributed any therapeutic advantage. Administration of vinblastine six hours prior to bleomycin, in an attempt to synchronize tumor cells for maximal destruction by bleomycin, has also been abandoned, and we now give vinblastine and bleomycin at the same time.

Seventy-nine patients were treated, from September 1976 to June 1978, as follows:

1. Platinum, 20 mg/m^2 for five days every three weeks, for three or four courses.

2. Bleomycin, 30 units i.v. weekly for 12 weeks.

3. Vinblastine, 0.4 mg/kg, 0.3 mg/kg, or 0.2 mg/kg every three weeks. Patients who received 0.2 mg/kg also received Adriamycin, 50 mg/m^2 every three weeks.

After 12 weeks of bleomycin, maintenance therapy was initiated on all three arms, consisting of vinblastine, 0.3 mg/kg monthly, for two years.

A partial remission was defined as a decrease of 50% or more in the sum of the products of diameters of all measurable lesions. A complete response was defined as a complete disappearance of all clinical, radiographic, and biochemical evidence of disease, including normal whole lung tomograms, serum human chorionic gonadotropin, alpha-fetoprotein, computerized abdominal tomography (CAT) scan, and ultrasonogram. Anything less was not considered a complete remission.

RESULTS

Since the results for the first group of patients have previously been reported (Einhorn and Donohue 1977), only the updated results will be discussed.

The complete remission rate was 70% (33 complete remissions in 47 evaluable patients). Five more patients (11%) were rendered disease free following surgical removal of residual disease. The tumors in three of these patients were found to have histologically converted from embryonal carcinoma to benign mature teratoma, and the patients remain free of disease 2½ to 3½ years postoperatively. The two patients who had persistent embryonal carcinoma surgically resected relapsed on maintenance vinblastine and died shortly thereafter.

Only six of these 33 patients with chemotherapy-induced complete remissions have relapsed. One patient relapsed on vinblastine maintenance therapy; subsequent therapy with Adriamycin, bleomycin, and vincristine was unsuccessful, and he died shortly after relapse. One patient refused maintenance therapy and was temporarily lost to follow-up; he returned moribund with massive pulmonary metastases and died within 24 hours of readmission. The other four patients relapsed on maintenance vinblastine. Although three of these four patients achieved a second remission with reinduction with platinum, Adriamycin, vincristine, and bleomycin, they all subsequently relapsed. Interestingly, two of these patients are in a third complete remission with platinum plus the epipodophyllotoxin derivative, VP-16. It is noteworthy that five of these six relapses occurred within nine months of chemotherapy administration, and the only other relapse occurred at 17 months.

The toxicity of this regimen has previously been described (Einhorn and Donohue 1977). The major serious toxicity was severe granulocytopenia. Eighteen patients required hospitalization for presumed sepsis. Seven of these patients had documented sepsis, and one died of sepsis.

Despite excellent complete remission and survival rates with this regimen, we were concerned about toxicity. Although platinum is potentially nephrotoxic, nephrotoxicity is only rarely a clinical problem when vigorous saline hydration is employed. Likewise, clinically significant bleomycin pulmonary fibrosis is an uncommon complication. Thus, the major serious toxicity is related to high-dose (0.4 mg/kg) vinblastine. Myalgia, constipation, and paralytic ileus were all troublesome side effects, but severe granulocytopenia and potential sepsis were the most worrisome toxicities.

Since there were no firm data indicating such high doses of vinblastine were required for optimal therapeutic effect, we started a random prospective trial in September 1976 comparing our standard platinum, vinblastine (0.4 mg/kg), bleomycin regimen with a similar regimen using a lower dose (0.3 mg/kg) of vinblastine. Because of encouraging results achieved with platinum and Adriamy-

Table 1. *Results With Platinum, Vinblastine, Bleomycin (PVB), and Optional Adriamycin*

Variable	PVB (0.3 mg/kg)	PVB (0.4 mg/kg)	PVB + Adriamycin	Total
Number of patients	27	26	26	79
Complete remissions	16 (59%)	18 (69%)	19 (73%)	53 (67%)
Partial remissions	10 (37%)	8 (31%)	6 (23%)	24 (30%)
Disease free after surgery	3 (11%)	5 (19%)	2 (8%)	10 (13%)
Relapses*	2/19 (10%)	4/23 (17%)	1/21 (5%)	7/63 (9%)
Number alive	22 (81%)	24 (92%)	21 (81%)	67 (85%)
Number currently NED	17 (63%)	18 (69%)	20 (77%)	55 (70%)

* Includes patients in complete remission and those rendered disease free following surgical removal of residual disease.

cin in patients who had progressed on vinblastine and bleomycin (Einhorn and Williams 1978), we decided to add a third arm to the random prospective study evaluating Adriamycin as first-line chemotherapy in combination with platinum, vinblastine, and bleomycin. Patients on all three arms received identical maintenance therapy (vinblastine 0.3 mg/kg every four weeks for a total of two years of therapy).

Seventy-nine patients have been entered on this random prospective study, and the results are summarized in Table 1. The complete remission rate (67%) and surgical resection rate for localized residual disease (13%) were remarkably similar to those with our original platinum, vinblastine, and bleomycin study (70% and 11%, respectively). The relapse rate remains low. There have been no drug-related deaths in these 79 patients; however, one patient died of a pulmonary embolus three months after laparotomy for removal of residual embryonal carcinoma. An autopsy failed to reveal any evidence of gross or microscopic carcinoma. Fifty-five patients (70%) remain continuously free of disease, and 67 patients (85%) remain alive.

DISCUSSION

Since the original report by Li et al. (1960) demonstrating activity of chemotherapy in disseminated testicular cancer, there have been numerous clinical trials evaluating a variety of drugs in testicular cancer. One point that is clear from the studies in the 1960s is that over 50% of these early complete remissions were apparent cures, and most relapses occurred during the first year of chemotherapy, with a smaller number in the second year (Li et al. 1960, Ansfield et al. 1969, MacKenzie 1966, Samuels and Howe 1970, and Kennedy 1970).

During the past five years, we have treated 129 patients with disseminated testicular cancer. One hundred one of these patients have achieved a disease-free status (86 with chemotherapy alone and 15 with chemotherapy and surgery). Only 15 of these patients have relapsed and all relapses occurred within one year of initiation of chemotherapy, except for one relapse occurring at 17 months.

Our experience with combination chemotherapy in patients with advanced testicular cancer allows us to suggest the following guidelines:

1. The goal of therapy in all patients should be complete remission; if a clinically complete remission is not achieved after three courses of cis-platinum in a responding patient, a fourth course should be given. We have not found any value in exceeding four courses.

2. If a clinically complete remission has not been achieved with chemotherapy, surgical excision of residual disease should be considered. The two clinical situations in which this is feasible include:

a. Complete disappearance of pulmonary metastases except for a solitary residual nodule or nodules confined to a single lobe of the lung; wedge resection is the preferred surgical approach.

b. Persistent abdominal disease. We do an exploratory laparotomy with removal of any residual tumor in patients who initially present with disseminated disease and achieve complete eradication of pulmonary metastases (confirmed by whole lung tomograms) but still have evidence of persistent abdominal disease (palpable abdominal mass or persistently abnormal abdominal CAT scan or ultrasonogram). It has not been necessary to do a laparotomy or retroperitoneal node dissection in any of the other patients in this series, despite the fact that many had evidence of abdominal disease initially.

3. The major toxicity with this therapeutic regimen has been the significant leukopenia and potential granulocytopenic sepsis secondary to vinblastine administration. However, preliminary results indicate that lower dosages of vinblastine will produce equivalent therapeutic results with less toxicity. Any patient who has received radiotherapy should have a 25% dosage reduction of vinblastine.

4. We hospitalize any patient with a temperature above 38.3° C and fewer than 1,000 granulocytes/mm^3, obtain appropriate cultures, and institute broad-spectrum antibiotic coverage with a cephalosporin and carbenicillin. We try to avoid aminoglycosides because of possible renal tubular damage caused by synergism between cis-platinum and aminoglycoside antibiotics. Some of the more significant transient nephrotoxicity in our earlier patients was seen in this clinical situation when aminoglycosides were used.

5. Vigorous attention is paid to saline hydration, regardless of the patient's oral intake. All patients receive 100 cc/hour normal saline intravenous hydration for 12 hours prior to institution of chemotherapy and for the entire five-day course of cis-platinum.

Platinum, vinblastine, and bleomycin with or without Adriamycin consistently produce a 60–70% complete remission rate, with a further 10–15% of patients rendered disease free following surgical removal of residual disease. Furthermore, chemotherapy can significantly alter the course of this disease, even when a complete remission is not seen, producing a more benign histologic form of tumor (teratoma) and perhaps accounting for the prolonged partial remissions seen in several cases.

The results of platinum combination chemotherapy regimens clearly indicate that disseminated testicular cancer is very responsive to chemotherapy, and a high percentage of patients are potentially curable, even with far-advanced disease. The complete remission rate of 65–70% and overall disease-free rate of 80% are as high as have been seen in any adult malignant disease treated with chemotherapy.

ACKNOWLEDGMENT

This investigation was supported in part by Public Health Service grant MO1 RROO 750–06.

REFERENCES

Ansfield, F. J., B. D. Korbitz, H. L. Davis, Jr., and G. Ramirez. 1969. Triple therapy in testicular tumors. Cancer 24:442–446.

Blum, R. H., S. Carter, and K. Agre. 1973. A clinical review of bleomycin—A new antineoplastic agent. Cancer 31:903–914.

DeVita, V. T., A. A. Serpick, and P. P. Carbone. 1970. Combination chemotherapy in the treatment of advanced Hodgkin's disease. Ann. Intern. Med. 73:881–895.

Einhorn, L. H., and J. P. Donohue. 1977. Cis-diamminedichloroplatinum, vinblastine, and bleomycin combination chemotherapy in disseminated testicular cancer. Ann. Intern. Med. 87:293–298.

Einhorn, L. H., and S. D. Williams. 1978. Combination chemotherapy with cis-diamminedichloroplatinum and Adriamycin in testicular cancer refractory to vinblastine plus bleomycin. Cancer Treat. Rep. 62:1351–1353.

Higby, D. J., H. J. Wallace, D. J. Albert, and J. F. Holland. 1974. Diamminedichloroplatinum: A phase I study showing responses in testicular and other tumors. Cancer 33:1219–1225.

Kennedy, B. J. 1970. Mithramycin therapy in advanced testicular neoplasms. Cancer 26:755–766.

Li, M. C., W. F. Whitmore, R. Golbey, and H. Grabstald. 1960. Effects of combined drug therapy on metastatic cancer of the testis. J.A.M.A. 174:145–153.

MacKay, E. N., and A. H. Sellers. 1966. A statistical review of malignant testicular tumors based on the experience of the Ontario Cancer Foundation Clinics, 1938–1961. Can. Med. Assoc. J. 94:389–399.

MacKenzie, A. R. 1966. Chemotherapy of metastatic testis cancer—Results in 154 patients. Cancer 19:1369–1376.

Rosenberg, B., L. VanCamp, and T. Krigas. 1965. Inhibition of cell division in *E. coli* by electrolysis products from a platinum electrode. Nature 205:678–699.

Samuels, M. L., and C. D. Howe. 1970. Vinblastine in the management of testicular cancer. Cancer 25:1009–1017.

Samuels, M. L., D. E. Johnson, and P. Y. Holoye. 1975. Continuous intravenous bleomycin therapy with vinblastine in stage III testicular neoplasia. Cancer Chemother. Rep. 59:563–570.

PROSTATIC CARCINOMA

Cancer of the Genitourinary Tract, edited by
D. E. Johnson and M. L. Samuels.
Raven Press, New York © 1979.

Prostatic Carcinoma: Significance of Histopathological Findings

F. K. Mostofi, M.D.

Department of Genitourinary Pathology, Armed Forces Institute of Pathology, Washington, D.C.

Histopathology plays a significant role in the correct diagnosis of carcinoma of the prostate, as well as in the clinical management of patients with this disease.

PATHOLOGICAL DIAGNOSIS OF CARCINOMA OF PROSTATE

We have discussed earlier the criteria for pathological diagnosis of carcinoma of the prostate and lesions that simulate carcinoma (Mostofi and Price 1973). Briefly, three criteria are used to diagnose prostatic carcinoma: cellular anaplasia, invasion, and disturbances of architecture.

Variations in size, shape, and staining of cells and nuclei and increased mitotic activity are generally used in diagnosing carcinoma. In prostatic carcinoma cells, vacuolization of the nucleus, coarse chromatin distribution, and a single, irregularly outlined nucleolus, if present, can help in the recognition of anaplasia. More frequently, the nucleus has a homogeneous, pale staining appearance. One reliable feature of malignant disease is variation in nuclear size.

Only 8% of prostatic tumors show marked anaplasia. In more than half of carcinomas anaplastic changes are moderate, while in 34% the anaplasia is slight or absent, and mitotic figures and giant cells are only rarely present. Thus, anaplasia is not always a dependable indicator of malignant disease in the prostate.

Invasion through the basement membrane is difficult to recognize in prostatic carcinoma. However, invasion of the stroma may be detected if the acini are in intimate relationship to the smooth muscle bundles. Transmission and scanning electron microscopy may also reveal invasion of the stroma.

Perineural invasion is a valuable pathognomonic feature of carcinoma; however, many transurethral resections (TUR) or needle biopsies, especially those that produce problematic results, do not show it. Perineural spaces are not

---

The opinions or assertions contained herein are the private views of the author and are not to be construed as official or as reflecting the views of the Department of the Army or the Department of Defense.

lymphatics; they are quite common in total prostatectomy specimens removed from patients with stage A and B tumors and have no prognostic significance (Byar and Mostofi 1972). Very rarely in TUR and only occasionally in needle biopsies does one see invasion of seminal vesicles or the capsule or periprostatic fibroadipose tissue. In such cases pathological recognition becomes easy, but the urologist should be informed of the periprostatic location of carcinoma in the diagnosis.

An area that has received little attention is intraprostatic lymphatic or vascular invasion, but this is often absent or undetected.

Thus, disturbances of architecture become the most important and frequently used criterion for diagnosing carcinoma of the prostate. Haphazard distribution of glands, glands closely packed together with little or no intervening stroma, small or microacinar glands, large glands without convolutions, small and large glands side by side, fused glands and glands in glands (cribriform), solid sheets, and columns and cords with little or no gland formation are manifestations of disturbances of architecture. The presence of one or more of these is diagnostic of carcinoma of prostate. It is the interpretation of these architectural disturbances, however, that often leads to disagreements in diagnosis.

In problem cases, we prepare additional sections and carefully search for nuclear changes and perineural invasion.

ROLE OF PATHOLOGY IN CLINICAL MANAGEMENT OF PROSTATIC CARCINOMA PATIENTS

About six years ago we undertook a systematic study of the histopathology of carcinoma of the prostate (Mostofi 1975, Harada et al. 1977) to determine if any one or combination of histological features had clinical significance. The material consisted of about 1,000 cases from the first Veterans Administration Cooperative Urological Research Group (1964), which involved 665 needle biopsies, 181 transurethral resections, and 141 total prostatectomies. Microscopic slides stained with hematoxylin and eosin were available for study. The clinical data and follow-up information were sent to Dr. David Byar of the National Cancer Institute, and a checklist was devised for pathological examination, which has since been published (Mostofi 1975). About 60 items could be grouped together under histological pattern, cytology, and associated lesions. Death rates were calculated by the number of deaths divided by total patient months of follow-up, expressed in deaths per 1,000 patient months. All patients were followed for at least five years. A preliminary report of the findings has been published (Harada et al. 1977) and a more detailed report is now being prepared.

I shall confine myself to three areas that appear to be of greatest prognostic significance.

Two major problems in basing a prognosis on histological grounds, as applied to carcinoma of the prostate, are defining differentiation and recognizing slight or moderate anaplasia. Differentiation and anaplasia have often been used synon-ymously or confused with each other (Mostofi 1976).

If we remember that normal development and maturation of the prostate result in the formation of tubuloacinar structures with large and small glands, tumors that produce such glands could justifiably be regarded as differentiated, and those that do not, as undifferentiated. Since the prostate normally consists of small and large glands, tumors that contain such glands could be regarded as well differentiated, those in which the glands are fused or cribriform, as moderately differentiated, and those that form no glands but consist of solid sheets or columns and cords, as undifferentiated.

We found that tumors that consisted of large or small glands were accompanied by extremely low death rates (2.7 and 1.2, respectively), tumors with fused glands and cribriform pattern, by a moderate death rate (9.5), and tumors that consisted of solid sheets or columns and cords, by a high death rate (17.2) (Table 1).

A second finding was that a critical level in the amount of various patterns in a given tumor seemed to be required for those patterns to have an effect on death rates. For example, up to 10% of the tumor could consist of cribriform pattern or solid sheets or columns and cords without seriously affecting the death rate (Table 1). This suggests that the amount of a pattern, rather than simply its presence, is important in prognosis, and that assigning equal values to both, as proposed by Gleason and Mellinger (1974), is not justified.

We have already defined anaplasia as slight, moderate, or marked variation of the nucleus from normal. The death rate for those with slight anaplasia was 1.24, with moderate anaplasia, 4.51, and with marked anaplasia, 14.88.

The study confirmed a previous observation Dr. Byar and I (Byar and Mostofi 1972) had made that perineural invasion has no prognostic significance, whereas

Table 1. *Death Rates Related to Pattern of Tumor*

Pattern	Percent of Tumor	Death Rate
Large glands	0–10	5.1
	11–50	2.7
Small glands	0–10	17.9
	11–30	7.8
	31–60	5.1
	61–100	1.2
Fused glands	0–10	3.9
	11–20	6.5
	21–50	7.9
	51–100	9.5
Cribriform	0–10	4.4
	11–40	5.8
	41–90	9.5
Medullary	0–10	3.5
Columns and cords	11–30	9.3
	31–100	17.2

invasion of the seminal vesicle, penetration of the capsule, and extension to the bladder neck carry a poor prognosis. A number of other factors, such as cell size, the presence of a nucleolus, the relationship of glands to stroma, and the presence of associated hyperplasia, atrophy, or inflammatory reaction, also affected death rates, but to a lesser extent. The two most important factors were differentiation and anaplasia.

In a recent conference held in Buffalo and chaired by Drs. Murphy and Whitmore, it developed that grading systems advocated by Farrow, Gaeta, Gleason, and Mostofi all worked, but none could be applied to individual patients, indicating that grading is of limited value in arriving at a prognosis in individual cases. This may be due to the fact that, in our preoccupation with devising a grading system, we have ignored two important areas: lymphatic and vascular invasion and the cell itself.

Although I have in the past (Mostofi 1952, Mostofi and Price 1973) called attention to lymphatic and vascular invasion as an important feature of carcinoma of the prostate, as far as I can determine there has been only one recent mention of such invasion (Catalona and Scott 1978). Why have we ignored lymphatic and vascular invasion in our reports on carcinoma of the prostate? There are several reasons for this, including the paucity of tissue, the shrinkage artifact, and the fact that at times the vessels are packed and almost completely obliterated by the tumor. These all make recognition of such invasion difficult. Furthermore, the erroneous impression has persisted that the prostate has no lymphatic vessels.

Surgical staging of carcinoma of the prostate by means of lymphadenectomy has shown that in 20–25% of stage A and B cancers, tumors that are locally confined to the prostate, there is regional lymph node metastasis (Whitmore 1973). Radioimmunoassays of prostatic acid phosphatase and various scanning methods have revealed that 5–20% of those stage A and B tumors have metastasized to the bone. So, based on the natural history of these untreated tumors, it is clear that lymphatic and vascular invasion does occur in carcinoma of the prostate. We pathologists must find a way to demonstrate this in the biopsy and alert the urologist. It may be that, by studying the cell itself, we will be able to determine if it can metastasize.

Until quite recently we had failed to recognize the pleomorphism of cell populations in carcinoma of the prostate. By the use of electron microscopy, Sinha et al. (1977) have recognized two cell types and Kastendieck and Altenähr (1976) have identified five. Stimulated by these studies, we have found that, by light microscopy, we can recognize as many as four different cell types in carcinoma of the prostate. What is the significance of such pleomorphism? We know that, in experimental animals, enzyme changes on the surface of the cell affect whether or not the tumor cell will metastasize and metastases will flourish. The need for studying receptor sites, surface enzymes, etc., cannot be overemphasized.

CONCLUSIONS

We have demonstrated that tumors that are well differentiated or show slight to moderate anaplasia are associated with a good prognosis, while those that are undifferentiated or show marked anaplasia carry a poor prognosis. We have not given adequate consideration to the tumor cell and its function. Light microscopy must be supplemented and greatly expanded by the application of newer techniques so that functional aspects of the cell can be incorporated into the diagnosis and management of patients with carcinoma of the prostate. It is not enough to say that the tumor is moderately differentiated and moderately anaplastic or that the sum of the Gleason principal and secondary patterns is six (Gleason and Mellinger 1974); we must be able to tell precisely what the cell population consists of, whether or not we are dealing with cells that are capable of metastasis or of resisting certain forms of therapy.

In his Health Memorial Award Lecture (Murphy 1979, see pages 5 to 24, this volume), Dr. Murphy said that none of the progress he reported in carcinoma of the prostate would have been possible without the organ site program support. I hope that pathologists and allied scientists can get the support they need to apply modern techniques to the study of carcinoma of the prostate so that five years from now, or whenever another M. D. Anderson Hospital conference is held on genitourinary tumors, we can report significant progress in individualizing the histopathology of carcinoma of the prostate and be able to say which tumors will respond to what forms of treatment.

REFERENCES

Byar, D. B., and F. K. Mostofi. 1972. Veterans Administration Cooperative Urological Research Group. Carcinoma of the prostate: Prognostic evaluation of certain pathologic features in 208 radical prostatectomies. Cancer 30:5–13.
Catalona, W. J., and W. W. Scott. 1978. Carcinoma of prostate: A review. J. Urol. 119:1–8.
Gleason, D. F., and G. T. Mellinger. 1974. Veterans Administration Cooperative Urological Research Group: Predictions of prognosis for prostatic adenocarcinoma and combined histological grading and clinical staging. J. Urol. 111:58–64.
Harada, M., F. K. Mostofi, D. K. Corle, D. P. Byar, and B. F. Trump. 1977. Preliminary studies of histologic prognosis in cancer of the prostate. Cancer Treat. Rep. 61:223–225.
Kastendieck, H., and E. Altenähr. 1976. Cyto- and histomorphogenesis of prostate carcinoma. Virchows Arch. (Pathol. Anat.) 370:207–224.
Mostofi, F. K. 1952. Criteria for pathological diagnosis of carcinoma of the prostate, in Proceedings of the Second National Cancer Conference. J. B. Lippincott Co., Philadelphia, pp. 332–343.
Mostofi, F. K. 1975. Grading of prostatic carcinoma. Cancer Chemother. Rep. 59:111–117.
Mostofi, F. K. 1976. Problems of grading carcinoma of prostate. Semin. Oncol. 3:161–169.
Mostofi, F. K., and E. B. Price, Jr. 1973. Atlas of Tumor Pathology. 2nd series, Fasc. 8. Tumors of the Male Genital System. Armed Forces Institute of Pathology, Washington, D.C.
Murphy, G. P. 1979. Prostatic cancer: Perspectives on progress, in Cancer of the Genitourinary Tract (The University of Texas System Cancer Center M. D. Anderson Hospital and Tumor Institute 23rd Annual Clinical Conference). New York, Raven Press, pp. 5–24.
Sinha, A. A., C. E. Blackard, and S. S. Ulysses. 1977. A critical analysis of tumor morphology

and hormone treatments in the untreated and estrogen treated responsive and refractory human prostatic carcinoma. Cancer 40:2836–2850.

Veterans Administration Cooperative Urological Research Group. 1964. Carcinoma of the prostate: Analysis of patient morbidity at the 6th month, 12th month, and 18th month follow-up examinations. J. Chron. Dis. 17:207–223.

Whitmore, W. F., Jr. 1973. The natural history of prostatic cancer. Cancer 32:1104–1112.

Cancer of the Genitourinary Tract, edited by
D. E. Johnson and M. L. Samuels.
Raven Press, New York © 1979.

Prostatic Irradiation: Iodine-125 Implantation

Willet F. Whitmore, Jr., M.D., Mostafa Batata, B.Ch., D.M.R.,* and Basil Hilaris, M.D.*

*Urologic Service, Department of Surgery, and *Department of Radiation Therapy, Memorial Sloan-Kettering Cancer Center, New York, New York*

Three factors have made evaluation of the impact of therapy upon the cure and/or survival of patients with prostatic cancer difficult: (1) the occurrence of the disease at a time in life when mortality from causes other than prostatic cancer is high, which is reflected in the fact that more patients die with prostatic cancer than of it; (2) the varied and unpredictable mode and rate of disease progression; and (3) the wide range of treatments that have been used in uncontrolled fashion in patients with various stages of the disease who have been selected by an ever changing and more discerning array of staging techniques. These considerations have made it possible logically to question the contribution of any form of therapy to the cure or survival of patients with any stage of the disease.

Evidence of favorable therapeutic effects from irradiation, limitations in the applicability of ablative surgical treatment, and possible functional advantages of irradiation over surgery and endocrine therapy have encouraged explorations of radiation techniques for the local and regional control of prostatic cancer. The use of iodine-125 for interstitial irradiation of selected prostatic cancers was initiated at the Memorial Sloan-Kettering Cancer Center in February 1970, and a series of publications has described the technique, complications, and early results (Barzell et al. 1977, Hilaris et al. 1972, 1974, 1975, 1977, 1978, Whitmore et al. 1972, 1974, Whitmore 1976). This report will be directed principally at experience in patients with regional lymph node metastases.

METHODS AND MATERIALS

In the years 1970–78, 429 patients underwent pelvic lymph node dissection and ^{125}I implantation for the management of prostatic cancer. This analysis is based upon the 135 (31%) patients who had histologically proven lymph node metastasis (N+).

Patient Selection and Evaluation

Patients were selected for ^{125}I implantation on the basis of the following criteria: (1) an estimated life expectancy, based on the patient's general health, of more than five years, (2) biopsy-proven prostatic cancer, and (3) stage B (T_1, T_2) or C (T_3, T_4) lesions. Patients with stage C lesions that extend beyond the prostatic capsule so as to make *palpable* definition of the apparent local extent of the disease difficult or impossible are not optimal candidates for ^{125}I implantation and may be better managed by external irradiation. This potential difficulty is a limitation because of the technical desirability of being able to palpate clearly the volume to be implanted. Such limitations make comparisons of the effectiveness of ^{125}I implantation and external irradiation, especially in the management of stage C lesions, difficult at best.

Evaluation of each patient included a complete medical history, complete physical examination, blood count, urinalysis, blood chemical screening profile, serum acid and alkaline phosphatase assays (Bodansky technique), intravenous pyelogram, and bone scan or skeletal survey, or both. Lymphangiograms were employed in about one third of the patients, but have been abandoned as a routine procedure. They were not used in determining stage. Bone scans have now replaced skeletal surveys in screening for bone metastases. An elevated serum acid phosphatase level did not exclude a patient from clinical stage C, provided there was no other evidence of distant metastasis. Cystoendoscopy was an invariable final staging technique carried out at the time of projected ^{125}I implantation. Bimanual palpation of the prostate and adjoining structures under anesthesia with and without the endoscope in place contributed to clinical evaluation of the local extent of the disease. Inspection of the bladder, bladder neck, and prostatic urethra provided important information relative to extension of the neoplasm into these areas. Evidence of trigonal or bladder neck invasion generally discouraged use of implantation in favor of external irradiation as a method of treatment.

Bladder outlet obstruction is a complication in patients otherwise suitable for ^{125}I implantation. No final judgment regarding the optimal technique of management has evolved to date. If a patient has an obstructing prostate, ^{125}I implantation may well produce at least a transient aggravation that results in urinary retention. Catheter management of this problem may be difficult because of intolerance of the catheter or urinary tract infection. Transurethral resection of the implanted prostate results in removal of a variable portion of the sources of therapeutic irradiation and leaves a prostatic fossa that must heal under the influence of the residual irradiation. A preliminary "prophylactic" trans-urethral resection removes a variable portion of the prostate, which was intended to support the implant, and thus interferes with the geometry of the implant. If an incomplete resection is done to reduce this effect, a poor functional result may ensue. Alternative methods of management include: (1) a transient trial of endocrine therapy to reduce the size of the obstructing prostate. The success of this depends on the extent to which the obstruction is due to neoplasm and the extent to which the neoplasm is endocrine responsive; (2) proceeding with ^{125}I implantation in the face of obstruction in the hope that implantation will result in sufficiently rapid reduction in prostatic size to obviate the impending obstruction; and (3) limited transurethral resection in conjunction with simultaneous ^{125}I implantation (including partial resection of the opposite prostatic lobe when the disease is clinically limited to one side of the gland). Although each maneuver has been at least occasionally successful, none has proved entirely satisfactory, and bladder outlet obstruction in the patient who is otherwise suitable for ^{125}I implantation remains a disconcerting problem.

Patients were followed at two- to six-month intervals postoperatively. The follow-up routines included evaluation of symptoms and physical findings and serum acid and alkaline phosphatase assays. Chest x-ray exams, bone scans, and intravenous pyelograms were performed at irregular one- to two-year intervals. Symptomatic abnormalities or abnormal physical findings were indications for appropriate specific investigations.

In general, follow-up prostatic biopsies were performed only if urinary symptoms or digital rectal examination suggested local recurrence. The clinical response of the prostate to ^{125}I implantation was judged by serial digital rectal examination and was considered favorable unless there was an increase in the size or degree of the preexisting abnormality. The arbitrary nature of this definition is recognized.

Technique

The patient is placed in a modified lithotomy position and a midline extraperitoneal incision made from the symphysis pubis to the umbilicus. A bilateral extraperitoneal lymph node dissection is carried out beginning just above the common iliac artery bifurcation and extending distally along the external iliac vessels to Poupart's ligament. The dissection includes excision of the fatty, areolar, and nodal tissues along and between the external iliac vessels laterally and the ramifications of the hypogastric vessels onto the bladder medially, including removal of the obturator nodes and vessels. After completion of this dissection, the endopelvic fascia is incised on either side of the prostate to permit palpation of the lateral aspects of the gland. Six-inch 17-gauge needles are then inserted in an anterior-posterior direction into the prostate, a finger in the rectum over an O'Connor drape permitting estimation of the depth of needle insertion and preventing rectal wall perforation. Iodine-125 is a relatively low energy, pure gamma-emitting radionuclide of iodine with a half-life of 60 days. The titanium capsules containing the radionuclide are 4.5 mm long and 0.8 mm in diameter, which permits them to traverse the 17-gauge implantation needles. The low energy of the irradiation reduces protection problems for personnel and leads to a rapid falloff in radiation dose outside the implanted volume. The relatively long half-life of the radionuclide provides a long shelf life and a protracted period of irradiation. Whether or not the latter is an advantage in the management of a generally slowly growing neoplasm such as prostatic cancer remains to be determined. A nomogram is used to determine the number of ^{125}I seeds required to deliver the desired dose, as well as the appropriate intervals between

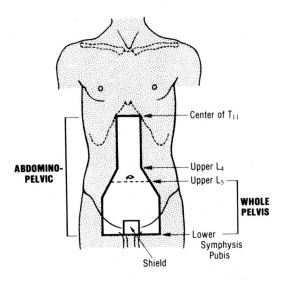

Figure 1. Portals for postoperative external irradiation.

the seeds. The seeds are implanted at the required intervals by means of a simple but specially designed instrument that controls introduction of the seeds as the needles are withdrawn.

Postoperative external irradiation was employed in 28 patients (Figure 1). Such treatment was based upon the possibilities that residual neoplasm near the pelvic lymph node dissection or in the undissected echelon of lymphatic drainage might account for the subsequent development of distal metastases and that appropriate irradiation might lessen this hazard. Irradiation was generally given through opposed, inverted T-shaped portals extending from Tll to the symphysis pubis, shielding the area of implantation (except in rare instances of suboptimal dose distribution) and including the areas of lymphatic drainage around the aorta and vena cava and the common and external iliac (including obturator) vessels. Midplane dosage ranged from 4,000 to 4,600 rads in four to seven weeks by means of megavoltage equipment.

External irradiation was employed in nonrandomized fashion. Patients with positive nodes in the pelvis were given the option of adjunctive pelvic or pelvic *and* para-aortic irradiation without any defined selection.

RESULTS

The results to be presented are based upon 135 patients, all of whom had regional lymph node metastases histologically demonstrated in the surgical specimens obtained during pelvic lymph node dissection. Of these patients, 123 have been followed for six months to seven years.

Lymphangiograms (LAG) were performed on 70 patients who were proven

Table 1. *Relation Between Clinical (T) and Pathological (N) Stage*

Clinical Stage	Pathological Stage		
	N_1	N_2	N_4
T_1 16	7	8	1
T_2 35	11	21	3
T_3 35	14	16	5
T_4 37	9	20	8
Total 123	41 (33%)	65 (53%)	17 (14%)

to have lymph node involvement. In 16 patients with grossly enlarged lymph nodes at operation, the LAG was interpreted as positive in five and negative in 11; in 54 patients with grossly unenlarged nodes at operation, the LAG results were considered positive in 17 and negative in 37. This disappointing 31% accuracy rate has led us to discontinue routine LAG in patients who are candidates for ^{125}I implantation.

The relation between clinical T category and pathologic extent of lymph node involvement revealed by pelvic lymph node dissection is shown in Table 1. The extent of lymph node involvement increases with the size of the primary tumor. Most patients with lymph node metastasis had relatively extensive involvement.

The relationship between T stage, N stage, and tumor grade is indicated in Table 2. Well-differentiated tumors tended to be of lower T and N stage than poorly differentiated lesions, although there were frequent exceptions.

The distribution of lymph node metastases in 123 patients is shown in Table 3. These data must be considered within the context of the dissection performed.

Survival (with and without evidence of prostatic cancer) at two and five years for the various T categories is shown in Table 4. In patients who developed evidence of distant metastases, endocrine therapy was usually initiated and contributed in an unquantitated manner to survival. Patients with low-stage tumors survived better than those with high-stage tumors, as anticipated.

Tables 5, 6, and 7 summarize survival without evidence of recurrence at two or more and five or more years relative to T stage, N stage, and histologic grade, respectively. The only unanticipated finding was the poor survival in

Table 2. *Relation Between Histologic Grade and T Stage and N Stage*

Histologic Grade*	Clinical Stage				Pathologic Stage		
	T_1	T_2	T_3	T_4	N_1	N_2	N_4
I 17	6	6	3	2	8	7	2
II 81	8	25	23	25	29	41	11
III 25	2	4	9	10	4	17	4

* I, well differentiated; II, moderately differentiated; III, poorly differentiated.

Table 3. *Distribution of Involved Lymph Nodes on Lymphadenectomy*

	Stage		
Involved Nodes	N_1 (41 patients)	N_2 (65 patients)	N_4 (17 patients)
Obturator	21	55	12
External iliac	20	44	12
Common iliac	0	0	15
Hypogastric	0	6	1
Para-aortic	0	0	2
Inguinal	0	0	1

Table 4. *Determinate Survival*

Clinical Stage		≥2 Years	≥5 Years
Low	T_1	11/11 (94%)	4/4 (71%)
	T_2	18/20	1/3
High	T_3	19/22 (74%)	5/8 (50%)
	T_4	24/36	10/22
Total		72/89 (81%)	20/37 (54%)

Table 5. *Determinate Survival Without Local or Distal Recurrence According to Clinical Stage*

Clinical Stage		≥2 Years	≥5 Years
Low	T_1	5/11 (58%)	0/4 (14%)
	T_2	13/20	1/3
High	T_3	11/22 (40%)	3/8 (20%)
	T_4	12/36	3/22
Total		41/89 (46%)	7/37 (19%)

Table 6. *Determinate Survival Without Local or Distal Recurrence According to Pathologic Stage*

Pathologic Stage	≥2 Years	≥5 Years
N_1	20/32 (63%)	2/8 (25%)
N_2	18/44 (41%)	4/21 (19%)
N_4	3/13 (23%)	1/8 (13%)

Table 7. *Determinate Survival Without Local or Distal Recurrence According to Histologic Grade*

Histologic Grade	≥2 Years	≥5 Years
I	3/10 (30%)	0/3 (0%)
II	30/57 (53%)	6/25 (24%)
III	8/22 (36%)	1/9 (11%)

the patients with low-grade lesions, but the number of cases is small. Whether the apparent freedom from recurrence at five or more years in the various categories reflects the success of therapy or the natural history of the disease is, of course, uncertain, but it is notable in any event, since all patients in all categories had proven lymph node metastasis.

The present status of 123 patients followed six months or more is shown in Table 8. The important feature is that a few patients who had positive nodes are alive five or more years later without evidence of recurrence.

In 51 (41%) of the 123 patients disease recurred; distant metastases alone occurred in 31, compared to local recurrence in seven and both distant metastases and local recurrence in 13. Treatment failure is related to the duration of follow-up in Table 9. The fact that a significant number of the treatment failures in this ongoing experience become evident more than two years after treatment is not surprising.

The clinical (T) and pathologic (N) stages for the 28 patients who received supplemental external irradiation to the pelvis alone or to pelvic and para-aortic areas are listed in Table 10. There was no apparent overall survival advantage at two or more and five or more years for those who did or did not receive irradiation (Table 11), nor was there any evidence of favorable effect of supplemental irradiation on the proportion of patients surviving without recurrence (Table 12). Furthermore, external irradiation did not demonstrably reduce distal or local recurrence in any of the T categories (Table 13). In Table 14 the relationship of N category to treatment failure in patients who did or did not receive external irradiation is indicated. Again, no advantage to supplemental external irradiation was demonstrated.

Table 15 indicates that complications of ^{125}I implantation and pelvic lymph

Table 8. *Status of Patients Followed Six Months or More*

Status	Years	No. of Patients	
Alive Without Recurrence	≥ 5	7	(58%)
	< 5	64	
With Recurrence	≥ 5	9	(25%)
	< 5	22	
Dead Without Recurrence	≥ 5	0	(1%)
	< 5	1*	
With Recurrence	≥ 5	4	(16%)
	< 5	16	

* Postoperative death.

Table 9. *Interval Between Treatment and Failure*

Type of Failure	6 Months	1 Year	2 Years	≥5 Years
Distant metastases only	3	9	25	31
Local recurrence only	—	—	4	7
Dist. mets. + loc. recurrence	—	2	6	13

Table 10. *Clinical and Pathologic Stages in Patients Treated With Postoperative External Irradiation*

	Pelvis Only			Pelvis + Para-aortic		
Stage	T_2	T_3	T_4	T_2	T_3	T_4
N_1 4	2	—	2	—	—	—
N_2 18	5	—	5	—	2	6
N_4 6	—	1	2	1	—	2
Total 28	7	1	9	1	2	8

Table 11. *Determinate Survival With and Without Postoperative External Irradiation*

External Irradiation	≥2 Years	≥5 Years
None	54/65 (83%)	13/34 (54%)
Pelvis only	12/14 (75%)	3/5 (54%)
Pelvis + para-aortic	6/10	4/8

Table 12. *Determinate Survival Without Local or Distal Recurrence With and Without External Irradiation*

External Irradiation	≥2 Years	≥5 Years
None	31/66 (47%)	5/24 (21%)
Pelvis only	6/14 (42%)	0/5 (15%)
Pelvis + para-aortic	4/10	2/8

Table 13. *Treatment Failure According to T Stage With and Without Postoperative External Irradiation*

External Irradiation	T_2	T_3	T_4
None	7/27 (26%)	10/32 (31%)	12/20 (60%)
Pelvis only	1/7 (25%)	1/1 (33%)	6/9 (71%)
Pelvis + para-aortic	1/1	0/2	6/8
Total	9/35 (26%)	11/35 (31%)	24/37 (65%)

Table 14. *Treatment Failure According to N Stage With and Without Postoperative External Irradiation*

External Irradiation	N_1	N_2	N_4*
None	10/37 (27%)	20/47 (43%)	6/11 (55%)
Pelvis only	2/4 (50%)	3/10 (39%)	3/3 (100%)
Pelvis + para-aortic	—	4/8	3/3
Total	12/41 (29%)	27/65 (42%)	12/17 (71%)

* Involved common iliac lymph nodes.

Table 15. *Treatment Complications With and Without Postoperative External Irradiation*

Complication	No Ext. Rad. 95 Patients	Ext. Rad. 17 Patients*	11 Patients†
Early			
Death	1	0	0
Wound infection and/or delayed healing	8 (14%)	0	1 (18%)
Thrombophlebitis or pulmonary embolism	4	0	1
Late			
Lymphedema of pubis, groin, or lower extremities	6	4	5
Bowel, bladder, urethral stenosis, ulcer, or bleeding	3 (18%)	1 (41%)	0 (55%)
Impaired sexual function‡	8	2	1

* Whole pelvis; † whole pelvis + para-aortic irradiation.
‡ Prior estrogen therapy in six.

node dissection were more frequent when supplemental external irradiation was employed. The complications of pelvic lymph node dissection and ^{125}I implantation have been discussed in detail elsewhere (Fowler et al., in press). There was one postoperative death from pulmonary embolism in the 135 patients included in this report. Lymphedema was infrequent and mild after surgery alone, but was a more significant problem in patients receiving supplemental irradiation. The bowel, bladder, and urethral complications after implantation were mild and transient.

DISCUSSION

Iodine-125 implantation has proved a technically feasible means of delivering radiation therapy to the prostate. Case selection involves particular attention to the extent of the local lesion, since a good implantation requires that the treatment volume be defined accurately by palpation. This means that cases must be more carefully selected for ^{125}I implantation than for external irradiation. Although the operative procedure has been generally well tolerated, it is not a minor one and some morbidity, and even mortality, must currently be anticipated.

The technique has provided significant information regarding regional lymph node metastases. Whether or not lymph node dissection has any therapeutic value remains to be determined; if not, prostatic cancer would be unique among visceral cancers since virtually all others have at least limited potential for cure when lymph node metastasis has occurred. Although the frequency of lymph node metastasis has been revealed by a wide range of experiences in the treatment of carcinoma of the prostate, the selection criteria involved in such programs, as in this experience with ^{125}I implantation, have not excluded the possibility that direct hematogenous dissemination occurs in some patients with prostatic cancer. In any event, this experience has clearly demonstrated the generally ominous significance of lymph node involvement, but has not excluded the possibility that some patients with nodal metastases may be cured by appropriate treatment (Barzell et al. 1977). The extent of nodal metastases increases with the clinical stage of the primary tumor. Although the obturator and external iliac nodes were the most frequently involved, such generalizations must be tempered by the nature of the sampling performed. At five years, more than three fourths of the patients with lymph node metastases have developed evidence of treatment failure. The criteria of tumor control used in this study leave open the question of whether or not the tumor has been locally destroyed by the treatment. Nevertheless, the local control rate, within the limitations of the definitions, implies either that the implantation of ^{125}I has some effect on local tumor control or that the local growth of prostatic tumors is often extremely protracted.

The data on the use of postoperative external irradiation, although not the results of a randomized trial, suggest that supplemental external irradiation to the pelvis or to the pelvis and para-aortic area in patients with positive nodes does not improve survival or reduce recurrence rates.

SUMMARY AND CONCLUSIONS

1. Analysis of an ongoing experience with ^{125}I implantation and bilateral pelvic lymph node dissection at MSK revealed histological evidence of regional lymph node metastases in 135 (31%) of 429 patients.

2. The operation is generally well tolerated, but is a major procedure and entails a definite risk of morbidity and mortality.

3. The logically anticipated correlations between clinical tumor stage, histologic grade, and regional lymph node involvement were generally observed.

4. Lymph node metastasis portends a 75% or greater probability of metastasis at five years, although some patients with lymph node metastasis are apparently well at that time.

5. Within the limitations of the follow-up intervals and the arbitrary definitions of local tumor control, the technique was associated with a 16% local failure rate.

6. A nonrandomized trial of supplemental external irradiation to the pelvis or pelvic and para-aortic areas has revealed no apparent advantages in terms of overall survival or disease-free survival and has apparently increased the frequency and severity of complications.

7. In the absence of control data, the relative contributions of the natural history of the disease and of the specific treatment to the results achieved remain uncertain.

REFERENCES

Barzell, W. E., M. A. Bean, B. S. Hilaris, and W. F. Whitmore, Jr. 1977. Prostatic adenocarcinoma: Relationship of grade and local extent to the pattern of metastases. J. Urol. 118:278–282.

Fowler, J. E., W. Barzell, B. S. Hilaris, and W. F. Whitmore, Jr. 1979. Complications of iodine[125] implantation and pelvic lymphadenectomy in the treatment of prostatic cancer. J. Urol. (in press).

Hilaris, B. S., W. F. Whitmore, Jr., M. Batata, and W. E. Barzell. 1977. Behavioral patterns of prostate adenocarcinoma following an I-I25 implanted pelvic node dissection. Int. J. Radiat. Oncol. Biol. Phys. 2:631–637.

Hilaris, B. S., W. F. Whitmore, Jr., M. A. Batata, W. Barzell, and N. Tokita. 1978. [125]I implantation of the prostate: Dose-response considerations. Front. Radiat. Ther. Oncol. 12:82–90.

Hilaris, B., W. F. Whitmore, M. Batata, and H. Grabstald. 1975. Carcinoma of prostate, *in* Handbook of Interstitial Brachytherapy, B. Hilaris, ed. Publishing Sciences Group, Inc., Acton, Mass., pp. 219–234.

Hilaris, B. S., W. F. Whitmore, Jr., M. A. Batata, and H. Grabstald. 1974. Radiation therapy and pelvic node dissection in the management of cancer of the prostate. Am. J. Roentgenol. 121:832–838.

Hilaris, B. S., W. F. Whitmore, H. Grabstald, and P. J. O'Kelly. 1972. Radical approach using interstitial and external sources. Clin. Bull. 2:94–99.

Whitmore, W. F., Jr. 1976. Retropubic implantation of I[125] in the treatment of prostatic cancer, *in* Prostatic Disease, H. Marberger, H. Haschek, H. K. A. Schirmer, J. A. C. Colston, and E. Witkin, eds. Alan R. Liss, Inc., New York, pp. 223–233.

Whitmore, W. F., B. S. Hilaris, and H. Grabstald. 1972. Retropubic implantation of iodine 125 in the treatment of prostatic cancer. J. Urol. 108:918–920.

Whitmore, W. F., Jr., B. Hilaris, H. Grabstald, and M. Batata. 1974. Implantation of I[125] in prostatic cancer. Surg. Clin. North Am. 54:887–895.

Cancer of the Genitourinary Tract, edited by
D. E. Johnson and M. L. Samuels.
Raven Press, New York © 1979.

Combined Interstitial and External Radiotherapy in the Definitive Management of Carcinoma of the Prostate

William Graham Guerriero, M.D., Marc T. Barrett, M.D., Thomas Bartholomew, M.D., C. Eugene Carlton, Jr., M.D., and Philip T. Hudgins, M.D.*

*The Roy and Lillie Cullen Department of Urologic Research, Division of Urology, Baylor College of Medicine, and the Urology Services of St. Luke's Episcopal Hospital, and *the Department of Radiology, The Methodist Hospital, Houston, Texas*

For more than half a century radical prostatectomy has been standard treatment for localized prostatic cancer. Developments in the management of this disease can be summarized as follows:

1911	Reports of treatment of prostatic carcinoma with induced radium (Rasteau 1911).
1922	Deming treats 100 cases of carcinoma of the prostate with radium (Deming 1922).
1941	Huggins and Hodges report on the effect of estrogens on carcinoma of the prostate (Huggins and Hodges 1941).
1952	Flocks reports the use of interstitial colloidal gold (^{198}Au) (Flocks et al. 1954).
1962	Bagshaw and Kaplan report success with external radiation (Bagshaw et al. 1965).
1965–67	Others confirm Bagshaw's report (George et al. 1965, Del Regato 1967).
1972	Whitmore reports the use of ^{125}I interstitial irradiation (Whitmore et al. 1972).
1972	Carlton uses combined interstitial and external radiotherapy (Cosgrove and Kaempf 1976).

However, radiotherapy provided by an interstitial or external source has, since 1952, become increasingly important in the treatment of locally extensive prostatic cancer. Radiotherapy for the treatment of less advanced prostatic malignant disease is being explored in a number of radiotherapy centers because of dissatisfaction with the results of radical prostatectomy. Increasingly, urologists are finding that prostatic cancer that was thought to be confined on the basis of clinical exam, is not when examined pathologically, and distant spread has been discovered in what was thought to be extremely localized cancer.

An analysis of the reports of Jewett (Jewett et al. 1968, Jewett 1975) reveals that prostatic cancer rarely is as localized microscopically as clinical examination suggests. Furthermore, results of radical prostatectomy for clinically localized tumor have not been as good as had been hoped.

McNeal (1969) and Byar and Mostofi (1972) have found that most prostatic cancer is multicentric or has spread throughout the gland when the tumor is examined histologically following surgery. In addition, Byar and Mostofi (1972) have demonstrated that surgical specimens examined by serial section contain cancer in the first one or two sections at the apex of the gland 50–75% of the time, suggesting that radical prostatectomy frequently may not remove all the local tumor. This fact argues against the practice of leaving a button of apical tissue to prevent incontinence.

McCullough and co-workers (1974) and Wilson and co-workers (1977), who have performed radical retropubic prostatectomies in conjunction with pelvic node dissection, have discovered that a significant number of clinical stage B and C patients have gross or microscopic lymphatic metastasis involving obturator or iliac nodes, or both.

Gleason and his colleagues (1974) have suggested that differentiation may be as important as surgical staging in selecting treatment and determining the prognosis of prostatic carcinoma. They have linked surgical stage and differentiation to form a category score that can predict the patient's future course.

In recognition of these factors, new staging systems, such as that of Jewett (1975), have been used to take these elements of the natural history of prostate cancer into account in selecting patients for radical prostatectomy. It has been suggested that diffuse stage A disease resembles diffuse stage B disease and should be treated aggressively. Small volume (focal) stage A disease should be observed. Stage B_1 disease, which most accurately could be described as a surgically staged Jewett nodule, appears to be more malignant than focal carcinoma and less malignant than carcinoma that diffusely involves the gland (stage A_2 and stage B_2) and should be treated for cure.

Reports of this kind have steadily increased the indications for radiotherapy at the expense of the radical operation.

In an attempt to evaluate the efficacy of radiotherapy in the treatment of locally extensive (stage C) prostate cancer, we previously reported our experience with combined interstitial and external radiotherapy for this tumor (Carlton et al. 1972, 1975). Those reports emphasized the usefulness of this form of treatment for stage C tumors less than 6 cm in diameter, which were classified as stage C_1, and suggested that this method of therapy might be useful in less advanced cases. But even though some localized tumors had been treated, meaningful survival data were not available at the time of those initial reports. This paper will update the series last documented in 1974, with greater emphasis on patients who have been treated for stage B and diffuse stage A carcinoma.

METHODS AND RESULTS

Five hundred forty-two patients treated for prostatic carcinoma with radiotherapy from 1965 to 1976 form the basis for this report. All patients have been followed for longer than one year. The distribution of cases as to clinical stage of disease is as follows: stage A, 97; B, 123; C_1, 151; C_2, 41; D_1, 103; and D_2, 27. Two hundred ninety-five patients have been staged surgically and followed for longer than one year. The average age of patients in this series is 64 years. The method of surgical staging and treatment has been described in detail (Carlton et al. 1975). Overall survival and durations of survival of these surgically staged patients are given in Table 1.

Criteria for surgical staging and combined interstitial radiation and external radiotherapy include expected survival of greater than five years, condition adequate to undergo lymphadenectomy and prostatic exploration, and prostatic carcinoma less than 6 cm in diameter with no evidence of distant metastasis. If bone scan, bone survey, and bone marrow biopsy are negative, an elevated acid phosphatase has not been a contraindication to the procedure. In our experience, patients of this type have positive pelvic nodes. The four patients we have treated in this manner to date have not yet developed bone metastasis.

We have staged our patients according to the procedure suggested by Whitmore (1956) and modified by Jewett (1975), except that stage C is divided into C_1 and C_2, depending on whether the tumor is less or more than 6 cm in diameter. The staging system can be summarized as follows:

A_1 Clinically occult carcinoma, small volume, fewer than three transurethral resection chips involved, focal.

A_2 Clinically occult carcinoma, multifocal or diffuse, more than three chips involved.

B   Clinically apparent carcinoma confined to the prostatic capsule by rectal exam.

C_1 Extensive carcinoma, less than 6 cm in diameter, penetrating prostatic capsule.

C_2 Extensive carcinoma, more than 6 cm in diameter, penetrating prostatic capsule.

Table 1. *Survival of Patients Treated by Radiotherapy for Carcinoma of the Prostate*

Stage	Total Number of Patients	Percent Surviving	Length of Survival	
			1–5 Years	5–10 Years
A_2	42	98%	30	11
B	82	85%	40	30
C_1	91	86%	62	16
D_1	80	79%	51	12

D_1 Positive pelvic nodes.

D_2 Bony metastasis or distant nodal metastasis; visceral metastasis.

Survival figures for surgical stage A, B, and C_1 patients are broken down according to length of follow-up in Tables 2, 3, and 4.

As would be expected, many more patients have been treated recently than in the early days of the series. This is illustrated graphically in Figure 1. The effect of differentiation on survival by stage is seen in Figure 2, while the effect of differentiation on the appearance of metastasis to the pelvic lymph nodes is seen in Table 5. A comparison of staging results with lymphadenectomy and clinical examination reveals that 24% of clinical stage A_2 cases, 19% of stage B cases, 31% of stage C_1 cases, and 86% of stage C_2 cases were surgical stage D_1.

Table 2. *Survival for Surgical Stage A_2 Patients*

Years Followed	Total Number of Patients	Alive with No Evidence of Disease	Alive with Disease	Dead with No Evidence of Disease	Dead with Disease
1–5	31	27 (87%)	3 (10%)	1 (3%)	0
5–10	11	7 (64%)	4 (36%)	0	0
Total	42	34 (81%)	7 (17%)	1 (2%)	0

Table 3. *Survival for Surgical Stage B Patients*

Years Followed	Total Number of Patients	Alive with No Evidence of Disease	Alive with Disease	Dead with No Evidence of Disease	Dead with Disease
1–5	49	31 (63%)	9 (18%)	9 (18%)	0
5–10	33	17 (52%)	13 (39%)	2 (6%)	1 (3%)
Total	82	48 (59%)	22 (27%)	11 (13%)	1 (1%)

Table 4. *Survival for Surgical Stage C_1 Patients*

Years Followed	Total Number of Patients	Alive with No Evidence of Disease	Alive with Disease	Dead with No Evidence of Disease	Dead with Disease
1–5	71	45 (63%)	17 (24%)	5 (7%)	4 (6%)
5–10	20	13 (65%)	3 (15%)	3 (15%)	1 (5%)
Total	91	58 (64%)	20 (22%)	8 (9%)	5 (5%)

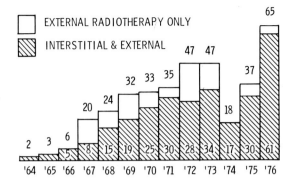

Figure 1. Number of patients treated per year, 1964–1976.

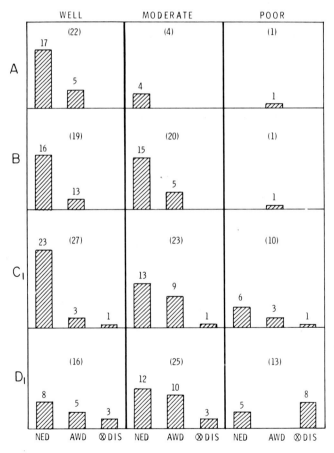

Figure 2. Survival of patients related to differentiation of tumor. (NED, no evidence of disease; AWD, alive with disease; ⊗ DIS, dead of disease.)

Table 5. *Relationship Between Histologic Differentiation and Appearance of Pelvic Lymph Node Metastasis*

Degree of Differentiation	Total Number of Patients	Nodal Metastasis as	
		% All Patients with Differentiation	% Patients with Stage D$_1$ Disease and Differentiation
Well	16	19%	30%
Moderately	25	35%	46%
Poorly	13	52%	24%

Surgical complications associated with pelvic lymphadenectomy included the following: lymphocele, <1% (prior to 1973, there had been a 10% incidence of lymphoceles); wound infection, 4%; persistent lymphatic drainage, 2%; phlebothrombosis, 10%; postoperative penile or lower extremity edema, 10%; and surgical mortality, <1% (one patient died from a pulmonary embolus). Late complications of radiotherapy and surgery are listed in Table 6.

DISCUSSION

Our objective in treating patients with prostatic cancer is to eradicate the primary lesion or control local spread of the disease. If that is not possible, we attempt to relieve symptoms of the tumor and prevent or delay onset of metastasis.

We feel that these objectives have been adequately met by combining interstitial and external radiotherapy. The isotope used for interstitial implantation is ^{198}Au, a potent beta and gamma emitter with greater tissue penetration than ^{125}I.

Table 6. *Percentages of Patients with Late Complications from Combined Interstitial and External Radiotherapy and Surgery (295 Patients)*

Complication	Mild	Moderate–Severe
Proctitis	12%	4%
Cystitis, urethritis	14%	3%
Rectal stenosis	2%	2%*
Stress incontinence	1%†	0
Impotence (29% unknown)	3%	2%
Penile or lower extremity edema	2%	0
Perineal irritation	1%	0
Hematuria (minor)	3%	0
Bladder neck contracture (after transurethral resection of the prostate)	25%	0

* Two patients required colostomies; one patient died of complications.
† Two patients after transurethral resection of the prostate.

The gold seeds are radiopaque and can be used as markers for external radiotherapy. The half-life of ^{198}Au is 2.7 days, resulting in a shorter, more intense period of treatment than with ^{125}I, a property that makes ^{198}Au admirably suited for use as an adjunct to external megavoltage therapy. Unlike ^{125}I, which is usually used as a single radiation source, ^{198}Au can be used to tailor combined therapy to the individual patient by placement of seeds where they are needed and modification of the amount of treatment to minimize complications and to permit therapy to the tolerance of each patient. The larger zone of penetration of interstitial radioactive gold and use of external beam therapy result in more assurance of homogeneity of radiation than does interstitial radiation therapy alone. A disadvantage of ^{198}Au implantation is the increased risk to the surgeon or radiotherapist inserting the gold grains, as the intensity of radiation with ^{198}Au is greater than that with ^{125}I.

The total dose given to the prostate gland by the use of adjunctive interstitial radiotherapy varies with the size of the gland and the number of seeds used, but usually is approximately 2,500 rads. Most of the radiotherapy dose is given via linear accelerator over one month starting two weeks after the surgical procedure. The maximum tumor dose is at least 6,500 to 7,000 rads in each patient, but again the total dose depends on the tolerance of the patient, the size of the tumor, and the period of time over which the treatment is given.

A number of our patients with stage A_2 disease discovered following complete transurethral resections have received external radiotherapy alone because little tissue was available for interstitial implantation. It is too early to evaluate the effectiveness of this form of therapy for stage A disease, and for this reason, these patients will form the basis for a later report.

A valid criticism of most reports of radiotherapy for prostatic carcinoma is that few patients have been treated for more than five years and most cancer deaths following radical prostatectomy occur between 7 and 15 years. Also, small tumors, usually moderately or well differentiated, are associated with an excellent prognosis, regardless of treatment. In addition, tumors in most radiotherapy and early surgical series have not been surgically staged. Surgical staging permits selection of those patients for treatment who would most likely survive longer periods of time, regardless of treatment.

Because of the number of such variables that enter into the survival of patients with prostatic carcinoma, we have presented our data in a number of ways. Probably the best method of presentation would be actuarial survival. Unfortunately, the number of patients treated for longer than five years available for analysis is too small to make such presentation meaningful. However, survival of those patients with stages A_2, B, C_1, and C_2 disease who have been followed for five years is better than would be predicted for men of the same age without prostate cancer. A comparison of survival data for patients with clinical and surgical stages A_2-C_1 disease shows little difference in survival (Table 7). This may be a result of the effectiveness of lymphadenectomy coupled with irradiation, or may reflect the generally good prognosis associated with predominantly well-

Table 7. *Survival by Stages of Patients Receiving Radiotherapy for Carcinoma of the Prostate*

Stage	Total Number of Patients	Percent Surviving	Length of Survival	
			1–5 Years	5–10 Years
A_2	53	94%	41	12
B	101	83%	62	39
C_1	131	86%	103	28

differentiated tumors. Fortunately, the percentage of patients in this series with poorly differentiated disease is small, only 11%. It is important to note, however, that these patients are surviving regardless of stage the same number of months as those with well and moderately differentiated carcinoma.

Length of follow-up is extremely important in evaluating the results of treatment of prostatic carcinoma. Of nine stage C_1 patients treated more than seven years ago, three are alive with disease and can be expected to die with cancer (Table 8). Two patients have died, both free of disease, for an overall survival rate of 78%. Twenty-three stage B patients have been followed more than seven years. Two (9%) have died, both with no evidence of disease, seven (30%) are alive with disease, and 14 (61%) are alive with no evidence of disease. These patients can best be compared with patients who have been surgically staged.

Our primary objective in treating patients with prostatic carcinoma is cure. We believe that this goal is attainable in patients with small tumors, stages A_2, B, and C_1, by means of radiotherapy. Cure is not sought in cases involving stage C_2 and D_1 disease, as the volume of tumor irradiated and the presence of distant metastasis make cure unlikely; however, the 67% five-year survival rate for patients with D_1 disease in our series is encouraging.

Whitmore and Bagshaw, among others, have emphasized the apparent radioresponsiveness of prostatic cancer. Ninety percent of patients treated by any of the popular forms of radiotherapy will evidence shrinkage of the tumor when examined 6–12 months later. Bagshaw et al. (1965) have emphasized that enlargement of the tumor after six months is a bad prognostic sign.

Table 8. *Survival for Patients with Surgical Stage C_1 Disease*

Years Followed	Total Number of Patients	Dead with Prostate Carcinoma	Dead with No Evidence of Disease	Alive with Disease	Alive with No Evidence of Disease
7	4	0	1	2	1
8	2	0	1	0	1
9	1	0	0	0	1
10	0	0	0	0	0
11	2	0	0	1	1
Total	9	0	2	3	4

We believe that the best method of evaluating patients following radiotherapy is a combination of clinical examination and needle biopsy examination of the treated prostate. Though it is sometimes difficult to obtain adequate tissue by needle biopsy, the presence of persistent carcinoma cells alerts the physician to the possibility of eventual failure of treatment.

It is heartening to find that 65% of our patients with stage B disease have negative prostate biopsies at one year. Our pathologist tells us that another 12% have positive biopsies with irradiation changes that suggest the tumor is nonviable. Follow-up biopsy results for the entire series are as follows: stage A, 13 negative out of 21 (62%); stage B, 28 out of 43 (65%); stage C_1, 28 out of 45 (62%); and Stage D_1, 12 out of 27 (44%).

Most of our patients had tumors that were well to moderately differentiated; however, in those patients with poorly differentiated tumors, local control of tumor growth has been as good as with the more differentiated tumors. Even though there is a higher incidence of lymph node metastasis in these patients with poorly differentiated tumors, overall survival for these patients is as good as that with the more favorable form of the disease in patients with stage D_1 cancer.

Complications have been few in the patients in this series. Most serious was the death from a pulmonary embolus of a patient who was on miniheparin therapy and wearing antiembolus stockings. Lymphedema, persistent lymphatic drainage, and wound infections, which occurred in less than 10% of our patients, generally resolved with proper treatment or time. No serious long-term surgical sequelae were noted. Irritative symptoms such as proctitis, cystitis, and urethritis occur in less than 20% of our patients and usually are mild and transient. However, rectal stenosis requiring colostomy did occur in two patients, both early in the series. One patient eventually died of multiple small bowel fistulae.

Early reports of our series (Carlton et al. 1972, 1975) suggested that impotence occurred in up to 25% of patients with this form of radiotherapy. For this report we again questioned each patient about potency. Impotence was rarely reported if the patient was potent preoperatively. Thus, we have been unable to confirm the 30% impotence figure reported by Bagshaw et al. (1965). The significance of this discrepancy from the data of the Stanford series and our own early figures is unknown. We would like to believe that minimal mobilization of the prostate and small, intense radiation fields have resulted in this improvement.

Radiotherapy is without question useful in the treatment of extensive prostatic carcinoma. The data presented indicate that radiotherapy has a place in diffuse disease confined to the prostate, whether occult or suspected. Although excellent results are reported in surgical series in which patients are adequately staged, radiotherapy offers equal if not better survival and an improved quality of life. Whether one chooses external therapy alone or combined megavoltage therapy and interstitial implantation, the patient can look forward to many years of freedom from the consequences of disseminated prostatic cancer and to the hope of cure.

REFERENCES

Bagshaw, M. A., H. S. Kaplan, and R. H. Sagerman. 1965. Linear accelerator supervoltage radiotherapy. VII. Carcinoma of the prostate. Radiology 85:121–129.

Byar, D. P., and F. K. Mostofi. 1972. Carcinoma of the prostate: Prognostic evaluation of certain pathologic features in 208 radical prostatectomies. Cancer 30:5–13.

Carlton, C. E., Jr., F. Dawoud, P. Hudgins, and R. Scott, Jr. 1972. Irradiation treatment of carcinoma of the prostate: A preliminary report based on 8 years of experience. J. Urol. 108:924–927.

Carlton, C. E., Jr., P. T. Hudgins, W. G. Guerriero, and R. Scott, Jr. 1975. Radiotherapy in the management of stage C carcinoma of the prostate. Trans. Am. Assoc. Genitourin. Surg. 67:70–74.

Cosgrove, M. D., and M. J. Kaempf. 1976. Prostatic cancer revisited. J. Urol. 115:79–81.

Del Regato, J. A. 1967. Radiotherapy in the conservative treatment of operable and locally inoperable carcinoma of the prostate. Radiology 88:761–766.

Deming, C. L. 1922. Cancer of the prostate and seminal vesicles—Results in one hundred cases of cancer of the prostate and seminal vesicles treated with radium. Surg. Gynecol. Obstet. 34:99–118.

Flocks, R. H., H. D. Kerr, H. B. Elkins, and D. A. Culp. 1954. Treatment of carcinoma of the prostate by interstitial radiation with radioactive gold (Au198): A preliminary report. J. Urol. 71:628–633.

George, F. W., C. E. Carlton, Jr., R. F. Dykhuizen, and J. R. Dillon. 1965. Cobalt-60 telecurietherapy in the definite treatment of carcinoma of the prostate—A preliminary report. J. Urol. 93:102–109.

Gleason, D. F., G. T. Mellinger, and the Veterans Administration Cooperative Urological Research Group. 1974. Prediction of prognosis for prostatic adenocarcinoma by combined histological grading and clinical staging. J. Urol. 111:58–64.

Huggins, C., and C. V. Hodges. 1941. Studies of prostatic cancer—Effect of castration, of estrogens and of androgen injection on serum phosphatases in metastatic carcinoma of the prostate. Cancer Res. 1:293–297.

Jewett, H. J. 1975. The present status of radical prostatectomy for stages A and B prostatic cancer. Urol. Clin. North Am. 2:105–124.

Jewett, H. J., R. W. Bridge, G. F. Gray, and W. M. Shelley. 1968. The palpable nodule of prostatic cancer—Results 15 years after radical excision. J.A.M.A. 203:115–118.

McCullough, D. L., G. R. Prout, and J. J. Daly. 1974. Carcinoma of the prostate and lymphatic metastases. J. Urol. 111:65–71.

McNeal, J. E. 1969. Origin and development of carcinoma in the prostate. Cancer 23:24–34.

Rasteau, D. 1911. Traitement du cancer de la prostate par le racium. Rev. Mal. Nutr. 363–398.

Whitmore, W. F. 1956. Symposium on hormones and cancer therapy: Hormone therapy in prostatic cancer. Am. J. Med. 21:697.

Whitmore, W. F., B. Hilaris, and H. Grabstald. 1972. Retropubic implantation of iodine-125 in the treatment of prostatic cancer. J. Urol. 108:918–920.

Wilson, C. S., D. S. Dahl, and R. G. Middleton. 1977. Pelvic lymphadenectomy for the staging of apparently localized prostatic cancer. J. Urol. 117:197.

Cancer of the Genitourinary Tract, edited by
D. E. Johnson and M. L. Samuels.
Raven Press, New York © 1979.

Experience With Limited-Field Irradiation for Adenocarcinoma of the Prostate

David H. Hussey, M.D.

*Department of Radiotherapy, The University of Texas System Cancer Center
M. D. Anderson Hospital and Tumor Institute, Houston, Texas*

In recent years, radiation therapy has become generally accepted as an effective treatment for patients with primary adenocarcinoma of the prostate. However, radiotherapy techniques for prostatic cancer vary, and the optimal tumor doses and field sizes for management of patients with this disease are not clearly established.

This paper is a review of the treatment experience with adenocarcinoma of the prostate by means of limited-field megavoltage radiotherapy at M. D. Anderson Hospital and Tumor Institute. The specific objectives are: (1) to present the results of limited-field radiation therapy in terms of local control, survival, and complication rates; (2) to correlate dose levels with control of the primary tumor and frequency of complications; and (3) to correlate field size with control of the cancer in the regional lymphatics.

CLINICAL MATERIAL

Between July 1966 and April 1974, 170 patients with adenocarcinoma of the prostate were treated with external-beam megavoltage irradiation at M. D. Anderson Hospital. The patient population ranged in age from 45 to 84 years, with an average age of 65 years. Many of the patients had undergone transurethral resections or needle biopsies of the prostate gland at other hospitals. In all cases, the diagnosis of adenocarcinoma was verified by M. D. Anderson Hospital pathologists. Although the biopsy specimens were not graded routinely, information regarding the histological grade was available for 102 patients.

Initial Evaluation and Clinical Staging

The initial clinical evaluation included a complete history and physical examination with digital examination of the prostate, complete blood count, urinalysis, blood urea nitrogen, liver function profile, and alkaline phosphatase and serum acid phosphatase determinations. Imaging studies included a chest x-ray, intravenous pyelogram, metastatic bone survey, and radionuclide bone scan. Although pedal lymphangiography now is performed routinely, only 18 patients had lymphangiograms during the period covered by this study.

The patients were staged clinically according to Del Regato's (1968) classification using a modification based on the bulk of the cancer:

Stage A   Occult carcinoma, one or two microscopic foci found incidentally at operation for benign disease or at autopsy.

Stage B   Carcinoma confined within the prostatic capsule with no elevation of the serum acid phosphatase.

Stage C   Carcinoma extending beyond the prostatic capsule, including the seminal vesicles, bladder, etc., or confined within the capsule with an elevated serum acid phosphatase.

Stage C_1 Moderately advanced—without pelvic wall fixation or invasion of the bladder or rectum.

Stage C_2 Massive—fixation to one or both pelvic walls, or direct invasion of the bladder or rectum.

Stage D   Bony or extrapelvic metastases.

The clinical stage distribution for this patient population is shown in Table 1. Five patients presented with stage B, 106 with stage C_1, and 59 with stage C_2. The allocation to stage C_1 or C_2 has been made retrospectively. This staging system shows good correlation with survival rates (Figure 1).

TREATMENT METHODS

At M. D. Anderson Hospital, most patients with stage B prostatic carcinoma have been treated by radical prostatectomy. Those who have refused surgery or have had medical contraindications to radical prostatectomy have been referred for radiation therapy. Most patients with stage C disease have been treated with radiation therapy, with or without hormonal manipulation. Those who have refused surgery and radiation therapy or have not been thought suitable for either have been treated with hormonal manipulation alone.

Table 1. *Clinical Stage Distribution*

Stage	By Tumor Dose		By Field Size		Total
	~6,500 rads	~7,000 rads	≤10 × 12 cm	>10 × 12 cm	
B	6% (3/48)	2% (2/122)	4% (5/139)	0% (0/31)	3% (5/170)
C_1	54% (26/48)	66% (80/122)	71% (99/139)	23% (7/31)	62% (106/170)
C_2	40% (19/48)	33% (40/122)	25% (35/139)	77% (24/31)	35% (59/170)

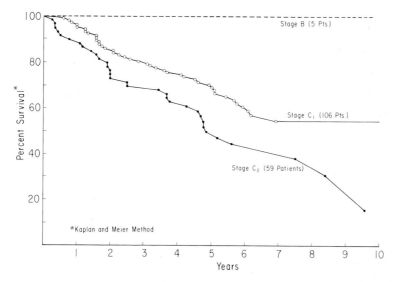

Figure 1. Actuarial survival by clinical stage for 170 patients treated with irradiation (minimum 4-year follow-up) (C_1 vs. C_2: Wilcoxon test, $p = 0.037$). (Reproduced with permission from Hussey, D. H. 1979. Prostate. *In* Fletcher, G. H. (ed.): *Textbook of Radiotherapy.* 3rd ed. Lea & Febiger, Philadelphia, in press.)

Radiotherapy Technique

Most patients were treated with 22- or 25-MeV x-rays through a four-field portal arrangement using 10×10 cm anterior and posterior portals and 10×8 cm lateral portals (Figure 2). A four-field portal arrangement with 25-MeV x-rays results in a uniform dose throughout the treatment volume (Figure 3 top). In contrast, ^{60}Co rotational therapy gives a nonuniform distribution of radiation, and a maximum tumor dose of 7,000 rads results in a minimum tumor dose of approximately 6,500 rads (Figure 3 bottom).

The fields usually extended from the ischial tuberosities to the inferior margins of the sacroiliac joints and encompassed most of the lesser pelvis (Figure 2). The posterior margin of the lateral portal was placed 1.5–2 cm posterior to the palpable disease as indicated by rectal examination. Slightly larger treatment portals were used for patients with more extensive neoplasms. However, no attempt was made to cover the common iliac or periaortic lymph nodes.

The total tumor dose ranged from 6,000 rads in six weeks to 7,000 rads in seven weeks. After a dose of 5,000 rads, the lateral portals were discontinued and an additional 1,000 to 2,000 rads were given through reduced anterior and posterior fields encompassing the primary tumor with minimal margins.

Hormonal Manipulation

Seventy-nine patients also received adjunctive hormonal treatment. Forty-one of these had been treated with estrogens or an orchiectomy prior to referral

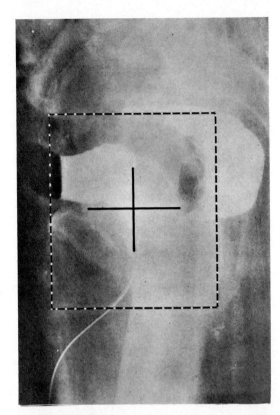
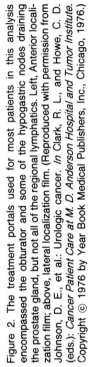
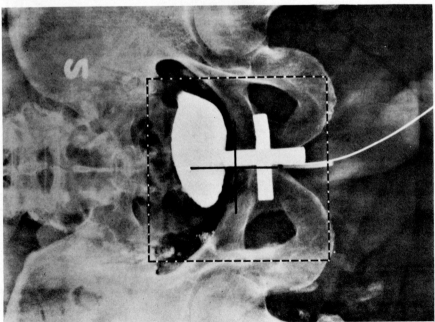

Figure 2. The treatment portals used for most patients in this analysis encompassed the obturator and some of the hypogastric nodes draining the prostate gland, but not all of the regional lymphatics. Left, Anterior localization film; above, lateral localization film. (Reproduced with permission from Johnson, D. E., et al.: Urologic cancer. *In* Clark, R. L., and Howe, C. D. (eds.): *Cancer Patient Care at M. D. Anderson Hospital and Tumor Institute.* Copyright © 1976 by Year Book Medical Publishers, Inc., Chicago, 1976.)

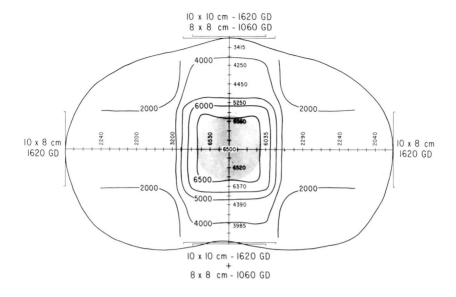

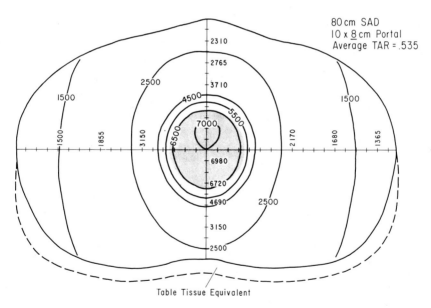

Figure 3. Representative isodose distributions for treating carcinoma of the prostate with (top) a four-field portal arrangement with 25 mV x-rays (100 cm source = skin distance), and (bottom) 360° ⁶⁰Co rotation. A circular tumor 7 cm in diameter is used for reference. The four-field portal arrangement (25 mV x-rays) results in a uniform dose of ~6,500 rads throughout the tumor volume. Cobalt-60 rotation therapy results in a nonuniform dose distribution, with 7,000 rads at the center of the tumor and ~6,500 rads at the periphery. (Abbreviations: GD = given dose; SAD = source-axis distance; TAR = tissue-air ratio.) (Reproduced with permission from Hussey, D. H. 1979. Prostate. *In* Fletcher, G. H. (ed.): *Textbook of Radiotherapy.* 3rd ed. Lea & Febiger, Philadelphia, in press.)

for radiation therapy. In most cases a daily dose of 5 mg of diethylstilbestrol was administered. After publication of the results of the Veterans Administration Cooperative Urological Research Group's study (Bailar et al. 1970), which showed an increased incidence of cardiovascular disease with estrogen administration, the dose was reduced in some instances to 1 to 2 mg daily. A previous analysis of the same clinical material (Neglia et al. 1977) showed that the local control and survival rates for prostatic cancer patients treated with radiotherapy are not improved by adjunctive hormonal therapy.

RESULTS

The patients were followed for four to 12 years. The average follow-up was six years nine months. Actuarial survival curves were computed using the Kaplan and Meier (1958) method. The patients were scored as having local failure if there was persistent disease centrally or within regional nodes. Central failure was defined as persistent nodularity or progressive growth on rectal examination, or histologic evidence of cancer at repeat biopsy or autopsy. Regional failure was defined as failure in the lymph nodes or at the pelvic sidewall, characterized by leg edema and/or sciatic pain.

Local Control, Survival, and Complications

The results show that radiation therapy is an effective treatment method for prostatic cancer localized to the pelvis. The actuarial 5- and 10-year survival rates were 64% and 42%, respectively (Figure 4). Local control of the disease was achieved in 84% of patients, and 8% developed major complications (Table 2). The most frequent complication, occurring in 6% of patients, was proctosigmoid injury, e.g., stricture, ulceration, and/or necrosis, requiring diverting colostomies. Most treatment failures resulted from hematogenous spread (Table 3).

Of the 102 patients whose primary tumors were histologically graded, 74 presented with well-differentiated tumors (grades I and II) and 28 with poorly differentiated tumors (grades III and IV). Histologic grading was an important prognostic indicator, since patients with well-differentiated neoplasms showed a significantly better survival than those with poorly differentiated cancers (Wilcoxon test, $p = 0.002$) (Figure 5).

Ten patients were treated with irradiation for residual or recurrent disease following radical prostatectomy. All 10 patients had local control of their disease following irradiation, and seven of these were alive with no evidence of disease at the time of analysis (four to eight years after irradiation). Two patients died of distant metastasis one year after radiation therapy, and one was alive at the time of analysis with distant metastasis.

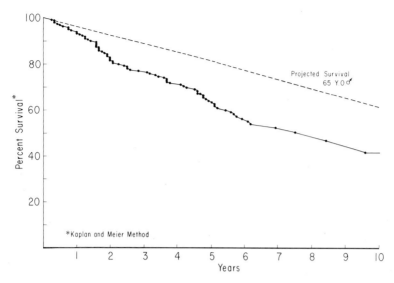

Figure 4. Actuarial survival for 170 patients with prostatic cancer treated with radiation therapy between July 1966 and April 1974 (minimum four-year follow-up). The expected survival for a normal population of 65-year-old men is shown for comparison. After six years, the survival parallels that for the general population of 65-year-old men. (Reproduced with permission from Hussey, D. H. 1979. Prostate. *In* Fletcher, G. H. (ed.): *Textbook of Radiotherapy.* 3rd ed. Lea & Febiger, Philadelphia, in press.)

Dose Relationships

To evaluate dose relationships, the clinical material was divided into two groups: (1) those patients who received a tumor dose of ~6,500 rads in 6½ weeks (range 6,000–6,750 rads), and (2) those who received a tumor dose of ~7,000 rads in 7 to 7½ weeks (range 6,750–7,250 rads). For early and moderately advanced cancers (stages B and C_1), there was no difference between the two

Table 2. *Results by Clinical Stage (Minimum Four-Year Follow-up)*

Stage	Local Control*	Survival*	Complications*
B	100%	100%	0%
	(5/5)	(5/5)	(0/5)
C_1	91%	61%	8%
	(96/106)	(65/106)	(9/106)
C_2	69%	44%	8%
	(41/59)	(26/59)	(5/59)
Total	84%	56%	8%
	(142/170)	(96/170)	(14/170)

* Local control, survival, and complication rates were computed at the time of analysis (mean follow-up 6 years, 9 months).

Table 3. *Sites of Failure*

Stage	Local Failure (with or without distant metastases)			Distant Metastasis (with or without local failure)
	Central	Regional	Central and Regional	
B	0% (0/5)	0% (0/5)	0% (0/5)	0% (0/5)
C_1	5% (5/106)	3% (3/106)	2% (2/106)	27% (29/106)
C_2	17% (10/59)	3% (2/59)	10% (6/59)	47% (28/59)
Total	9% (15/170)	3% (5/170)	5% (8/170)	34% (57/170)

groups in terms of local control and survival (Table 4). For massive tumors (stage C_2), the local control and survival rates with ~7,000 rads were superior to those achieved with ~6,500 rads.

A significantly greater incidence of major complications was observed with higher doses (Table 4). Only one of 33 patients treated with a dose of ~6,500 rads developed a major complication. This patient was treated with a large-field, 360° rotation technique using ^{60}Co, which carried a high likelihood of complications. However, 12 of 110 patients treated with doses of ~7,000 rads developed major complications.

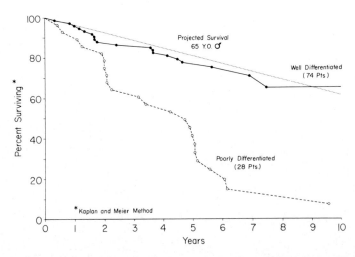

Figure 5. Survival by histologic grade, July 1966–April 1974. Minimum four-year follow-up. Information regarding the histologic grade of the prostatic carcinoma was available for 102 of 170 patients treated. The expected survival of a normal population of 65-year-old men is shown for comparison. (Reproduced with permission from Hussey, D. H. 1979. Prostate. *In* Fletcher, G. H. (ed.): *Textbook of Radiotherapy.* 3rd ed. Lea & Febiger, Philadelphia, in press.)

Table 4. Local Control, Survival, and Complication Rates by Tumor Dose* (Minimum Four-Year Follow-up)

Stage	Local Control†		Survival†		Complications†	
	~6,500 rads	~7,000 rads	~6,500 rads	~7,000 rads	~6,500 rads	~7,000 rads
B	100% (3/3)	100% (2/2)	100% (3/3)	100% (2/2)	0% (0/3)	0% (0/2)
C_1	94% (16/17)	92% (68/74)	65% (11/17)	64% (47/74)	6%‡ (1/17)	11% (8/74)
C_2	62% (8/13)	79% (27/34)	31% (4/13)	56% (19/34)	0% (0/13)	12% (4/34)
Total	82% (27/33)	88% (97/110)	55% (18/33)	62% (68/110)	3% (1/33)	11% (12/110)

* Excluding 27 patients diagnosed >6 months before radiotherapy.

† Local control, survival, and complication rates were computed at the time of analysis (mean follow-up 6 years, 9 months).

‡ The only complication in the group receiving ~6,500 rads was in a patient treated with large fields using a rotation technique with ^{60}Co.

Volume Relationships

Most patients in this study were treated with limited portals. These fields included the obturator and some of the hypogastric nodes draining the prostate gland, but not all the regional lymphatics. Even the larger portals used for more advanced disease (stage C_2) did not encompass the common iliac or periaortic nodes. A high incidence of regional node metastases has been reported from most lymphadenectomy series (Bagshaw et al. 1977, Flocks et al. 1959, and Hilaris et al. 1977). Because of this, the patients were studied to determine whether or not recurrences were developing at the regional level.

A significant failure rate in the regional lymph nodes was not observed clinically (Table 3). Only five of 170 patients (3%) developed clinical evidence of regional metastasis with central local control, although some patients may have died of distant metastasis before regional nodal failures became apparent. Whether or not these patients could have been cured with extended-field irradiation is uncertain.

DISCUSSION

Lymphadenectomy studies have shown that the incidence of regional metastasis varies from 7% to 29% for stage B, and from 38% to 61% for stage C (Bagshaw et al. 1977, Flocks et al. 1959, and Hilaris et al. 1977). The most frequent sites of regional nodal metastasis are the obturator, external iliac, and hypogastric lymph nodes, in that order (Table 5). Presacral, common iliac, and periaortic nodes are involved less frequently, but these areas have usually not been dissected in most reported series. When the common iliac and periaortic areas have been dissected by means of a transperitoneal approach, the common iliac and periaortic nodes have been found to be involved in approximately 20% of patients (Bagshaw et al. 1977).

The critical question is whether or not patients with lymph node metastases

Table 5. *Incidence of Regional Metastasis by Nodal Group*

Nodal Group	Retroperitoneal Pelvic Lymphadenectomy*	Transperitoneal Lymphadenectomy†
Obturator	30%	39%
External iliac	27%	27%
Hypogastric	5%	32%
Common iliac	5%	21%
Periaortic	—	22%

* Dissection of the external iliac and obturator nodes and partial dissection of the common iliac and hypogastric nodes. The presacral and periaortic nodes were not dissected (128 patients with stage B and 80 with stage C) (Hilaris et al. 1977).

† Dissection of the obturator, external iliac, hypogastric, common iliac, and periaortic nodes (1 patient with stage A, 32 with stage B, and 33 with stage C) (Bagshaw et al. 1977).

can be salvaged by radiation therapy. Experience with carcinoma of the cervix (Wharton et al. 1976) has shown that a small percentage of patients with metastases to the pelvic nodes can be cured with radiation therapy, but when the common iliac and/or periaortic nodes are involved, almost all patients die of distant metastases. The preliminary results from Stanford (Bagshaw et al. 1977) show a similar pattern for carcinoma of the prostate. In the Stanford study, a significant number of patients with nodal metastases confined to the pelvis were alive with no evidence of disease (NED) in the early follow-up period. However, the NED rate was markedly diminished when the periaortic lymph nodes were involved because of the early appearance of hematogenous spread.

Most patients in this study were treated with relatively small treatment portals. Although the obturator and some of the hypogastric nodes draining the prostate were encompassed, not all of the primary lymphatic drainage was included. Nevertheless, a significant failure rate in the regional lymphatics was not observed clinically (Table 3). It is possible that some of the regional nodal failures remained occult in patients who later developed distant metastases. Whether or not these patients would have been salvaged with larger treatment portals is a matter of conjecture.

Experience at M. D. Anderson Hospital has shown that over 90% of small to moderately advanced adenocarcinomas of the prostate (stages B and C_1) can be locally controlled with doses of ~6,500 rads in 6½ weeks. However, with massive tumors (stage C_2), the local control rate is improved when doses in the range of 7,000 rads are employed. In the M. D. Anderson series, the cancer was locally controlled in 79% of patients with stage C_2 disease with doses of ~7,000 rads, compared to only 62% of patients receiving doses in the range of 6,500 rads (Table 4).

The treatment portals for stage C adenocarcinoma of the prostate have recently been increased slightly to ensure better coverage of the obturator, external iliac, and hypogastric lymph nodes. If the lymphangiogram is negative, the initial treatment portals usually measure 12×14 cm anteriorly and posteriorly and 12×8 cm laterally. The treatment portals are reduced after 4,500 rads in 4½– 5 weeks. The total dose is determined by the bulk of the disease and the volume irradiated. For stage C_1, a dose of 6,500 rads in 6½–7 weeks is usually sufficient. For massive disease, a dose of 7,000 rads in 7–7½ weeks is usually employed. The treatment portals are not extended to include the common iliac or periaortic areas unless there is lymphangiographic evidence of regional nodal metastases because of the increased risk of complications associated with large treatment portals.

ACKNOWLEDGMENT

This investigation was supported in part by grant CA 06294, awarded by the National Cancer Institute, Department of Health, Education and Welfare.

REFERENCES

Bagshaw, M. A., D. A. Pistenma, G. R. Ray, F. S. Freida, and R. L. Kempson. 1977. Evaluation of extended field radiotherapy for prostatic neoplasm: 1976 progress report. Cancer Treat. Rep. 61:297–307.

Bailar, J. C., III, D. P. Byar, and the Veterans Administration Cooperative Urological Research Group (VACURG). 1970. Estrogen treatment for carcinoma of the prostate: Early results with 3 doses of diethylstilbestrol and placebo. Cancer 26:257–261.

Del Regato, J. A. 1968. Radiotherapy for Carcinoma of the Prostate: A Report from the Committee for Cooperative Study of Radiotherapy for Carcinoma of the Prostate. Colorado Springs, Penrose Cancer Hospital.

Flocks, B., D. Culp, and R. Porto. 1959. Lymphatic spread from prostatic cancer. J. Urol. 81:194–196.

Hilaris, B. S., W. F. Whitmore, M. Batata, and W. Barzell. 1977. Behavioral patterns of prostate adenocarcinoma following an ^{125}I implant and pelvic node dissection. Int. J. Radiat. Oncol. Biol. Phys. 2:631–637.

Hussey, D. H. 1979. Prostate, *in* Textbook of Radiotherapy, G. H. Fletcher (ed.). 3rd ed. Lea & Febiger, Philadelphia (in press).

Johnson, D. E., R. B. Bracken, S. Wallace, M. L. Samuels, D. H. Hussey, L. S. Miller, and A. G. Ayala. 1976. Urologic cancer, *in* Cancer Patient Care at M. D. Anderson Hospital and Tumor Institute, R. L. Clark and C. D. Howe, eds. Year Book Medical Publishers, Chicago, pp. 361–414.

Kaplan, E. L., and P. Meier. 1958. Nonparametric estimations from incomplete observation. Am. Statist. Assoc. J. 53:457–480.

Neglia, W. J., D. H. Hussey, and D. E. Johnson. 1977. Megavoltage radiation therapy for carcinoma of the prostate. Int. J. Radiat. Oncol. Biol. Phys. 2:873–882.

Wharton, J. T., H. W. Jones, T. G. Day, F. N. Rutledge, and G. H. Fletcher. 1976. Preirradiation celiotomy and extended field irradiation for invasive carcinoma of the cervix. Obstet. Gynecol. 49:333–338.

Cancer of the Genitourinary Tract, edited by
D. E. Johnson and M. L. Samuels.
Raven Press, New York © 1979.

Extended-Field Radiation Therapy for Prostatic Adenocarcinoma: Status Report of a Limited Prospective Trial

David A. Pistenma, M.D., Malcolm A. Bagshaw, M.D., and Fuad S. Freiha, M.D.*

*Division of Radiation Therapy, Department of Radiology, and * Division of Urology, Department of Surgery, Stanford University School of Medicine, Stanford, California*

Initially, irradiation of prostatic carcinoma at Stanford was restricted to the prostate gland and the immediately adjacent periprostatic tissue (Bagshaw et al. 1965, Ray et al. 1973). After 1971 treatment volumes in many patients were extended to include the obturator and the internal, external, and common iliac lymph nodes. In some patients with proven extensive adenopathy, the para-aortic lymph nodes were also treated.

Ninety-six of approximately 230 patients who had been treated with extended-field radiation therapy since 1971 were entered into a controlled prospective trial (Bagshaw et al. 1975, 1977). These patients were followed frequently in a joint urology-radiotherapy clinic by means of appropriate examination to detect asymptomatic metastases and needle biopsies to evaluate the status of the prostate after irradiation.

The goals of the study were as follows:

1. To determine whether or not radiotherapy directed to known areas of disease plus apparently uninvolved contiguous lymph nodes (extended-field treatment) results in better survival than treatment restricted to known areas of disease (limited-field treatment);

2. To assess the morbidity produced by the extended-field treatment compared to the potential therapeutic gain;

3. To accumulate data on histologic grading and diagnostic procedures (such as lymphangiograms, bone scans, and acid phosphatase determinations) for improving the precision and usefulness of staging systems;

4. To compare the accuracy of clinical staging (including lymphography) with surgical staging;

5. To relate survival or disease progression to pretreatment parameters; and

6. To follow the status of the primary tumor with posttreatment prostatic biopsies.

This report will be limited to a description of the current status of these 96 patients 15 months to seven years after treatment.

MATERIALS AND METHODS

Patient Selection

Criteria for admission to the protocol included: (1) histopathologic confirmation of the diagnosis by the Division of Surgical Pathology at Stanford, (2) no prior definitive surgery except transurethral resection of the prostate, (3) no castration, (4) no antiandrogenic therapy for more than two months prior to consultation, (5) patient under 71 years of age and medically and psychologically able to undergo lymph node biopsy or dissection, (6) no evidence of metastases to bone or viscera, (7) informed consent by the patient, and (8) agreement by the referring physician.

Of the total patient pool of 558 patients seen for adenocarcinoma of the prostate, 324 were excluded from the clinical trial protocol for the following reasons: consultation only, 68; over 70 years of age, 89; surgery contraindications, 59; prior definitive treatment, 61; distant metastases, 39; and second primary, eight. Of the 234 eligible for the protocol, 111 did not join because the patient or physician refused, 24 because of laparotomy off protocol, and three because distance precluded follow-up. Thus, 96 (41%) of those eligible actually joined the study. The criteria of informed consent by the patient and agreement by the referring physician were difficult to satisfy because of concerns related to lymph node sampling and/or dissection and to the determination of treatment by random allocation.

Three of the original 96 patients were dropped from the protocol after entry for medical reasons (one had distant metastases, one had a medical condition discovered after acceptance, and one was found to have a second primary at laparotomy).

The mean age at entry was 60.4 years. To date, 86 of the original 96 have been followed from 15 months to seven years.

Clinical Evaluation

The preoperative diagnostic evaluation included complete history and physical examination, complete blood count, reticulocyte count, platelet count, erythrocyte sedimentation rate, urinalysis, serum creatinine, complete chemical screening panel, and serum acid phosphatase (total and tartrate inhibited). The preoperative radiographic evaluation included routine chest radiographs, metastatic bone survey, intravenous pyelogram, and bipedal lymphangiography. Radioisotope bone scans were performed on all patients.

Clinical staging by digital rectal examination was expressed according to a TNM system derived specifically for this protocol (Bagshaw et al. 1975). T

Table 1. *Stanford Clinical Staging System (T Stage Only) (Feb. 1975 Revision)*

T Stage of Primary Tumor	Definition Based on Digital Rectal Exam (Except for T0)	Approximate American Urologic Stage
TX	Characteristic anatomic relationships distorted and/or absent secondary to major surgical intervention, i.e., radical prostatectomy.	A
T0	Latent carcinoma: Incidental finding of carcinoma in the operative specimen. x. Percent of gland involved unknown. a. TURP: < than 5% of chips involved by tumor. b. TURP: > 5% of chips involved by tumor.	A
T1	Palpable tumor limited by the prostatic capsule and not distorting the superior or lateral anatomic boundaries. a. Solitary nodule equal to or less than 1 cm in diameter, surrounded by normal compressible prostatic tissue (lesion amenable to radical prostatectomy). b. Palpable tumor greater than 1 cm, occupying less than 50% of a lobe. c. Palpable tumor occupying 50% or more of a lobe, multiple nodules limited to one lobe or involvement of both lobes.	B_1 B_2 B_2
T2	Palpable tumor limited by the prostatic capsule, causing minimal distortion of, but not obliterating, a lateral sulcus or invading the seminal vesicles. a. Palpable tumor occupying less than 50% of a lobe. b. Palpable tumor occupying 50% or more of a lobe, multiple nodules limited to one lobe, or involvement of both lobes.	B_2
T3	Palpable tumor extending beyond the prostatic capsule and definitely obliterating a lateral sulcus and/or invading the seminal vesicles. a. Tumor involving less than 50% of a lobe. b. Palpable tumor occupying 50% or more of a lobe, multiple nodules limited to one lobe, or involvement of both lobes.	C
T4	Palpable tumor extending beyond the prostatic capsule and invading the rectum, bladder, or both pelvic sidewalls. Patients with IVP findings suggestive of bladder involvement will undergo cystoscopy and, if indicated, biopsy.	D

categories are outlined in Table 1. This staging system antedates the International Union Against Cancer (UICC) and American Joint Committee TNM systems, which are currently under trial, and, although grossly similar as to major T categories, includes a finer breakdown within these categories. We have continued to use this system to accumulate data that might be of value in future refinements of the American Joint Committee and UICC TNM systems.

Surgical Lymph Node Staging

After completion of the preoperative evaluation, 93 of the 96 patients underwent selected lymph node biopsies or lymph node dissections. In the first 46 patients a transperitoneal approach was used to obtain biopsy specimens of selected high para-aortic and pelvic lymph nodes and to examine the liver, while in the last 47 patients a retroperitoneal approach was used. Initially, selected lymph node biopsies were performed in both groups, using the lymphogram as a guide, whereas in the last two years essentially complete dissections of the obturator, internal and external iliac, common iliac, and low para-aortic nodes have been performed.

Randomization of Patients

Following completion of the laparotomy, the pathologic stage was determined at a joint conference that included the operating surgeons, diagnostic radiologists, radiotherapists, and pathologists. The patient was randomly assigned to one of several treatment options, depending upon the proven extent of lymph node disease. When the disease was limited to the prostate (N = 54), patients were randomized between two groups; one received definitive radiation therapy to the prostatic region only (N = 26), while the other received definitive radiation therapy to the pelvic lymph node groups as well as the prostate (N = 28). If metastases were found in the pelvic lymph nodes (N = 18), patients were again assigned to receive definitive radiotherapy to the entire regional lymph node-bearing area in the pelvis as well as the prostate gland (N = 11), or to the prostate, the pelvic lymph nodes, plus the para-aortic lymph nodes (N = 7). If metastases were found in both the pelvic and para-aortic lymph node regions (N = 14), the patients received radiation to the prostate, pelvic lymph nodes, and para-aortic lymph nodes. (Seven patients are not included above because they have been followed less than 15 months.)

Radiation Therapy Technique

The treatment volumes have been constant throughout the period of the study. However, the total doses and number of fields treated per day have been changed slightly. The patients were treated isocentricly with a 4-MeV linear accelerator at a source–axis distance of 80 cm.

The prostatic region only was treated consistently by bilateral 120° arc moving beam therapy to a total dose of 7,400–7,600 rads in 7½ weeks given in five 200-rad fractions per week.

The simultaneous irradiation of pelvic lymph nodes and prostate was accomplished by a four-field technique (anterior, opposed posterior, right and left lateral) encompassing lymph nodes from the L4–5 interspace superiorly to the ischial tuberosities inferiorly. Initially, 5,500 rads in 200-rad fractions were delivered via two fields per day over 5½ weeks, followed by a 1,500-rad boost in 1½ weeks to the region of the prostate gland only. Because of unacceptable morbidity to the small bowel with that treatment scheme, the irradiation of the pelvic lymph nodes was modified to deliver 2,600 rads in 13 fractions with four fields per day over 2½ weeks. This was followed by a 2,000-rad boost to the prostate gland only, after which the pelvic node irradiation was completed with an additional 2,400 rads in 12 fractions over 2½ weeks to the same volume described above. This gave total doses of 5,000 rads to the nodes and 7,000 rads to the prostate over seven weeks.

The para-aortic lymph nodes were treated with AP and PA crossfire supplemented by opposed lateral or opposed oblique fields. Initially, a dose of 5,500 rads in 5½ weeks was given via two fields per day. Again, because of unacceptable morbidity, the total dose was reduced to 5,000 rads over 7 weeks at a rate of 200 rads per day with two or four fields per day.

Histologic Grading of Prostate Tissue Specimens

All prostatic biopsy specimens were graded by R. L. Kempson according to a modified Broder's classification (Kempson and Levine 1974). They were graded as well differentiated, moderately differentiated, or poorly differentiated. In addition, all specimens were graded by D. L. Gleason according to his five-grade method (Gleason 1966). With this method, each of the major and minor glandular patterns is assigned a number grade 1 through 5, and the two scores are summed to give a pattern score ranging from 2 to 10. The pattern score has been shown in other studies to correlate well with survival and other factors. In addition, Gleason and Mellinger have suggested that numerical values could be assigned to the clinical stage and added to the pattern scores to arrive at a category score (Gleason et al. 1974). We have adapted the Gleason and Mellinger clinical stage subdivisions to the Stanford T staging system (e.g., T0 = 1, T1a–T1b = 2, T1c = 3, T2b = 4, and T3 = 5) to arrive at modified Gleason categories. Thus, our category scores range from 3 to 15.

RESULTS

Clinical Stage and Histologic Grade

Table 2 shows the distribution of patients according to clinical stage and histologic grade of the primary tumor. Note the distinct concordance between regressive differentiation and advancing clinical stage.

Lymph Node Metastases

We will show in a later section that the presence of lymph node metastases before treatment has a profound influence on the outcome of therapy in this

Table 2. *Distribution of Patients According to Clinical Stage and Differentiation of Primary Tumor*

Amer. Urol. Stage	Stanford TNM Stage	Number of Patients	Differentiation of Primary Tumor		
			Well Diff.	Moderately Diff.	Poorly Diff.
A	T0	3	1 (33%)	1 (33%)	1 (33%)
B	T1,T2	52	8 (15%)	39 (75%)	5 (10%)
C	T3	41	1 (2%)	23 (56%)	17 (41%)
Total		96	10 (10%)	63 (66%)	23 (24%)

group of patients. For this reason, extra attention has been paid to a detailed correlation of the results of surgical staging with clinical stage, histologic grade, and pretreatment acid phosphatase levels in an effort to help identify predictors of lymph node metastases that are less invasive than laparotomy.

Distribution of Adenopathy

The distribution of adenopathy according to lymph node group is presented in Table 3. These data clearly underestimate the true incidence of adenopathy, since 46 of the patients underwent biopsies of suspicious nodes only.

Lymphograms

Table 4 illustrates the lymphographic-histologic correlation in 89 patients who underwent complete studies. The relatively high percentage of false-positive and false-negative studies detracts from the routine usefulness of lymphography as a diagnostic tool. The false-negative studies were due to microscopic foci below the threshold of detection by current lymphographic techniques or, occasionally, to complete replacement of the lymph node by tumor. In high-risk patients to be described later, however, the lymphogram identified lymph node involvement in nine of 14 patients.

Table 3. *Incidence of Lymph Node Involvement by Tumor (93 Patients)*

Lymph Node Group	Number of Patients Undergoing Biopsy	Number (%) With Tumor	Percent Opacified*
Para-aortic	74	13 (18%)	93
Common iliac	76	13 (17%)	95
External iliac	74	16 (22%)	94
Internal iliac	63	15 (24%)	87
Obturator	51	16 (31%)	94

* Refers to histologic evidence of retained contrast material within the lymph node specimen.

Table 4. *Lymphographic-Histologic Correlation in 89 of 93* Patients With Prostatic Carcinoma*

Lymphogram	Histologic Examination		Total
	Positive	Negative	
Positive	15	7	22
Negative	15	52	67
Total	30	59	89

Overall accuracy = 67/89 (75%), True-negative rate = 52/59 (88%), True-positive rate = 15/30 (50%), False-negative rate = 15/67 (22%), False-positive rate = 7/22 (32%).

* Two patients did not have lymphograms for medical reasons; in two others, biopsies were not performed on lymphographically positive nodes.

Clinical Stage and Adenopathy

The incidence of lymph node metastases as a function of clinical stage is tabulated in Table 5. Note the orderly progression from 0% lymph node involvement in stage T0 to 56% for T3 tumors.

Clinical Stage, Histologic Grade, and Adenopathy

The incidence of lymphadenopathy according to the clinical stage and histologic grade of the primary tumors is shown in Table 6. Only one of nine patients with well-differentiated tumors had lymph node metastases, while 16 of the 61 patients with moderately differentiated and 16 of 23 with poorly differentiated tumors had metastases to lymph nodes.

Gleason Grading System and Adenopathy

Table 7 shows the distribution of node metastases relative to clinical stage and the Gleason grading system. The Gleason pattern scores are arranged according to the modified T staging system for the 93 patients who had lymph node biopsies. Note that only one of 15 patients (7%) with Gleason pattern scores of 5 or less had lymph node metastases, whereas 16 of 21 patients (76%) with pattern scores of 8 to 10 had lymphadenopathy.

Modified Gleason-Mellinger Categories and Adenopathy

If numbers are arbitrarily assigned to the T stages and these numbers are added to the pattern scores, one arrives at the modified Gleason-Mellinger categories, which range from 3 through 15. The incidence of lymph node metastases in our protocol patient group segregated according to the modified Gleason-Mellinger categories is shown in Table 8. None of the 15 patients falling into categories 3 through 8 had lymph node metastases. From category 9 through 15 there is a systematic progression in incidence of lymph node metastases from 20% to 100%.

Table 5. Correlation Between Clinical Stage and Lymph Node Biopsy Results

Clinical Stage		Lymph Node Biopsy Results				
Amer. Urol. Stage	Stanford (Mod. TNM)	Negative Nodes	+Regional Nodes Only	+PA Nodes Only	+Regional and PA Nodes	Positive Total
A	T0	3	0	0	0	0/3 (0%)
B	T1a,T1b	10	1	0	0	1/11 (9%)
	T1c	10	0	0	2	2/12 (17%)
	T2a	4	1	0	0	1/5 (20%)
	T2b	15	6	0	0	6/21 (29%)
Subtotal		42	8	0	2	10/52 (19%)
C	T3a	2	0	0	0	0/2 (0%)
	T3b	16	11	0	12	23/39 (59%)
Subtotal		18	11	0	12	23/41 (56%)
Total		60	19	0	14	33/93 (35%)

Table 6. Distribution of Patients With Metastases to Lymph Nodes According to Clinical Stage and Histologic Grade of Primary Tumor

Amer. Urol. Stage	Stanford TNM Stage	Number of Patients	Differentiation of Primary Tumor*			Ratio of Patients With + Nodes to Total
			Well Diff.	Moderately Diff.	Poorly Diff.	
A	T0	3	0/1 (0%)	0/1 (0%)	0/1 (0%)	0/3 (0%)
B	T1,T2	49	1/7 (14%)	7/37 (19%)	2/5 (40%)	10/49 (20%)
C	T3	41	0/1 (0%)	9/23 (39%)	14/17 (82%)	23/41 (56%)
Totals		93	1/9 (11%)	16/61 (26%)	16/23 (70%)	33/93 (35%)

* Patients with metastases to lymph nodes/patients in subgroup.

Table 7. Distribution of Patients With Lymph Node Metastases According to Clinical Stage and Gleason Histologic Pattern Score of the Primary Tumor

Amer. Urol. Stage	Stanford TNM Stage	Gleason Pattern Score of Primary Tumor*									Total
		2	3	4	5	6	7	8	9	10	
A	T0		0/2						0/1		0/3
B	T1a,T1b			0/1	0/2	0/5	1/3				1/11
B	T1c		0/1		0/2	0/4	1/3	0/1	1/1		2/12
B	T2a			0/1		1/2	0/2				1/5
B	T2b			0/1		2/10	4/9	0/1			6/21
C	T3			0/1	1/4	2/8	5/11	6/8	7/7	2/2	23/41
Total		0	0/3	0/4	1/8	5/29	11/28	6/10	8/9	2/2	33/93
Percent with metastases			0%	0%	13%	17%	39%	60%	89%	100%	35%

* Patients with metastases to lymph nodes/patients in subgroup.

Table 8. *Incidence of Lymph Node Metastases (LNM) According to Modified Gleason-Mellinger Categories*

Modified Gleason Category	No. LNM/ No. in Category (%)
3	— (—)
4	0/2 (—)
5	— (—)
6	0/2 (—)
7	0/3 (—)
8	0/8 (—)
9	2/10 (20%)
10	4/20 (20%)
11	6/18 (33%)
12	6/13 (46%)
13	6/8 (75%)
14	7/7 (100%)
15	2/2 (100%)
Total	33/93 (35%)

Clinical Stage, Histologic Grade, and Acid Phosphatase Levels Combined

The incidence of lymph node metastases according to clinical stage and histologic grade for patients presenting with normal or elevated total serum acid phosphatase levels is shown in Table 9. Only one of 23 patients (4%) with state T0, T1, or T2 tumors and normal serum acid phosphatase levels had node metastases. At the other extreme, 13 of 14 patients (93%) with poorly differentiated T3b tumors and elevated serum acid phosphatase levels had lymph node metastases.

Current Patient Status

Of the 86 patients followed from 15 months to seven years, 76 (88%) are living and 50 (58%) have no evident disease. Because the number of patients

Table 9. *Ratio of Patients With Positive Lymph Nodes vs. Stage, Grade, and Acid Phosphatase*

Stage			Acid Phosphatase*	
Modified TNM	Amer. Urol.	Differentiation	Normal	Elevated
T0 T1a, T1b,T1c T2a,T2b }	A & B	Well	0/4	1/4
		Moderately	1/16	6/22
		Poorly	0/3	2/3
T3a,T3b	C	Well	—	0/1
		Moderately	3/8	6/15
		Poorly	1/3	13/14

* Using p-nitrophenyl phosphate as substrate. Normal range ($\pm$ 2 SD) is 0.13–0.64 Bessey-Lowry (BL) units.

Table 10. Current Status of Patients Followed 15 Months to Seven Years After Treatment

Status of Pretreatment Lymph Nodes	Protocol Group X-ray Therapy	No. Pts.	Pts. Aš		Pts. Ac̄			Pts. Dc̄			Di
			No. (%)	−Biop.	No. (%)	M	Only +Biop.	No.	M	Only +Biop.	
Negative	Prostate only	26	21 (81%)	3	5 (19%)	3	2	0	—	—	0
	Prostate + pelvic	28	20 (71%)	7	6 (21%)	2	4	2	2(2)	—	0
Positive pelvic	Prostate + pelvic	11	4 (36%)	1	3 (27%)	1(1)	2	4	4(1)	—	—
	Prostate, pelvic, + para-aortic	7	3 (43%)	1	4 (57%)	4(3)	—	0	—	—	0
Positive pelvic and para-aortic	Prostate, pelvic, + para-aortic	14	2 (14%)	1	8 (57%)	7	1	3*	2(2)	1	1†
Total		86	50 (58%)	13	26 (30%)	17(4)	9	9 (10%)	8(5)	1	1 (1%)

Abbreviations: Aš = alive without cancer, Ac̄ = alive with cancer, Dc̄ = Died with cancer, Di = Died intercurrent disease, M = bone metastases, + Biop = positive postirradiation biopsy of prostate, − Biop = negative postirradiation biopsy of prostate, ( ) = number with metastases who also had apparently viable tumor in the prostate.
* One died of diffuse histiocytic lymphoma with diffuse prostatic metastases.
† Died of lung cancer at one year, no postmortem exam, clinically NED.

in each cell is small and the period of follow-up relatively short, survival curves are inadequate. Therefore, the results to date are tabulated for each of the five treatment groups according to survival with or without known or suspected disease (Table 10).

Patients with suspected disease are currently being recalled for posttreatment prostatic needle biopsy; to date, only one third of the biopsies have been completed. Of the 32 completed, 17 (53%) were considered positive and 15 (47%) negative. Although the sample for biopsy data is incomplete and the findings subject to the vagaries of interpretation of postirradiated tissue, most of the positives have occurred in patients with tumors that involved the entire gland, with or without extension beyond the prostate.

For those patients without positive lymph nodes on initial evaluation, the disease-free survival rates are 81% for those with radiation to the prostate only and 71% for those with both prostatic and pelvic irradiation. Elective treatment of the regional lymph nodes does not appear to improve the survival rate.

Seven of 18 patients with positive pelvic nodes are surviving without evident disease for 15, 23, 33, 36, 42, 60, and 66 months. Two others are surviving with apparently positive prostatic biopsies. The issue of whether or not it is worthwhile to irradiate the next higher echelon of nodes in such patients remains unsettled. Unfortunately, the number of patients is too small to expect to demonstrate significant differences between those who received regional irradiation only and those who received treatment to the next echelon of lymph nodes as well. Although no patients have died in the extended treatment group, four are living with apparent bone metastases. Conversely, among the patients who received regional irradiation only, four have died with metastatic disease and three others are living with disease, including one with osseous metastases and two with apparently positive prostatic disease. In summary, four of 11 patients who received regional treatment only and three of seven who received extended field treatment are living without evident disease.

The results to date demonstrate the potentially grave consequences of positive adenopathy, particularly when there is involvement of both the pelvic and the para-aortic lymph nodes. In this group of patients, only two of the original 14 survive without evident disease. One other is surviving with a positive prostatic biopsy. Seven others are living with bone metastases. Three who died had bone metastases, and one died with neoplasm in the prostate only.

Complications of Treatment

One major goal of this study was to document the value of extended-field therapy relative to possible morbidity due to lymph node biopsies or dissections. Two complications found to be important in this regard were small bowel obstruction and lymphedema.

Small Bowel Obstruction

During the first two years of the study, we observed that patients receiving extended-field treatments were experiencing unduly high rates of small bowel obstructive symptoms. Of 26 patients treated, 21 had extended fields, including 14 (67%) with serious symptoms. Eight patients required surgical correction of the obstruction. One third of the patients who had positive pelvic nodes only and were symptomatic required corrective surgery, while all five patients with positive para-aortic nodes required it.

Starting in November 1973, the following action was taken to reduce these sequelae of extended treatment: (1) the extent of sampling of the pelvic and para-aortic nodes was reduced, (2) the total radiation dose to the lymph node regions was reduced from 5,500 rads (in 5½ weeks) to 5,000 rads (in 7 weeks) by inserting the coned-down prostatic boost dose (2,000 rads in 2 weeks) at the midpoint of the regional or extended-field irradiation, and (3) the number of fields treated per day was increased from two to four to improve homogeneity of delivery of each day's dose to both pelvic and para-aortic node regions.

In the subsequent 18-month period (11/73–4/75), 20 additional patients underwent transperitoneal lymph node biopsy with the above modifications. Extended fields were used in 12 of these. Only two had symptoms, one of whom required surgical intervention and was found to have an obstruction caused by adhesions that were probably not due to radiation.

In the final period (4/75–6/77), all lymph node biopsies were performed extraperitoneally. Of the 47 patients treated in this period, 30 had extended-field irradiation. Only one had partial small bowel symptoms and he was managed conservatively, without surgery.

In addition to the reduction in morbidity due to small bowel complications, the extraperitoneal method of exploration resulted in shorter hospital stays and reduced immediate complications of surgery (Freiha 1977).

Lymphedema

With the change to extraperitoneal biopsy of lymph nodes in April 1975, a more extensive sampling of nodes and a resultant new complication of edema of the penis, scrotum, suprapubic area, or legs, or any combination of these, was observed.

Of the 47 patients treated in this period, 26 (55%) had one or more of these complications. Of those treated with only limited fields (prostate only), seven of 17 (41%) had symptoms, but all occurred prior to radiation. Of those treated with extended fields, 19 of 30 (63%) experienced symptoms of this type. In contrast to the previous group, in five (26%) symptoms occurred prior to radiation and in 14 (74%) after treatment. These observations indicate that the larger radiation volume had an additive effect with the surgery on the production of this complication.

DISCUSSION

The similarity in disease-free survival between patients with surgically proven negative lymph nodes who received prostatic irradiation and those who received total pelvic irradiation is not surprising, since the only patients who could have been helped would have been those with occult lymph node metastases that might have been missed by the staging procedure. This situation became increasingly unlikely as the dissections became more extensive during the course of the study. Therefore, it appears that there is no need to follow a negative lymph node dissection with irradiation. In fact, to do so simply increases the possibility of posttreatment lymphedema. Among those 54 patients with disease limited to the prostate, two have died, both with persistence of disease in the prostate and osseous metastases, and five others are living with osseous metastases in the absence of demonstrable adenopathy. Six others who are surviving had apparently positive prostatic biopsies. Whether their disease is biologically active is uncertain in view of several series that have demonstrated reversion of positive biopsies to negative on subsequent specimens (Sewell et al. 1975, Kagan et al. 1977, Cox and Stoffel 1977). We were, however, sufficiently impressed with the apparent viability of tumor in several of these and several nonprotocol patients to carry out ^{125}I implants as a second attempt at definitive therapy (Goffinet et al., in preparation).

The patients with proven pelvic adenopathy might have provided the best test of the efficacy of elective irradiation extended to the next lymph node echelon, the para-aortic nodes, but their numbers were too small to derive a statistical comparison. Inspection of Table 10, however, reveals little apparent difference in status between those patients who received radiation to the prostate and pelvic lymph nodes and those also irradiated in the para-aortic lymph nodes except that there have been no deaths in the latter group, while there have been four deaths in the former. This observation, however, is tempered by the fact that four patients treated electively in the para-aortic region are living with apparent bone metastases and might be expected to eventually succumb to their disease.

Most of the third group of patients, those with biopsy-proven para-aortic lymph nodes, are manifesting more bone metastases with longer survival.

The most striking feature of the study is the profound adverse effect on total and disease-free survival of the presence of lymphadenopathy. Histologically involved lymph nodes were found in 36% of the patients. Among the 32 patients with proven adenopathy followed longer than 15 months, 18 (56%) have manifest bone metastases (Table 10). This is in remarkable agreement with the observations of Hilaris et al. (1977), who found a 40% incidence of positive lymph nodes among their 208 surgically staged patients, 69% of whom developed osseous metastases within five years.

The adverse influence of adenopathy on overall survival was demonstrated when we pooled these protocol patients with nonprotocol patients who had been surgically staged and treated during the same interval (Bagshaw, in press). The probability of survival (Kaplan-Meier) at five years was 0.95 for patients with no adenopathy and 0.58 for those with proven adenopathy.

These observations prompted the detailed correlations of clinical stage, histologic grade, and serum acid phosphatase described earlier to identify, if possible, diagnostic parameters that might be associated with risk of lymph node metastases. Table 11 details three risk groups. The low-risk (4% chance of lymph node metastases) and high-risk (93% chance of lymph node metastases) groups are well defined. Patients identified as at low risk may not require laparotomy for the evaluation of lymph nodes. Patients at low risk for adenopathy could receive irradiation to the prostate and pelvic lymph nodes in an attempt to eliminate nodal metastases in those who have positive lymph nodes, since postirradiation complications in the absence of surgical staging have been virtually eliminated with the radiation technique described. Patients in the high-risk group are likely to have extensive adenopathy amenable to visualization by lymphograms. Whether or not they should receive extended-field irradiation is moot. In this series there are only three potential disease-free survivors among 14 with proven para-aortic adenopathy. The intermediate group, i.e., those with a 35% chance of lymph node metastases, is poorly defined and lymph node biopsy is probably justified for adequate staging.

A remarkably similar definition of risk groups can be derived from the modified Gleason-Mellinger categories, which take into account only stage and grade (Table 12).

Lymphography was generally disappointing in the low- and intermediate-risk groups; however, involved lymph nodes were identified by lymphograms

Table 11. *Functional Grouping of Patients Based Upon Clinical Stage, Histologic Grade, and Total Serum Acid Phosphatase Levels*

Risk Group	Amer. Urol. Stage	Stanford TNM Stage	Grade	Acid Phosphatase	Ratio of Patients With Positive Lymph Node Biopsies to Total Group
Low	A,B	T0,T1a,T1b	1,2	Nl. or Abn.	1/13
	B	T1c,T2a,T2b	1,2	Nl.	0/12
Subtotal					1/25 (4%)
Intermediate	A,B	T0,T1a,T1b	3	Nl. or Abn.	0/1
	B	T1c,T2a,T2b	1,2	Abn.	7/21
	B	T1c,T2a,T2b	3	Nl. or Abn.	2/5
	C	T3a,T3b	1,2,3	Nl.	4/11
	C	T3a,T3b	1,2	Abn.	6/16
Subtotal					19/54 (35%)
High	C	T3a,T3b	3	Abn.	13/14 (93%)
Total					33/93 (35%)

Abbreviations: Nl = Normal, Abn = abnormal.

Table 12. *Functional Grouping of Patients Based Upon Clinical Stage and Modified Gleason-Mellinger Categories*

Risk Group	Modified Gleason-Mellinger Categories	No. of Patients (%)	Ratio of Patients With Lymph Node Metastases to Total Group (%)
Low	3–8	15 (16%)	0/15 (0%)
Intermediate	9–12	61 (66%)	18/61 (30%)
High	13–15	17 (18%)	15/17 (88%)
Total		93 (100%)	33/93 (35%)

in nine of the 14 high-risk patients. Lymphography combined with fine-needle aspiration was used in one patient to prove para-aortic metastases (Goldstein et al. 1977, Pereiras et al. 1978). This combination could avert a useless laparotomy in patients in the high-risk group with para-aortic lymph nodes demonstrated by lymphography.

Although we have not observed frank recurrence of neoplasms in treated lymph node-bearing regions, our ability to detect recurrence in these regions is limited.

Although posttreatment prostatic biopsy was an original feature of this protocol, aggressive implementation was delayed due to a number of factors, the most important being the reluctance of patient and physician alike to intervene when the prostate appeared normal clinically. During the last two years, after it became apparent that a second attempt at definitive treatment with ^{125}I implants could be carried out, we were obligated to pursue this with more vigor. Consequently, the first biopsies have generally been performed in patients who appeared, on the basis of clinical examination, to have persistent disease. This raises the obvious questions of when and to whom radiation by interstitial implant should be administered.

Approximately 135 patients were treated contemporaneously off protocol. They were excluded for the reasons stated earlier. Their records are available for analysis of prognostic factors and status, but we decided not to include them with the protocol group because a review of the pretreatment histopathologic grading is incomplete. Since most of these patients have not undergone a staging laparotomy, it will be of interest to compare their response to treatment with that of the protocol patients once they can be matched according to age, stage, grade, and pretreatment acid phosphatase levels.

This analysis of a small but carefully staged group of patients perhaps raises more questions than it answers. Although some patients with proven adenopathy are surviving without evident disease for a reasonably long period, clearly a large fraction of patients with lymph node metastases later develop bone involvement.

SUMMARY AND CONCLUSIONS

Patients with prostatic carcinoma apparently localized to the prostate and with no adenopathy demonstrable by lymph node dissection appear to derive no benefit from supplemental treatment of regional lymph nodes by radiation therapy.

The presence of histopathologically proven lymphadenopathy by sampling or dissection of regional lymph nodes appears to have such an adverse influence on disease-free survival, particularly with reference to subsequent manifestations of bone metastases, that it is unlikely that a potential improvement in outcome by elective irradiation of the next higher lymph node echelon can be demonstrated.

In the presence of histopathologically proven lymphadenopathy, regional lymphatic irradiation in addition to irradiation of the prostate may be efficacious, as nine of 32 patients are surviving without evidence of disease and three others are surviving with apparently positive prostatic biopsies. In view of the small number of patients and the restricted term of the follow-up, however, this cannot be concluded with certainty at this time.

Clinical stage, pathologic grade, and pretreatment acid phosphatase levels taken together appear to be useful predictors of the probability of lymph node involvement. Patients may be subdivided into low-, intermediate-, and high-risk groups on the basis of these three variables.

Because of a relatively high incidence of false-negative and false-positive studies, current lymphographic techniques are unreliable for detecting lymphadenopathy in the low- and intermediate-risk groups. In the high-risk category, however, lymphography successfully demonstrated lymphadenopathy in nine of 14 patients.

ACKNOWLEDGMENTS

The authors wish to thank Richard L. Kempson, M.D., of the Division of Surgical Pathology at Stanford University School of Medicine and Donald F. Gleason, M.D., of the Department of Pathology, Fairview Hospital, Minneapolis, Minnesota, who graded all initial prostatic biopsy specimens by their respective methods. This investigation was supported by grants CA-05838 and CA-15455 awarded by the National Cancer Institute, Department of Health, Education and Welfare.

REFERENCES

Bagshaw, M. A. 1979. Perspectives on radiation treatment of prostate cancer: History and current focus, *in* Prostatic Cancer, G. P. Murphy, ed. PSG Publishing Co., Littleton, Mass. (in press).

Bagshaw, M. A., H. S. Kaplan, and R. H. Sagerman. 1965. Linear accelerator supervoltage radiotherapy. VII. Carcinoma of the prostate. Radiology 85:121–129.

Bagshaw, M. A., D. A. Pistenma, G. R. Ray, F. S. Freiha, and R. L. Kempson. 1977. Evaluation of extended-field radiotherapy for prostatic neoplasm: 1976 progress report. Cancer Treat. Rep. 61:297–306.

Bagshaw, M. A., G. R. Ray, J. R. Salzman, and E. Meares, Jr. 1975. Extended-field radiation therapy for carcinoma of the prostate: A progress report. Cancer Chemother. Rep. 59:165–173.

Cox, J. D., and T. J. Stoffel. 1977. The significance of needle biopsy after irradiation for stage C adenocarcinoma of the prostate. Cancer 40:156–160.

Freiha, F. S. 1977. Surgical staging of prostatic cancer: Transperitoneal versus extraperitoneal lymphadenectomy. J. Urol. 118:616–617.

Gleason, D. F. 1966. Classification of prostatic carcinoma. Cancer Chemother. Rep. 50:125–128.

Gleason, D. F., G. T. Mellinger, and the Veterans Administration Cooperative Urological Research Group. 1974. Prediction of prognosis for prostatic adenocarcinoma by combined histologic grading and clinical staging. J. Urol. 111:58–64.

Goldstein, H., J. Zornoza, and S. Wallace. 1977. Percutaneous fine needle aspiration biopsy of pancreatic and other abdominal masses. Radiology 123:319–322.

Hilaris, B. S., W. S. Whitmore, M. Batata, and W. Barzell. Behavioral patterns of prostate adenocarcinoma following an ^{125}I implant and pelvic node dissection. 1977. Int. J. Radiat. Oncol. Biol. Phys. 2:631–637.

Kagan, A. R., J. Gordon, J. F. Cooper, H. Gilbert, H. Nussbaum, and P. Chan. 1977. A clinical appraisal of post-irradiation biopsy in prostatic cancer. Cancer 39:637–641.

Kempson, R. L., and G. Levine. 1974. The relationship of grade to prognosis in carcinoma of the prostate. Front. Radiat. Ther. Oncol. 9:267–273.

Pereiras, R. V., W. Meiers, B. Kunhardt, M. Troner, D. Hutson, J. S. Barkin, and M. Viamonte. 1978. Fluoroscopically guided thin needle aspiration biopsy of the abdomen and retroperitoneum. Am. J. Roentgenol. 131:197–202.

Ray, G. R., J. R. Cassady, and M. A. Bagshaw. 1973. Definitive radiation therapy of carcinoma of the prostate. Radiology 106:407–418.

Sewell, R. A., V. Braven, S. K. Wilson, and R. K. Rhamy. 1975. Extended biopsy follow-up after full course radiation for resectable prostatic carcinoma. J. Urol. 113:371–373.

Cancer of the Genitourinary Tract, edited by
D. E. Johnson and M. L. Samuels.
Raven Press, New York © 1979.

Chemotherapeutic Treatment on a National Randomized Trial Basis by the National Prostatic Cancer Project

Gerald P. Murphy, M.D., D.Sc.

Director, National Prostatic Cancer Project, Roswell Park Memorial Institute, Buffalo, New York

The National Prostatic Cancer Project instituted goals for the use of chemotherapy in 1973. Before commenting on the numerous objective results that have been obtained, the validity of the observations, and the correctness of this approach, I would like to discuss certain aspects of those goals that have occasionally been blurred or perhaps ignored to reemphasize our approach and to demonstrate our progress.

For over 30 years, many patients with metastatic prostate cancer in the United States have received valid, appropriate treatment for their primary disease. Most of these patients have subsequently undergone hormonal palliation by means of castration, administration of estrogenic compounds or derivatives, or both. Those patients who then relapse present a dilemma for the urologist. They are frequently bedridden, with severe pain and all the other signs and symptoms of total clinical degeneration, and have a very poor prognosis. I need not cite references to support this statement for you all know its validity. All the patients in our early studies and trials had progressive disease, in the opinion of the participating physicians. They were no longer responding to hormonal therapy, and exhibited pain, weight loss, debility, and other subjective and objective indications of degeneration.

Since such patients are not likely to live long, the goals of treatment are (1) to alleviate signs and symptoms of disease, (2) to prolong survival, if possible, and (3) to compare the course of disease in patients receiving new forms of treatment with that in untreated or conventionally treated individuals. All these goals have been met since trials were instituted in 1973 (Scott et al. 1975). Our immediate aims in testing various estrogenic compounds in such patients were to detect activity, to determine if such activity was reproducible, on a randomized basis in many centers and in subsequent trials, and to discover whether or not such activity could be initiated in earlier phases of the disease. At the same time, we wished to benefit patients who had little or no hope. I will submit evidence to you today that indicates all these goals have been achieved.

In our trials, a distinction had to be made between patients who had been irradiated and thus had compromised bone marrow reserves and patients who had not (Scott et al. 1975, Murphy et al. 1977). The types of agents used had to be modified accordingly. Our results (Scott et al. 1975, Murphy et al. 1977) demonstrate that, even with this limitation, active agents can be found that are better than the so-called standard, randomized treatment (Scott et al. 1975, Murphy et al. 1977).

The criteria of response employed in these trials are definitive and reproducible, and are now being applied on an international basis by other groups with similar results.

The criteria for objective complete response include all of the following:

1. Tumor masses, if present, totally disappeared and no new lesions appeared.
2. Elevated acid phosphatase, if present, returned to normal.
3. Osteolytic lesions, if present, recalcified.
4. Osteoblastic lesions, if present, disappeared.
5. If hepatomegaly is significant, complete reduction in liver size, and normalization of all pretreatment abnormalities of liver function.
6. No significant cancer-related deterioration in weight (>10%), symptoms, or performance status (became or remained ambulatory).

The criteria for objective partial regression include all of the following:

1. At least one tumor mass, if present, reduced by >50% in cross-sectional area.
2. Elevated acid phosphatase, if present, returned to normal.
3. Osteolytic lesions, if present, undergo recalcification in one or more, but not in all.
4. Osteoblastic lesions, if present, do not progress.
5. If hepatomegaly is significant, reduction in liver size and *at least* a 30% improvement in all pretreatment abnormalities of liver function.
6. No increase in any other lesion and no new areas of malignant disease.
7. No significant cancer-related deterioration in weight (>10%), symptoms, or performance status (improved or remained the same).

The criteria for objectively stable include all of the following:

1. No new lesions, and no lesions measurably present increased more than 25% in cross-sectional area.
2. Acid phosphatase level decreases, though need not return to normal.
3. Osteolytic lesions, if present, do not appear to worsen.
4. Osteoblastic lesions, if present, remain stable.
5. Hepatomegaly, if present, does not worsen by more than 30% and symptoms of hepatic abnormalities do not worsen.
6. No significant cancer-related deterioration in weight (>10%), symptoms, or performance status (improved or remained the same).

The criteria for objective progression include any of the following:

1. Significant cancer-related deterioration in weight (>10%), symptoms, or performance status (at least one score level).
2. Appearance of new areas of malignant disease.
3. Increase in any previously measurable lesion by greater than 25% in cross-sectional area.
4. Development of recurring anemia secondary to prostate cancer (not treatment related—Protocols 500 and 600).
5. Development of ureteral obstruction (Protocols 500 and 600). An increase in acid or alkaline phosphatase *alone* is not considered an indication of progression. That should be used in conjunction with other criteria.

The criteria of response for a patient with advanced disease who has undergone all the standard treatments are understandably different from those for a patient with newly diagnosed or stable disease. In other areas, such as in adjuvant trials following primary treatment with radiation or surgery, these criteria obviously must be altered. I would like to emphasize again that all the patients in this study had progressive disease, but none had had prior chemotherapeutic treatment. Moreover, they had been off other treatment for a sufficient length of time prior to randomization to permit determination of progression and response to treatment (Scott et al. 1975, Murphy et al. 1977).

Patients who achieved stability in these trials differed from conventionally thought of stable patients in other randomized trials dealing with, for example, leukemias or solid tumors. These patients all had progressive disease, and when the progression stopped they were termed stable. Unless we recognize this difference and report our results in terms of stable disease, partial regression, and complete regression, our definitions and criteria can be misleading.

The principal investigators in the National Prostatic Cancer Project include: Gerald P. Murphy (Roswell Park Memorial Institute), Douglas E. Johnson (M. D. Anderson Hospital and Tumor Institute), William W. Scott (Johns Hopkins Hospital, Brady Urological Institute), George R. Prout, Jr. (Massachusetts General Hospital), Mark S. Soloway (University of Tennessee Center for the Health Sciences), Robert P. Gibbons (Virginia Mason Medical Center), Stefan A. Loening (University of Iowa Hospitals and Clinics), Joseph D. Schmidt (University of California Medical Center, University Hospital), Jean B. deKernion (Tulane School of Medicine), and J. Edson Pontes (Wayne State University).

The program seems to have reached an effective size, based on peer review and other commentaries. The procedures for patient randomization and follow-up are summarized in Figure 1. Reevaluation of data, correlation of histological findings, and centralization of acid and alkaline phosphatase special tests for rechecking have been hallmarks of this project from the beginning. Data review has led to significant conclusions, but the quality of the evaluation has always been the primary concern. Figure 2 indicates the increase in the number of patients participating in this project since its inception in 1973. The expansion

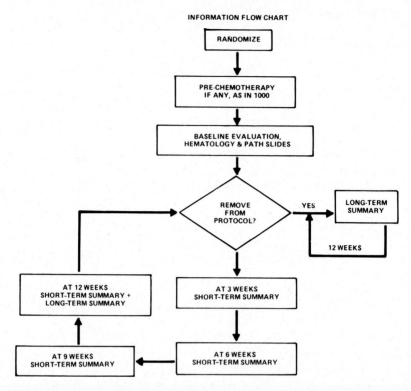

Figure 1. Processing of randomized patients in the National Prostatic Cancer Project. The long-term and short-term summary forms should cover only the period since the last report. At death a final long-term summary is sent. For Protocols 900 and 1000, the intervals between short forms will vary between treatment arms.

of the group, the creation of the protocols, and continuing follow-up have resulted in impressive progress.

Stratification of patients according to whether or not they had received radiation therapy, and thereby had compromised bone marrow reserve, is shown in Figure 3, which also gives an overview of the various protocols. Protocol

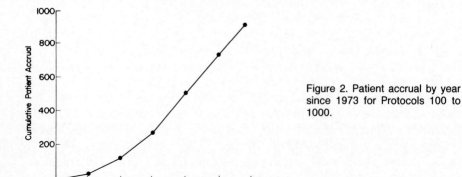

Figure 2. Patient accrual by year since 1973 for Protocols 100 to 1000.

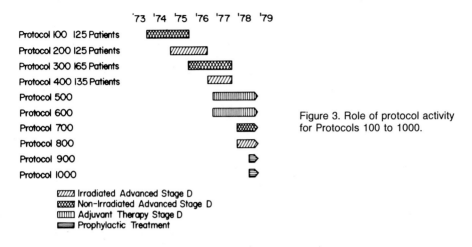

'73 '74 '75 '76 '77 '78 '79

Protocol 100 125 Patients
Protocol 200 125 Patients
Protocol 300 165 Patients
Protocol 400 135 Patients
Protocol 500
Protocol 600
Protocol 700
Protocol 800
Protocol 900
Protocol 1000

Figure 3. Role of protocol activity for Protocols 100 to 1000.

⬚⬚⬚ Irradiated Advanced Stage D
▨▨▨ Non-Irradiated Advanced Stage D
⬚⬚⬚ Adjuvant Therapy Stage D
▭ Prophylactic Treatment

100 identified the activity of 5-fluorouracil and Cytoxan (Scott et al. 1975), while the effectiveness of Estracyt was determined in Protocol 200. Protocol 300, which compared Cytoxan, procarbazine, and dimethyl triazeno imidazole carboxamide (DTIC), has also been completed (Schmidt et al. 1979), and DTIC and Cytoxan were identified as effective single agents. Protocol 400 compared the effects of prednimustine plus Estracyt to prednimustine alone, and found no difference in activity between the two (Murphy et al. 1977). Phase II studies have identified the mechanism of action of prednimustine (Catane et al. 1978).

Our goals in Protocols 500 and 600 will take longer to achieve. These protocols include newly diagnosed patients (Protocol 500) (Figure 4) and patients with stable disease (Protocol 600) (Figure 5). The role of chemotherapy in combination with hormonal treatment is undergoing evaluation on a randomized basis in

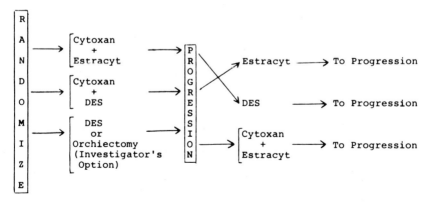

Figure 4. Protocol 500 treatment schema, used in patients with early metastatic stage D disease: Cytoxan (1 gm/m² i.v. every three weeks) plus Estracyt (600 mg/m² p.o. daily in three divided doses), Cytoxan (1 gm/m² i.v. every three weeks) plus diethylstilbestrol (DES) (1 mg t.i.d. p.o.), DES (1 mg t.i.d. p.o.) alone, or orchiectomy. Patients whose disease progresses after the initial 12 weeks of therapy are crossed over.

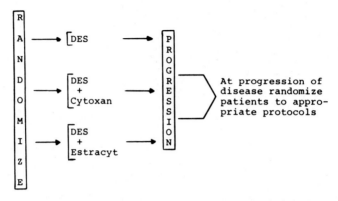

Figure 5. Protocol 600 treatment schema, used in stable stage D patients: DES (1 mg t.i.d. p.o.), DES (1 mg t.i.d. p.o.) plus Cytoxan (1 gm/m² i.v. every three weeks), or DES (1 mg t.i.d. p.o.) plus Estracyt (600 mg/m² p.o. daily in three divided doses).

these studies. No patient will enter or complete either protocol without having had one course of chemotherapy and exposure to conventional hormonal treatment. This represents an application of the results of Protocols 100 through 400 to an earlier stage of the disease.

Protocols 700 and 800 represent a continuing search for new agents to employ at the end stage of the disease. Nonirradiated patients with advanced disease, similar to those in Protocols 100 and 300, are undergoing treatment in Protocol 700 (Figure 6) with hydroxyurea, 1-(chlorethyl)-3-(4-methyl-cyclohexyl)-1-nitro-

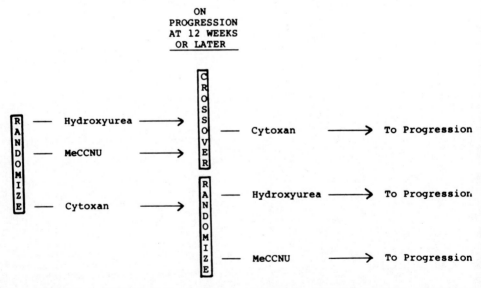

Figure 6. Protocol 700 treatment schema, used in nonirradiated, relapsing stage D patients: Hydroxyurea (3 gm/m² p.o. every three days in three divided doses), MeCCNU (175 mg/m² p.o. every six weeks), or Cytoxan (1 gm/m² i.v. every three weeks).

sourea (MeCCNU), or Cytoxan. Similarly, patients who have received similar forms of radiotherapy are receiving Estracyt, vincristine, or a combination of the two agents in Protocol 800 (Figure 7).

Protocols 900 and 1000 represent our adjuvant treatment trials; patients receiving definitive surgery and surgical staging are evaluated in Protocol 900 (Figure 8) and those receiving primary radiotherapy for so-called localized lesions are seen in Protocol 1000 (Figure 9). These protocols indicate the beginning, continuation, and ultimate goals of the National Prostatic Cancer Project.

Follow-up of the patients entered into these protocols generates a considerable amount of data, which are summarized in Table 1. There have been relatively few violations of the initial protocol, considering the number of patients entered and the newness and diversity of the group. All patients are followed, even if they represented protocol violations, received no treatment, or received less than three weeks of treatment. There were not many such patients and they have not altered greatly the ease of assessment or the validity of the conclusions. The number of evaluable patients depends on whether the protocol is completed, as in Protocols 100 through 400, or is still open, as in Protocols 500 through 1000. In addition, a number of patients are still undergoing treatment, and many others are currently being followed.

In all clinical trials, especially those for this type of disease, the rates of entries into current protocols are important. Those rates are summarized for this project in Table 2. There can be no "ideal entry rate" for clinical investigation. This project began with four participating centers, and now consists of 9

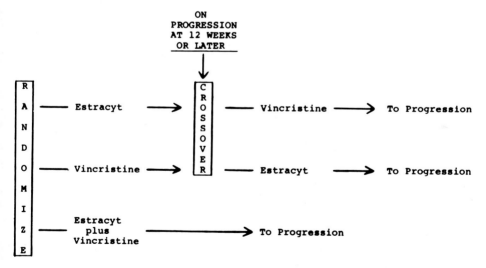

Figure 7. Protocol 800 treatment schema, for irradiated, advanced relapsing stage D patients: Estracyt (600 mg/m² p.o. daily in three divided doses), vincristine (1 mg/m² i.v. once every two weeks), or Estracyt (600 mg/m² p.o. daily in three divided doses) plus vincristine (1 mg/m² i.v. once every two weeks).

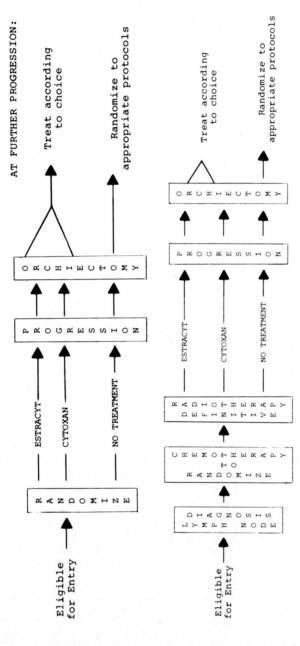

Figure 8 (top). Protocol 900 treatment regimens, for surgically treated primary prostate cancer patients: Estracyt (600 mg/m² p.o. daily in three divided doses), cyclophosphamide (1 gm/m² i.v. every three weeks), or no treatment.

Figure 9. Protocol 1000 treatment regimen, for stage D primary prostate cancer patients: Prior definitive radiotherapy and lymph node diagnosis by pelvic lymph node dissection or lymphangiogram with fine-needle biopsy, followed by randomized adjuvant chemotherapy with Estracyt (600 mg/m² p.o. daily in three divided doses), cyclophosphamide (1 gm/m² i.v. every three weeks), or no treatment.

Table 1. Number of Patients Entered and Status for National Prostatic Cancer Project Protocols as of August 11, 1978

Patients	Protocol										
	100	200	300	400	500	600	700	800	900	1000	Total
Entered	125	125	165	135	98	77	73	87	12	4	901
Excluded											
Protocol violations	4	2	2	5	1	3	0	0	0	0	17
No treatment	4	6	7	6	1	0	3	3	0	0	30
Received <3 weeks of treatment	8	12	25	8	8	6	3	3	0	0	73
Insufficient information for evaluation	0	0	2	0	36	28	39	45	12	4	166
Evaluable	109	105	129	116	52	40	28	36	0	0	615
Currently on treatment*	1	2	8	4	71	43	40	47	11	4	231
Currently being followed	3	6	19	17	81	56	50	63	12	4	311

* May include crossover treatment.

Table 2. *Entry Rates in Current Protocols Before and After Last Evaluation*

Current Protocol	Date Activated	Entered Through 11-14-77	Entry Rate Per Week	Entered 11-5-77 Through 8-11-78*	Entry Rate Per Week
500	7-1-76	58	.83†	40	1.00
600	7-1-76	43	.61†	34	.85
700	5-24-77	35	1.52§	38	.95
800	5-24-77	35	1.52§	52	1.30
900	5-1-78	0	.00	12	.80‡
1000	5-1-78	0	.00	4	.27‡
Total		171	2.44	180	4.50

* 40 weeks.   § 23 weeks.
† 70 weeks.   ‡ 15 weeks.

or 10, depending on the particular protocols. The patient entry rates have been influenced over time by this factor. The numbers for this table have not been updated since May 1978, but an improved rate of entry will be noted in subsequent reports.

There has been some concern that patients with slow-growing and well-differentiated tumors might be selected for primary chemotherapeutic trials, while those with more poorly differentiated and thus less responsive tumors are selected for standard treatment (Coune 1978). This has not proven to be the case, as is shown in Table 3, which summarizes the findings on most of the slides available on all the patients in completed Protocols 100 through 400. These do not represent all the findings, but do represent those that are definable within the criteria of tumor screening applied by Dr. John Gaeta, the referee pathologist for the National Prostatic Cancer Project. As shown here, no preference can be found in any of the arms. Quite the contrary, in fact; in some cases the more poorly or at least moderately differentiated tumors were found in the chemotherapeutic groups.

Other protocols will have been initiated by the time this report is presented, but since they are still in the evaluatory stage, it would be premature to discuss them. Similarly, it would be premature to discuss protocols in which patient entry, follow-up, and evaluation are still ongoing.

SUMMARY

We have found that Cytoxan, 5-fluorouracil, DTIC, Estracyt, and prednimustine can improve the lot of patients with advanced prostatic cancer who have relapsed following appropriate hormonal treatment. These agents have a limited degree of toxicity in terms of symptoms and objective laboratory findings (Scott et al. 1975, Murphy et al. 1977, Schmidt et al. 1978, Catane et al. 1978). The results have constantly been reviewed by our own groups, as well as those of

Table 3. *Primary Tumor Grade According to Treatments on Protocols 100–400*

| Tumor Grade | Protocol 100 | | | | | | Protocol 200 | | | | | | Protocol 300 | | | | | | Protocol 400 | | | |
| | Standard | | 5-FU | | Cytoxan | | Standard* | | Estracyt | | Strepto-zotocin | | Cytoxan | | DTIC | | Procar-bazine | | Predni-mustine + Estracyt | | Predni-mustine | |
	No.	%	No.	%	No.	%	No.	%	No.	%	No.	%	No.	%	No.	%	No.	%	No.	%	No.	%
Well differentiated	1	3	4	11	2	5	0	—	2	4	1	2	0	—	0	—	1	2	2	4	4	8
Moderately differentiated	17	46	11	31	11	27	6	29	17	39	20	50	11	35	18	36	13	32	12	24	16	31
Poorly differentiated	18	49	20	56	26	63	14	67	25	57	19	48	20	64	32	64	24	60	36	72	31	60
Anaplastic	1	3	1	3	2	5	1	5	0	—	0		0		0		2	5	0	—	1	2
Total	37		36		41		21		44		40		31		50		40		50		52	
Unknown	0		3		4		1		0		2		2		6		4		2		2	

* Distribution of grading significantly different ($p < 0.05$) from that for patients on streptozotocin by Wilcoxon test.

others (Schmidt et al. 1976). Continuing evaluation of the ongoing protocols will doubtless provide additional important knowledge.

Combinations of drugs have not been tested extensively and have not shown increased benefit. Other trials comparing hormonal treatment to early primary chemotherapeutic treatment in newly diagnosed metastatic prostate cancer patients and in patients with so-called stable metastatic prostate cancer are under way and important differences are anticipated. Adjuvant trials involving patients treated primarily with surgery or radiotherapy for cure provide an opportunity for early comparison of various adjuvants.

ACKNOWLEDGMENT

This investigation was supported by grant 50175–04 from the National Cancer Institute, Department of Health, Education and Welfare.

REFERENCES

Catane, R., J. H. Kaufman, S. Madajewicz, A. Mittleman, and G. P. Murphy. 1978. Prednimustine therapy for advanced prostatic cancer. Br. J. Urol. 50:29–32.

Coune, A. 1978. Carcinoma of the prostate, in Randomized Trials in Cancer: A Critical Review by Sites, M. J. Staquet, ed. Raven Press, New York, pp. 389–409.

Murphy, G. P., R. P. Gibbons, D. E. Johnson, S. A. Loening, G. R. Prout, J. D. Schmidt, D. S. Bross, T. M. Chu, J. F. Gaeta, J. Saroff, and W. W. Scott. 1977. A comparison of estramustine phosphate and streptozotocin in patients with advanced prostatic carcinoma who have had extensive irradiation. J. Urol. 118:288–291.

Schmidt, J. D., D. E. Johnson, W. W. Scott, R. P. Gibbons, G. R. Prout, and G. P. Murphy. 1976. Chemotherapy of advanced prostatic cancer: Evaluation of response parameters. Urology 7:602–610.

Schmidt, J. D., W. W. Scott, R. P. Gibbons, D. E. Johnson, G. R. Prout, Jr., S. A. Loening, M. S. Soloway, T. M. Chu, J. F. Gaeta, N. H. Slack, J. Saroff, and G. P. Murphy. 1979. Comparison of procarbazine, DTIC and cyclophosphamide in relapsing patients with advanced carcinoma of the prostate. J. Urol. 121:185–189.

Scott, W. W., D. E. Johnson, J. E. Schmidt, R. P. Gibbons, G. R. Prout, J. R. Joiner, J. Saroff, and G. P. Murphy. 1975. Chemotherapy of advanced prostatic carcinoma with cyclophosphamide or 5-fluorouracil: Results of first national randomized study. J. Urol. 114:909–911.

Cancer of the Genitourinary Tract, edited by
D. E. Johnson and M. L. Samuels.
Raven Press, New York © 1979.

Chemotherapy of Prostatic Cancer

David F. Paulson, M.D., William R. Berry, M.D.,*
Edwin B. Cox, M.D.,* and John Laszlo, M.D.*

*Departments of Urology and *Medicine, Duke University Medical Center,
Durham, North Carolina*

Two major problems in assessing the impact of chemotherapy programs for disseminated prostatic carcinoma are the identification of stratification indices defining the relative biologic hazard of disseminated disease within a single patient, and the identification of those indicators of disease response that accompany prolonged survival. The study to be described was undertaken not only to define the response of endocrine-unresponsive prostate adenocarcinoma patients to multiagent chemotherapy, but also to identify stratification indices and indicators of disease response.

METHODS

Between May 1973 and September 1977, 88 patients with hormone-resistant stage IV prostatic carcinoma were studied according to a phase II protocol that used a five-drug chemotherapy program. Hormone resistance was defined as progressive bone pain, weight loss, or increase in tumor size or extent following therapy with orchiectomy, estrogens, or both. A treatment course included melphalan, 2 mg p.o. daily, methotrexate (MTX), 25 mg p.o. weekly, 5-fluorouracil (5-FU), 500 mg p.o. weekly, and vincristine, 1 mg i.v. weekly for four weeks. This drug combination was repeated every four months. In addition, patients were given prednisone, 40 mg daily for two weeks, and the dose was then reduced by 5 mg weekly to a maintenance dose of 10 mg daily. Patients who had previously received radiation of >4,000 R to the spine and pelvis were started on one-half the dose of melphalan, methotrexate, and 5-FU. Patients with known peptic ulcer disease or glucose intolerance were not given prednisone.

Patients were excluded from the study if their prechemotherapy leukocyte count was <3,000/mm^3, platelet count was <100,000/mm^3, or creatinine was >2.5 mg/dl. No patient was excluded because of poor performance status or limited life expectancy. Patients with active infections were first treated with antibiotics and thereafter entered into the study.

Prior to therapy, all patients were evaluated by means of a complete history and physical examination, blood count, blood chemistries, serum acid phosphatase, carcinoembryonic antigen (CEA), urinalysis, chest x-ray exam, bone scan, bone x-ray exams, liver-spleen scan, intravenous pyelogram (IVP), and measurements of luteinizing hormone (LH), follicle-stimulating hormone (FSH), prolactin, and testosterone. Only the last 24 patients underwent bone marrow aspiration and/or biopsy. Patients with pleural effusions had cytologic examinations performed to determine malignancy, but suspected parenchymal lung, liver, or lymph node metastases were not biopsied unless these were the only evidence of metastases. After onset of chemotherapy, the following data were systematically collected according to the protocol: weekly—complete blood counts; every four weeks—history and physical examination, blood chemistries, acid phosphatase, and CEA; every 12 weeks—urinalysis, chest x-ray exam, bone scan, liver-spleen scan, IVP, serum LH, FSH, prolactin, and testosterone.

All patients were followed through the entire course of their illness and were continued on therapy until disease progression or drug intolerance or toxicity. Progression was defined as increasing bone pain, progressive weight loss, or any increase in objective measurement of tumor masses. Secondary therapy in the form of such agents as intravenous estrogen, diethylstilbestrol diphosphonate, and other single-agent chemotherapy was used in a few patients. Data for three patients who clearly responded to increased estrogen doses, even though they were initially thought to be unresponsive to hormones, are included in the data reported.

Drug dosage was adjusted to minimize toxicity on the following basis: If the white blood count was $<3,000/mm^3$ or platelets $<100,000/mm^3$ on the day the patient was to receive 5-FU and MTX, all drugs except prednisone were suspended for a week and then resumed at the same doses. If two consecutive episodes of leukopenia or thrombocytopenia occurred, the doses of melphalan, 5-FU, and MTX were cut in half. If patients developed a white count of $\leq 3,000$ or platelets of $\leq 100,000$ on half-dose therapy, the drugs were omitted for one week and then resumed. The reduced doses were given as often as counts permitted.

All prospectively collected data were maintained in the Duke Comprehensive Cancer Center Data Management Unit, where they could be reviewed and analyzed interactively by means of a graphics system. Curves representing nonparametric estimates of survival were generated using the Kaplan-Meier method (Kaplan and Meier 1958). On the survival graphs, the median survival is the point at which the time curve intersects the line representing 50% survival. Censored survival values representing patients still alive at the time of last follow-up are represented by single verticle bars on the graphs. When the longest survival value is a censored one, the curve is divided into two parts, representing upper and lower boundaries of survival estimates beyond the last death. Survivals of pairs of subgroups were tested for difference by the Cox-Mantel test (Cox 1972).

RESULTS

Demographic Data

There were 64 white and 22 black patients in our study. No difference was found in survival between the two groups (Table 1). No limits were set on the amount of radiation previously received, although doses of myelotoxic drugs were reduced by 50% for patients who had received >4,000 R to the spine or pelvis. There was no difference in survival between patients who had had prior radiation and those who had not (Table 1). Toxicity was the same in both groups: 25 of 49 patients with prior radiation experienced leukopenia (WBC <3,000), compared to 18 of 39 with no prior radiation.

All patients had stage IV disease. Of the 88 patients, 85 had bony metastases, while three had only soft tissue metastases. Twenty-two of these 85 patients had metastases to soft tissues (i.e., lung, liver, and/or lymph nodes) in addition to their bony metastases. Those patients who had soft tissue as well as bony metastases had a shorter survival than those who had only bony metastases (Figure 1 and Table 1).

Of patients with soft tissue metastases, five had nodular lung metastases, four patients had lymphangitic lung metastases, nine had malignant pleural effusion, four had palpable lymph node metastases, and 13 had abnormal liver scans felt to be attributable to tumor. The only specific site of metastasis for which a poor prognosis was noted was the pleura (Table 1).

An elevation of lactic acid dehydrogenase (LDH) (63 patients) or serum glutamic oxaloacetic transaminase (SGOT) (21 patients) was significantly associated with shortened survival ($p < 0.003$ and $p < 0.006$, respectively) (Figure 2 and Table 1). If both LDH and SGOT were abnormal (11 patients), the association

Table 1. *Prognostic Value of Initial Patient Characteristics*

Variable	Trait A (number)		Median Survival (weeks)	Trait B (number)		Median Survival (weeks)	p
Race	White	(64)	39.2	Black	(22)	44.2	.789
Age	>65	(43)	28.8	<65	(45)	57.0	.014
Prior radiation	No	(39)	39.0	Yes	(49)	39.6	.653
Sites of metastases	Bone + other organ	(22)	28.9	Bone only	(63)	45.6	.012
Malignant pleural effusion	Yes	(9)	24.5	No	(79)	41.9	.041
Liver scan	Abnormal	(13)	27.0	Normal	(75)	40.3	.058
LDH	>200 U	(63)	29.1	≤200 U	(35)	62.7	.003
SGOT	>50 U	(21)	27.2	≤50 U	(67)	48.5	.006
Alkaline phosphatase	>110 U	(71)	35.4	≤110 U	(17)	75.9	.013
Acid phosphatase	>5 U	(32)	26.5	≤5 U	(56)	51.7	.010

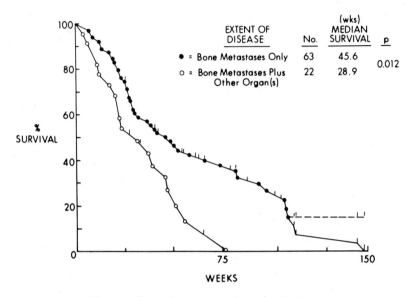

Figure 1. Survival based on extent of metastases.

was even greater ($p < 0.002$), although the median survival was about the same as if either were abnormal (27.2 weeks).

Any initial elevation of alkaline phosphatase was associated with decreased survival. Seventy-one of the 88 patients had elevated values and their median survival time was less than half that of those having normal values (35.4 weeks, compared to 75.9 weeks, $p < 0.013$) (Table 1, Figure 3). Higher initial levels

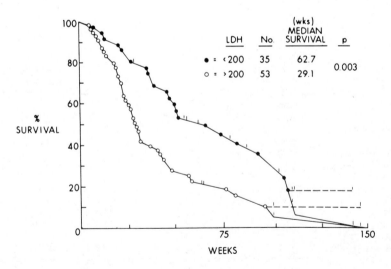

Figure 2. Survival based on value of serum LDH.

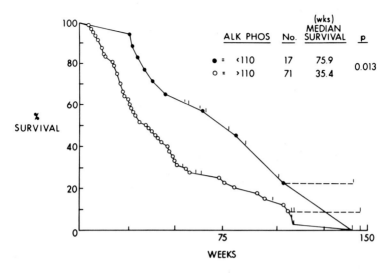

Figure 3. Survival based on value of serum alkaline phosphatase.

of alkaline phosphatase did not have any greater effect on survival; i.e., the median survival for all subgroups (patients with initial values of 110–500 U, 500–1,000 U, or >1,000 U) did not differ significantly.

Sixty-eight of 88 patients had elevated acid phosphatase levels (>0.8 U) as performed by the colorimetric assay. Elevated initial values of acid phosphatase were associated with a poor prognosis only when patients with values of >2.0 U were compared to those with levels below 2.0 U ($p > 0.04$) (Table 1, Figure 4).

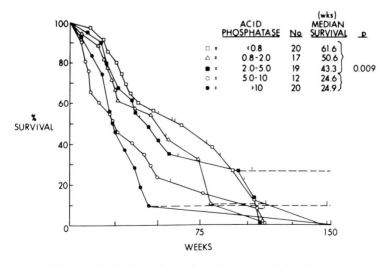

Figure 4. Survival based on value of serum acid phosphatase.

Thirty-five patients had initially low albumin levels (<3.5 gm/dl), and the presence of hypoalbuminemia was associated with short survival. Low albumin had no correlation with abnormal liver scans.

Response to Therapy

Acid Phosphatase

Sixty-seven of 84 patients had elevated levels of acid phosphatase (APT) prior to therapy. A fall in APT levels of more than 50% or to normal, maintained for at least two months, was assessed in relation to survival, and 24 of 67 patients whose elevated levels of APT fell more than 50% experienced a longer median survival time (MST) than those whose values did not fall 50% (Figure 5). Moreover, the 11 patients whose values fell by more than 50% but not to normal had a MST of 34.0 weeks, compared to 26.5 weeks for those whose values did not fall more than 50% ($p = 0.309$). The 13 patients whose elevated levels of APT fell to normal experienced a MST of 98.0 weeks, as compared to 28.4 weeks for all the other patients with elevated values that did not fall to normal ($p = 0.007$) (Figure 6). Prolonged survival was thus noted only in those patients whose elevated APT values fell to normal.

Alkaline Phosphatase

Seventy patients had elevated levels of serum alkaline phosphatase (ALKP) prior to treatment. Twenty-four patients whose elevated values fell more than

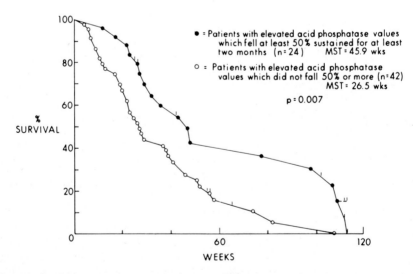

Figure 5. Survival of patients whose APT values fell more than 50% versus those patients whose values did not.

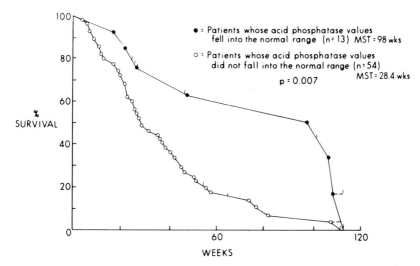

Figure 6. Survival of patients whose acid phosphatase value fell to normal versus those patients whose acid phosphatase did not fall to normal.

50% for at least two months experienced a MST of 47.6 weeks, while the MST was 25.1 weeks for those whose values did not fall 50% ($p > 0.03$). Twelve patients whose ALKP values fell by more than 50% but not to normal had a MST of 32.0 weeks, compared to 25.1 weeks for those whose values did not fall 50% ($p = 0.44$). The MST for the 12 patients whose elevated values fell to normal was 75.1 weeks, compared to 27.7 weeks for all patients with initially elevated enzyme levels that did not return to normal ($p = 0.012$) (Figure 7).

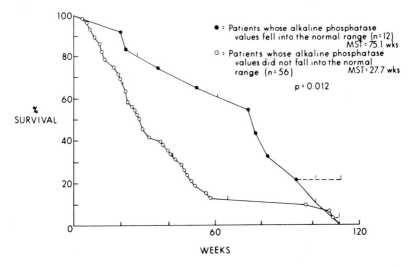

Figure 7. Survival of patients whose ALKP values fell to normal compared to those patients whose values did not.

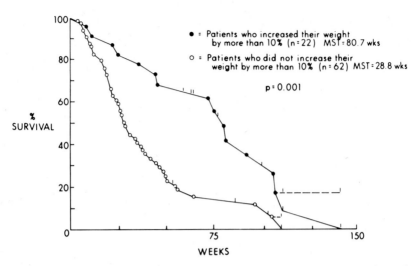

Figure 8. Survival for patients who increased their weight by 10% or more compared to patients who did not.

Thus, a fall in elevated ALKP levels was associated with prolonged survival only if the levels returned to normal.

Weight Gain

Twenty-two patients increased their weight by 10% or more over their on-study weight. These 24 patients had a MST of 80.7 weeks, compared to 28.8 weeks for those patients who did not increase their weight by more than 10% ($p = 0.001$) (Figure 8).

Evaluable Metastatic Disease

Bone Lesions

Seventy-two patients had osteoblastic metastases by standard bone x-ray exam and in none were these resolved with therapy. Four patients had mixed lytic-blastic bone lesions, none of which recalcified with therapy.

Bone scans were abnormal in 82 patients. Three patients had normal scans but blastic disease by bone x-ray. No scan showed resolution with therapy.

Soft Tissue Lesions

Seven of 85 patients had measurable soft tissue disease, either pulmonary nodules or palpable lymph nodes. Three of these seven showed a greater than

50% reduction in measurable tumor mass and normalization of acid or alkaline phosphatase, or greater than 10% weight gain. The four without tumor shrinkage demonstrated no acid or alkaline phosphatase response or weight gain.

Prostatic size could not be used as a measurable indicator of disease because of variability in results produced by serial rectal examination.

Overall Treatment Response

Thirty-three of 84 patients showed normalization of either acid phosphatase or alkaline phosphatase or a weight gain of greater than 10%, and three patients had normalization of both acid and alkaline phosphatase and a weight gain of greater than 10%. The three patients who demonstrated this combined response have maintained their response for 15, 27, and 29 months from the initiation of therapy.

Normalization of the serum marker proteins, acid phosphatase or alkaline phosphatase, or a weight gain of greater than 10% was associated with prolonged survival, with a MST of 76.1 weeks, compared to 28.2 weeks for those who did not respond (Figure 9). These response indicators shown to be associated with prolonged survival were identified in 33 of 84 patients, for a response rate of 37.9% (excluding three patients who responded to high-dose estrogens after failing chemotherapy).

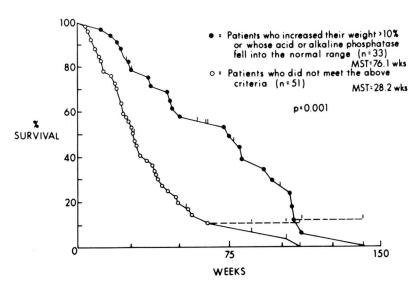

Figure 9. Survival for patients whose acid and/or alkaline phosphatase values fell to normal and/or who increased their weight by at least 10% compared to patients who met none of these criteria.

DISCUSSION

Demographic Data

The Cancer Surveillance, Epidemiology and End Results (SEER) Program of the National Cancer Institute has reported that black patients with prostate cancer have a poorer prognosis than white patients (Heise 1976). We could detect no significant difference in survival between blacks and whites. Perhaps the data in the SEER study represent the effect of socioeconomic factors on the delivery of health care, rather than any biologic difference in the tumor between these groups.

Schmidt et al. (1976) have reported that prior radiation therapy is a predictor of poor prognosis for patients subsequently treated with chemotherapy. We failed to demonstrate any difference in survival between those who had received radiation and those who had not, and we see no reason to exclude from chemotherapy any patient who has had prior radiation, although the initial dose of drugs may have to be modified for those with extensive pelvic and spinal radiation.

Extent of Disease

The overwhelming majority of patients with stage IV prostate cancer have bony metastases. Some patients, however, develop soft tissue metastases. This has been reported by the Veterans Administration Cooperative Urological Research Group and others to be associated with poor prognosis, as judged by survival (Gutman 1959, Ishibe 1977). Patients who had soft tissue metastases (palpable lymph nodes, lung or pleural metastases, and/or abnormal liver scans apparently due to tumor) in addition to bony metastases fared less well than those with only bony disease. However, patients with soft tissue metastases are more likely to have measurable tumor masses and are therefore more likely to be admitted to protocol studies. Because of this selective factor, such studies are not necessarily accurate for the entire group of patients with stage IV prostate cancer. Thus, it is very important to stratify patients according to the presence of soft tissue metastases when these patients enter protocol studies.

Serum LDH and SGOT have received little attention in research on prostatic carcinoma. Neither was felt to be a significant factor by the National Prostatic Cancer Project (Prout 1969). An abnormality in either enzyme was associated with a poor prognosis in this study.

Alkaline phosphatase is more often abnormal in patients with prostate cancer than in patients with any other tumor that metastasizes to the bone (Gutman 1959). Although it has been discussed as a parameter of response with hormonal therapy, it has not been reported to be of prognostic significance (Ishibe 1977, Prout 1969). Alkaline phosphatase elevation was quite common in our study and was associated with a poor prognosis. There was, however, no relationship between extent of alkaline phosphatase elevation and survival, since any elevation of the enzyme carried a poor prognosis. The enzyme elevation is probably an indirect indicator of the metabolic activity of the tumor.

The correlation of elevated levels of serum acid phosphatase with poor prognosis was reported as early as 1956 (Ganem 1956) and has been noted in patients at all stages in hormonal therapy, but before chemotherapy. This study reaffirms the importance of acid phosphatase as a prognostic factor.

Response to Therapy

The data reported here indicate that there are biochemical and physiological indicators of response to chemotherapy that can be correlated with prolongation of survival and reduction of soft tissue lesions when these are present. Normalization of either of the biochemical markers of extended disease, acid phosphatase and alkaline phosphatase, can be associated with prolonged survival. The data clearly demonstrate that a reduction short of normal levels, however, is not associated with extended survival. Although others have used varying degrees of acid or alkaline phosphatase reduction as indicators of response, any change short of normalization did not indicate benefit (Hurst et al. 1973, Sanford et al. 1976, Collier and Soloway 1976, Nilsson and Gosta 1976, Eagan et al. 1975, Kane et al. 1977, Coune 1975, Scott et al. 1975). Previous prostatic chemotherapy trials have used weight as an indicator of treatment response, some researchers citing the absence of additional weight loss as a therapeutic response, and others requiring a 5% or 10% weight gain. In the present study, weight gain of less than 10% could not be correlated with enhanced survival. While other chemotherapy programs may affect body weight to varying degrees, the data presented here indicate that this physiological response can be assessed and a value established that indicates treatment benefit.

In summary, there appear to be historical, physical, and biochemical factors that not only permit stratification of patients with prostatic carcinoma, but also permit assessment of response to treatment.

REFERENCES

Collier, D., and M. S. Soloway. 1976. Doxorubicin hydrochloride, cyclophosphamide, and 5-fluorouracil combination in advanced prostate and transitional cell carcinoma. Urology 8:459–464.

Coune, A. 1975. Carcinoma of the prostate: Prognostic factors and criteria of response, in Cancer Therapy: Prognostic Factors and Criteria of Response, M. J. Staquet, ed. Raven Press, New York, pp. 269–287.

Cox, D. R. 1972. Regression models and life tables. J. R. Stat. Soc. 34:187–202.

Eagan, R. T., D. C. Utz, and R. O. Myers. 1975. Comparison of adriamycin (NSC-123127) and the combination of 5-fluorouracil (NSC-19893) and cyclophosphamide (NSC-26271) in advanced prostatic cancer: A preliminary report. Cancer Chemother. Rep. 59:203–207.

Ganem, E. J. 1956. The prognostic significance of an elevated serum acid phosphatase level in advanced prostatic carcinoma. J. Urol. 76:179–181.

Gutman, A. B. 1959. Serum alkaline phosphatase activity in disease of skeletal and hepatobiliary systems. Am. J. Med. 27:875–901.

Heise, H. W. 1976. Cancers of the male genital organs, *in* Cancer Patient Survival, Report No. 5, DHEW publication no. (NIH) 77–992, L. M. Axtell, A. J. Asire, and M. H. Myers, eds. U.S. Government Printing Office, Washington, D.C., pp. 190–205.

Hurst, K. S., D. P. Byar, and the Veterans Administration Cooperative Urological Research Group. 1973. An analysis of the effects of changes from the assigned treatment in a clinical trial of treatment for prostatic cancer. J. Chron. Dis. 26:311–324.

Ishibe, T. 1977. Alkaline phosphatase in serum of patients with prostatic carcinoma. Urology 10:227–232.

Kane, R. D., L. H. Stocks, and D. F. Paulson. 1977. Multiple drug chemotherapy regimen for patients with hormonally-unresponsive carcinoma of the prostate: A preliminary report. J. Urol. 117:467–471.

Kaplan, E. L., and P. Meier. 1958. Non-parametric estimation from incomplete observations. J. Am. Stat. Assoc. 53:457–480.

Nilsson, T., and J. Gosta. 1976. Primary treatment of prostatic carcinoma with estramustine phosphate: Preliminary report. J. Urol. 115:168–169.

Prout, G. R. 1969. Chemical tests in the diagnosis of prostatic carcinoma. J.A.M.A. 209:1699–1700.

Sanford, E. J., J. R. Drago, and T. J. Rohner, Jr. 1976. Aminoglutethamide medical adrenalectomy for advanced prostatic carcinoma. J. Urol. 115:170–174.

Schmidt, J. D., R. P. Gibbons, D. E. Johnson, G. R. Prout, W. W. Scott, and G. P. Murphy. 1976. The National Prostate Cancer Project. Chemotherapy of advanced prostatic cancer—evaluation of response parameters. Urology 7:602–610.

Scott, W. W., R. P. Gibbons, and D. E. Johnson. 1975. Comparison of 5-fluorouracil (NSC-19893) and cyclophosphamide (NSC-26271) in patients with advanced carcinoma of the prostate. Cancer Chemother. Rep. 59:195–201.

Cancer of the Genitourinary Tract, edited by
D. E. Johnson and M. L. Samuels.
Raven Press, New York © 1979.

Hormonal Therapy for Prostatic Carcinoma

Prince D. Beach, M.D.

*Section of Urology, Veterans Administration Hospital and Baylor College of Medicine,
Houston, Texas*

The opinions expressed in this paper are based on the work of the Veterans Administration Cooperative Urological Research Group (VACURG) and the current literature, but some of my conclusions go beyond those reported in our studies. I agree with the reported studies as far as they go, but believe future developments will bear out the opinions expressed in this presentation.

First, I would like to explain my concept of the progression of prostate cancer; while it differs from that used at M. D. Anderson Hospital, it is the most commonly recognized model in prostate carcinoma. Dr. Whitmore (1973) has pointed out that while breast cancer seems to follow an orderly progression from stage A to D (Figure 1), such is most likely not the case with prostate cancer. Because the prostate is derived from both the wolffian and müllerian systems and is highly responsive to many male and female hormones, prostatic cancer is more likely to progress in the manner illustrated in Figure 2. Tumors may remain for long periods in their original stage, move on to the next, or jump ahead to a more advanced stage.

The problem with this system is that it is based primarily, in the earlier stages, on rectal palpation of the prostate. It has become apparent that this system has a defect in the stage A, or I, group, as studies demonstrating the importance of cellular differentiation to patient survival (Gleason et al. 1974) and the use of pelvic lymphadenectomy in surgical staging (McCullough et al. 1974) have brought out. Most urologists and pathologists now agree that there is a stage A_1, which consists of a focus of tumor cells, usually well-differentiated, and a much more significant stage A_2, which consists of many areas of carcinoma that are diffusely disseminated throughout the prostate and range from well to poorly differentiated. We now know, through surgical staging by lymphadenec-

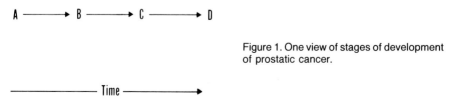

Figure 1. One view of stages of development of prostatic cancer.

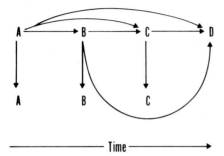

Figure 2. Alternate view of stages of development of prostatic cancer.

tomy, that poorly differentiated stage A_2 tumors are accompanied by a 20–30% incidence of positive nodes, which means that a significant number of clinically stage A (I) patients are surgically stage C (III) and D (IV) (McCullough et al. 1974). This is important because these patients require a different hormone therapy approach. In one series, 80% of stage A patients were stage A_2, with large, diffuse carcinomas, and 88% of those who died were in this group (Heaney et al. 1977).

Palliative hormonal therapy for prostate cancer was first developed by Huggins and co-workers (1941). Much subsequent work has confirmed the route of action of estrogens depicted in Figure 3. The key hormone is estrogen, which functions through the pituitary axis via the luteinizing hormone (lh) and the follicular stimulating hormone (fsh) to control the output of testosterone in the testis. It is now well confirmed that testosterone is essential to the survival of the prostate cell. Testosterone is converted to dihydrotestosterone at the cell membrane through interaction with 5α-reductase. Dihydrotestosterone is then conveyed through the cytoplasm to the cell nucleus, where it is bound to chromatin and activates transcription to form messenger RNA (Moore and Wilson 1972).

Estrogen acts primarily by decreasing the amount of testosterone available to the prostate cell. However, in the last six years evidence has accumulated that estrogen also has a direct effect on the prostate cells that bear estrogen receptors (Yanihara and Troen 1972, Shimazaki et al. 1971). This is still unsettled because estrogen can stimulate and inhibit prostate growth, as well as promote the release of prolactin, which is a known stimulator of prostate growth. There is also evidence that estrogen can inhibit both DNA polymerase and 5α-reductase activity, indicating a direct nuclear site inhibition (Shimazaki et al. 1971).

The antiandrogen cyproterone acetate acts through the adrenal axis. Spironolactone does also, but further down the sequence with less disruption of other adrenal steroidogenesis. Flutamide, however, apparently acts directly at the cell nucleus by blocking the binding of dihydrotestosterone to the nuclear receptor, and it can apparently also block the effect of adrenal androgens on the prostate cell (P. C. Walsh 1975). Prolactin, which is known to stimulate prostate growth, can also be blocked by L-dopa, apparently at the receptor level.

The above makes clear that the "target organ responsiveness of hormonally

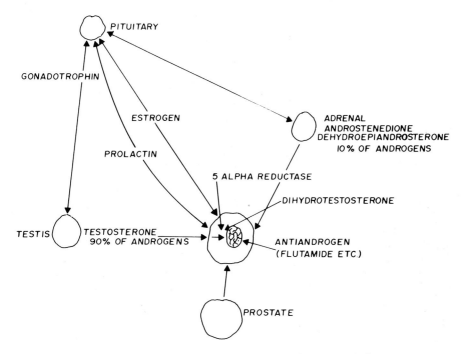

Figure 3. Route of action of estrogens on the prostate cell.

responsive tumors is related to *receptor* content and suggests that the clinical application of this method [measurement of steroid receptors in the tumor] to the study of patients with metastatic carcinoma of the prostate may enable us to predict which patients will respond to therapy" (Walsh 1975, p. 138). We have great need for a method that will allow us to select therapy appropriate to individual patients, because we have made little progress in some 30 years of hormone treatment of patients with this cancer.

Diethylstilbestrol (DES) remains the estrogen agent of choice, but the appropriate dosage is still debated. The VA studies have shown that 5 mg or more of DES carries a real risk of cardiovascular complications, at least in patients with a history of cardiovascular problems. The studies have also shown that a 1-mg dose of DES has the same effect on the carcinoma as a 5-mg dose, without any apparent cardiovascular risk (Byar 1973). The problem is to find parameters to measure the effect of DES on individual patients' cancers. The markers we now have for this carcinoma are ineffectual compared to those available for testis tumors.

Plasma testosterone levels can be used as a guide to appropriate DES dosages. Studies have shown that 1 mg of DES will suppress plasma testosterone to castration levels in most patients (Kent et al. 1973). However, over a period of several weeks, this level will be maintained in only 40% of patients so treated

(Shearer et al. 1973). On the other hand, 3 mg DES will produce and maintain castration levels in 100% of patients, and an increase to 5 mg of DES or any higher dose has no additional effect on the plasma testosterone levels (Robinson and Thomas 1971). Thus, the evidence is accumulating that 3 mg of DES is the appropriate dose for the average patient. Although VA researchers intend to pursue this further to determine the cardiovascular risk with this dose, a retrospective look has not yet revealed a significant increase in risk.

Some centers, including M. D. Anderson Hospital, use 5-mg doses for stage D (IV) patients. The indication for doses greater than 3 mg seems to be when a rapid estrogen effect is needed for selected patients, such as those with spinal cord compression or significant ureteral obstruction (P. C. Walsh 1975).

Another indicator of treatment response is prostatic acid phosphatase, but 20% of prostate cancer patients do not have elevated acid phosphatase levels, regardless of their stage or grade. The VA researchers have found that, for those who do show an elevation, a drop of at least 50% in the initial level (regardless of whether from two to one or from 100 to 50) indicates that the patient is responding to DES (Byar 1973). Likewise, if the level does not drop or drops and then rises by 50%, the patient is not hormone responsive or is no longer responding. In this context, prostatic acid phosphatase can be a useful indicator for selecting hormone therapy or judging the need for another mode of therapy.

The place for orchiectomy in treatment for prostatic carcinoma is still debated. Another VA study (Blackard et al. 1973) indicates that orchiectomy alone or with DES offers no advantage over DES alone. Some investigators agree, while others still insist orchiectomy should be the primary treatment. If plasma testosterone levels are used as indicators of hormone effectiveness, it is difficult to justify orchiectomy. On the other hand, orchiectomy can be useful in treating patients who cannot tolerate DES or who cannot be depended upon to take their medication. There is also the rare patient in pain while on DES who responds to orchiectomy, although relief is almost always short-lived.

Tace should also be mentioned briefly. A dose of 24 mg of Tace daily does not lower testosterone levels, so this agent is a less effective indicator of response than DES. However, since some patients do respond, response occurs through a different mechanism (Shearer et al. 1973).

Stilphostrol is widely used, usually in stage D (IV) patients who no longer respond to DES or initially failed to respond. This agent is thought to be effective on such patients because the intravenous dose of 1 gm a day for five days has an additional antiandrogen effect directly on the cell nucleus, rather than entirely through the pituitary axis. Evidence is accumulating that it sometimes produces more rapid relief of ureteral obstructions than radiotherapy.

The effect of orchiectomy on the adrenal androgens must also be considered. In some patients the adrenal androgens increase 100-fold after orchiectomy. Although these androgens are 10 times less effective than testosterone, such an increase can have an adverse effect. Such patients may subsequently respond to adrenalectomy or hypophysectomy.

Another basic concern in palliative treatment for prostate cancer is the timing for initiating hormone therapy. One VA study found no adverse effect from delaying hormone therapy in patients without symptoms, and those patients subsequently responded to estrogen therapy in spite of the delay (Byar 1973). Therefore, we generally recommend no hormone therapy for asymptomatic patients. However, in the stage D (IV) patient hormone therapy is indicated, regardless of symptoms, in most instances. For instance, a subsidiary VA study in which x-ray exams were used to evaluate metastatic bone lesions to determine prognosis showed that a patient with a lesion of the femur has only a six-month expected survival, as compared to those without, who have a 12-month (Byar 1973).

Finally, I would like to focus again on stage A_2 patients with diffuse undifferentiated tumors. Surgical staging by lymphadenectomy has shown a 23% incidence of positive nodes in patients in this group, which places them in the stage C or D category. These are the patients who have been undertreated in the past and deserve aggressive treatment. If they are not candidates for prostatectomy or irradiation, they should be put on aggressive hormone therapy even if they are asymptomatic, because such a diffuse, undifferentiated, clinically benign tumor is an aggressive cancer.

The basic point is that the old routine of automatic orchiectomy and large doses of estrogen for all prostate cancer is passé. Palliative hormone therapy should be adapted to the individual patient who is fighting his own cancer. The average patient responding to estrogen therapy does so for three to four years. Since Byar (1973) found no adverse effect from delaying hormone therapy, a firm basis has been established for delaying palliative hormone therapy until the patient is symptomatic. The only exceptions are patients with stage A_2 or D disease.

The antiandrogens will play an increasing role in hormone therapy for prostatic cancer patients. Research shows that the response to estrogen depends on the availability of estrogen receptors in the prostate cancer cell. Some clones of cells have adequate estrogen receptors and others are devoid of such receptors. It would appear that the latter clones will respond to such antiandrogens as flutamide. Therefore, I think a combination of estrogen and an antiandrogen will be the most efficacious palliative treatment for patients with this cancer in the future.

REFERENCES

Blackard, C. E., D. P. Byar, and W. P. Jordan. 1973. Orchiectomy for advanced prostatic carcinoma—A re-evaluation. Urology 1:553–560.

Byar, D. P. 1973. The Veterans Administration Cooperative Urological Research Group's studies of cancer of the prostate. Cancer 32:1126–1130.

Gleason, D. F., G. T. Mellinger, and the Veterans Administration Cooperative Urological Research Group. 1974. Prediction of prognosis for prostatic adenocarcinoma by combined histological grading and clinical staging. J. Urol. 3:58–64.

Goland, M., ed. 1975. Normal and Abnormal Growth of the Prostate. Charles C Thomas, Publisher, Springfield, Ill. 941 pp.

Heaney, J. A., H. C. Chang, J. J. Daly, and G. R. Prout, Jr. 1977. Prognosis of clinically undiagnosed prostatic carcinoma and the influence of endocrine therapy. J. Urol. 118:283–287.

Huggins, C., and C. V. Hodges. 1941. Studies on prostatic cancer: Effect of castration, of estrogens and of androgen injection on serum phosphatases in metastatic carcinoma of the prostate. Cancer Res. 1:293–297.

Kent, J. R., A. J. Bischoft, L. J. Ardnino, G. T. Mellinger, D. P. Byar, M. Hill, and X. Kosbur. 1973. Estrogen dosage and suppression of testosterone levels in patients with prostatic carcinoma. J. Urol. 109:858.

McCullough, D. L., G. R. Prout, Jr., and J. J. Daly. 1974. Carcinoma of prostate and lymphatic metastases. J. Urol. 111:65–71.

Moore, R. J., and J. D. Wilson. 1972. Localization of the reduced nicatomide adenine dinucleotide phosphate Δ 4-3-ketosteroid 5a-oxidoreductase in the nuclear membranes of the rat ventral prostate. J. Biol. Chem. 247:958.

Robinson, M. R. G., and B. S. Thomas. 1971. Effect of hormonal therapy on plasma testosterone levels in prostatic carcinoma. Br. Med. J. 4:391–394.

Shimazaki, J., T. Horaguchi, and Y. Ohki. 1971. Properties of testosterone 5a-reductase of purified nuclear fraction from ventral prostate of rats. Endocrinol. Jpn. 18:179.

Shearer, R. J., W. F. Hendry, I. F. Sommerville, and J. D. Ferguson. 1973. Plasma testosterone: An accurate monitor of hormone treatment in prostatic cancer. Br. J. Urol. 45:668–677.

Walsh, P. C. 1975. Physiological basis for hormonal therapy in carcinoma of the prostate. Urol. Clin. North Am. 2:125–138.

Whitmore, W. F., Jr. 1973. The natural history of prostatic cancer. Cancer 32:1104–1112.

Yanihara, T., and P. Troen. 1972. Studies of the human testis. III. Effect of estrogen on testosterone formation in human testis in vitro. J. Clin. Endocrinol. 34:968–973.

GENITOURINARY TRACT SARCOMAS

Cancer of the Genitourinary Tract, edited by
D. E. Johnson and M. L. Samuels.
Raven Press, New York © 1979.

Sarcomas of the Genitourinary Tract: Case Histories

Joseph G. Sinkovics, M.D., Carl Plager, M.D., Andrew von Eschenbach, M.D.,* and Douglas E. Johnson, M.D.*

*Departments of Medicine and *Urology, The University of Texas System Cancer Center M. D. Anderson Hospital and Tumor Institute, Houston, Texas*

The prognosis of patients with sarcomas arising in visceral organs in adulthood remains grave. Sarcomas of the extremities or trunk are discovered relatively early and can readily be managed by wide excision followed by radiotherapy, while sarcomas of visceral organs usually have infiltrated neighboring tissues by the time of diagnosis and are seldom amenable to complete surgical removal.

This retrospective review of patients treated in the solid tumor service of the Department of Medicine and in the Department of Urology will show that sarcomas of the genitourinary tract in adults carry a very poor prognosis and require multimodal treatment, and the optimum method of treatment will have to be determined by prospectively randomized clinical trials.

PRIMARY SARCOMAS OF THE KIDNEY

In the young adult, late-onset Wilms' tumor should be distinguished from primary sarcoma of the kidney. Table 1 summarizes the data on eight patients with primary sarcomas of the kidney. Patient 1's disease was unusually protracted. Her chemotherapy originally consisted of drugs primarily used to treat patients with acute myelogenous leukemia, but she did not respond to these or other drugs (vincristine and cyclophosphamide). Only two patients (7 and 8) responded; the CyVADIC regimen was used in both cases. Patient 8 began chemotherapy with a huge, inoperable, local recurrence and achieved complete remission after the small residual tumor was surgically resected and radiotherapy was administered to the tumor bed (Krutchik et al. 1978) (Table 2).

Two more patients are currently undergoing treatment. Patient 9 underwent a nephrectomy for leiomyosarcoma of the right kidney in 1978 and has remained clinically tumor free for eight months while receiving adjuvant chemotherapy with vincristine, actinomycin-D, and cyclophosphamide. Patient 10 developed fibrosarcomatous metastases after a nephrectomy for kidney carcinoma in 1978. An especially large metastasis was found in the right thigh and inguinal region. He has received two courses of chemotherapy with vincristine, cyclophospha-

Table 1. *Data on Patients With Primary Sarcoma of the Kidney*

Patient	Sex	Birthdate	Clinical Data	Outcome
1	F	1912	Leiomyosarcoma R kidney. Nephrectomy '59. R infraclavicular metastases excised '62. Lung metastases excised '64. Local recurrence. Lung metastases '66. Ara-C, 6-MP, VCR, CTX.	Death 1968
2	M	1928	Leiomyosarcoma L kidney. Nephrectomy '66. Local recurrence. Lung metastases '66. XRT, CTX, procarbazine.	Death 1967
3	M	1941	Poorly differentiated fibrosarcoma R kidney. Lung & bone metastases '71. Adria, DTIC.	Death 1971
4	F	1915	Poorly differentiated sarcoma L kidney. Nephrectomy '71. Local recurrence. Intraabdominal spread '71. Adria, DTIC.	Death 1972
5	M	1921	Leiomyosarcoma L kidney '73. Lung & bone metastases '73. CyVADIC.	Death 1975
6	F	1910	Leiomyosarcoma R kidney. Nephrectomy '74. VCR, Act-D, CTX. Local recurrence '75. Adria, DTIC. Lung metastases.	Death 1976
7	F	1927	Leiomyosarcoma L kidney. Nephrectomy '75. Local recurrence. Lung metastases. CyVADIC, DTIC, Act-D.	CR, alive 1978
8	M	1920	Renal carcinoma with fibrosarcomatous stroma. Nephrectomy '76. Local recurrence. CyVADIC PR. Resection, XRT.	CR, alive 1978

Abbreviations: VCR = vincristine; CTX = cyclophosphamide; 6-MP = 6-mercaptopurine; Ara-C = cytarabine; Adria = Adriamycin; DTIC = dacarbazine; CyVADIC = cyclophosphamide, vincristine, Adriamycin, dacarbazine; Act-D = actinomycin-D; XRT = radiotherapy; CR = complete remission; PR = partial remission.

mide, Adriamycin, and dacarbazine with only minimal tumor response. We are considering replacing Adriamycin with actinomycin-D after 450–500 mg/m^2 of Adriamycin has been administered. Surgical removal of the metastatic tumor (especially if it decreases after chemotherapy), radiotherapy to the metastatic tumor (if response to chemotherapy does not occur), or both, are contemplated.

The grave prognosis that accompanies this tumor suggests the optimum treatment is nephrectomy followed by radiotherapy to the tumor bed and adjuvant combination chemotherapy. Mucositis and intestinal toxicity may be expected if radiotherapy and Adriamycin or actinomycin-D are used together. However, these two antibiotics are indispensable in treating patients with sarcomas.

Primary sarcomas of the kidney are well-established entities with a high mortality rate (Niceta et al. 1974). Fibrosarcoma (34%), leiomyosarcoma (31%),

Table 2. *Patient 8, With Sarcomatous Renal Cell Carcinoma*

1976	May	Renal cell carcinoma in fibrosarcomatous stroma. Nephrectomy
	Aug.	Large local recurrence. Inoperable.
	Sept.	VCR 2 mg, CTX 1 gm, Adria 100 mg, DTIC 2.5 gm. 9 monthly courses (Adriamycin total dose 900 mg). BCG sarcoma lysates.
1977	May	Complete remission.
	June	VCR 2 mg, CTX 750 mg, Act-D 1.2 mg, DTIC 1.8 gm in 3 monthly courses.
	Sept.	Local recurrence. Resection.
	Oct.	4,500 rads irradiation.
1978	Sept.	Complete remission.

and liposarcoma (20%) are the most common (Richaud et al. 1977), but primary osteosarcoma of the kidney is also known to occur (Axelrod et al. 1978).

PRIMARY SARCOMAS OF THE URINARY BLADDER

The most common primary sarcoma of the urinary bladder is leiomyosarcoma. Two of four patients in our experience with this tumor are tumor free today (Table 3). Patient 13 had residual tumors after surgery, but became clinically tumor free during two years of chemotherapy with vincristine, actinomycin-D, and cyclophosphamide; she remains in complete remission two years after discontinuation of chemotherapy (Table 4). Patient 14 developed hematuria in 1970. After transurethral resection of what was diagnosed as a bladder sarcoma,

Table 3. *Data on Patients With Sarcomas of the Urinary Bladder*

Patient	Sex	Clinical Data	Outcome
11	M	Leiomyosarcoma invasive '75. VCR, CTX, Adria, DTIC, MeCCNU, Act-D.	Death 1976
12	M	Leiomyosarcoma invasive '70. VCR, CTX, Adria, DTIC, XRT (fast neutrons).	PR, alive with tumor 1978
13	F	Leiomyosarcoma invasive '74. VCR, Act-D, CTX.	NED 1978
14	M	Leiomyosarcoma '70. Recurrent after excision and radiotherapy '74. Metastatic to scalp after cystectomy and ileal conduit '77. VCR, Act-D, CTX.	NED 1978 (Possible stable lung metastases)

Abbreviations: NED = no evidence of disease; MeCCNU = methyl CCNU (semustine).

Table 4. *Patient 13, With Leiomyosarcoma of Urinary Bladder*

1974	Leiomyosarcoma of urinary bladder invading perivesical fat and small intestine. Surgical excision. Residual tumor.
1974–76	VCR 49 mg, CTX 33.6 gm, Act-D 30 mg in 12 courses.
1978	NED. Needs hormone replacement (Premarin and Provera).

he received radiotherapy with 7,000 rads. In 1974 a local recurrence developed and a tissue diagnosis of leiomyosarcoma was established. Total cystectomy (including prostatectomy and seminal vesiculectomy) with an ileal loop diversion was performed. In 1977 a metastatic lesion in the scalp was resected. The patient began a two-year treatment program in February 1977 with vincristine, actinomycin-D, and cyclophosphamide for five days a month, with bacillus Calmette-Guérin (BCG) scarifications on days 17 and 24 after each course of chemotherapy. After 20 courses of treatment, he remains tumor free.

Most reviews of cases involving sarcomas originating in the urinary bladder or prostate evaluate patients treated with outdated modalities of radiotherapy and chemotherapy and do not clearly distinguish between tumors occurring in childhood and those occurring in adulthood (Narayana et al. 1978; for references, see Sinkovics, in press). Sarcomas occurring in children carry a better prognosis than those occurring in adults, and sarcomas of the urinary bladder are less aggressive than those of the prostate. The efficacy of chemotherapy regimens containing Adriamycin has not been well evaluated.

PRIMARY PARATESTICULAR RHABDOMYOSARCOMA

Primary paratesticular rhabdomyosarcoma is a highly malignant tumor with a clear tendency to invade retroperitoneal lymph nodes and spread hematogenously. However, patient 15 remains tumor free after radical orchiectomy without any chemotherapy or radiotherapy (Table 5). Patient 18 has also achieved prolonged tumor-free status.

Patient 19 had large unresected retroperitoneal lymph nodes obstructing the right kidney, which completely receded while he was on chemotherapy. Resection of possible recurrent nodes and radiotherapy may be used in the event of relapse. Chemotherapy will be discontinued after two years if the patient remains tumor free. Patient 20 was clinically tumor free after surgery and receives vincristine, actinomycin-D, and cyclophosphamide as adjuvant chemotherapy.

Patients 21, 22, and 23 presented with hypercalcemia and widely metastatic rhabdomyosarcoma. Hyperuricemia and azotemia were also present. The mechanism of the hypercalcemia is not clear. Only patient 23's parathormone and prostaglandin levels have been investigated. His parathormone levels were not elevated, and blood for prostaglandin level determinations has been deep frozen. Indomethacin appears to have temporarily controlled the hypercalcemia in this case.

Patient 24 did not receive chemotherapy and died within one year of diagnosis.

Table 5. *Data on Patients With Testicular and Paratesticular Rhabdomyosarcomas*

Patient	Birthdate	Clinical Data	Outcome
15	1947	Embryonal, R spermatic cord '67. Radical orchiectomy.	NED 1978
16	1956	Embryonal, L epididymis '72. Metastases to subcutaneous tissues, retroperitoneal lymph nodes, liver. VCR, Act-D, CTX, progression. VCR, CTX, Adria, DTIC.	Dead 1973
17	1954	Embryonal, L testis '71. Metastases to para-aortic nodes. XRT, VCR, Act-D, CTX, progression.	Dead 1972
18	1950	L paratesticular '72. Radical orchiectomy 0/42 nodes. VCR, Act-D, CTX, 1 year.	NED 1978
19	1959	Alveolar, R spermatic cord '76. Retroperitoneal nodes with hydronephrosis. Radical orchiectomy. VCR, CTX, Adria/Act-D, DTIC.	NED 1978
20	1956	L paratesticular, '77. Radical orchiectomy. XRT, VCR, Act-D, CTX.	NED 1978
21	1946	Embryonal, R testis '65. Widely metastatic. Hypercalcemia.	Dead 1965
22	1954	Embryonal, L testis '71. Para-aortic nodes. Widely metastatic. Hypercalcemia.	Dead 1973
23	1959	Embryonal, R testis '77. Radical orchiectomy. Bone metastases. Hypercalcemia '78. XRT, VCR, CTX, Adria/Act-D, DTIC.	Alive with residual tumor 1978
24	1951	Embryonal '66. Orchiectomy.	Dead 1967
25	1952	Embryonal '73. Radical orchiectomy. VCR, Act-D, CTX. Bone, brain, testicular metastases. XRT, Adria, DTIC, BCG, sarcoma lysates. Progression.	Dead 1974
26	1954	Embryonal (vs. extraosseous Ewing's) '77. Lung, bone, brain metastases. VCR, Act-D, CTX. Progression. XRT, Adria, DTIC. Progression.	Dead 1977

Patients 25 and 26 were treated aggressively, but both rapidly succumbed to widely disseminated tumors (Figures 1 and 2). Three more patients recently began adjuvant treatment. Patient 27 receives chemotherapy with vincristine, actinomycin-D, and cyclophosphamide; patients 28 and 29 receive the CyVADIC regimen. After orchiectomy, there was no clear evidence of retroperitoneal spread or distant metastases in these cases. All three patients remain tumor free in the first three to six months of adjuvant chemotherapy.

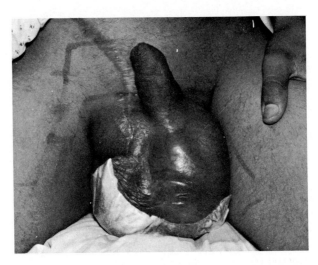

Figure 1. Patient 26. Large testicular tumor diagnosed as extraosseous Ewing's sarcoma.

Two modalities of investigational immunotherapy may also be beneficial in such cases (Sinkovics et al. 1977a,b, 1978): nonspecific immunostimulation with BCG scarification twice monthly (on days 17 and 24 of each course of chemotherapy, with chemotherapy on days 1–5 of 28-day intervals as bone marrow reserves permit), and tumor-specific immunization with sarcoma lysates (viral oncolysates).

While the optimal treatment for rhabdomyosarcoma of the testis or paratesticular tissues is not known, it appears that surgery alone cures only an occasional

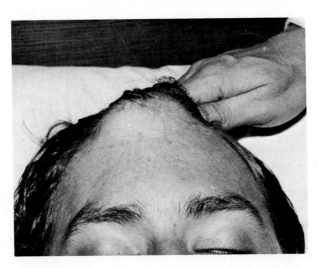

Figure 2. Metastasis of the tumor to the frontal bone and invading the brain.

patient. The present consensus of opinion is that if retroperitoneal nodes contain metastases, the nodes should be dissected and the area irradiated. Since rhabdomyosarcoma is known to be sensitive to radiotherapy and chemotherapy, chemotherapy is essential for treating metastatic disease and appears to be justified as adjuvant treatment for subclinical metastatic disease. One form of adjuvant treatment is a combination of vincristine, actinomycin-D, and cyclophosphamide administered for one year, with Adriamycin and dacarbazine held in reserve for relapse. Another option is the full CyVADIC regimen (cyclophosphamide, vincristine, Adriamycin, and dacarbazine) for two years, with replacement of Adriamycin by actinomycin-D after 500 mg/m^2 of Adriamycin has been given. The latter regimen is also recommended for metastatic disease. There is no proven effective treatment for sarcomas resistant to these regimens, but high-dose methotrexate with leucovorin rescue, cis-platinum, or the nitrosoureas may be tried.

Patient 22 was tested for immune reactions to cultured allogeneic rhabdomyosarcoma cells. His lymphocytes showed selective cytotoxicity toward sarcoma cells, and this cytotoxicity persisted despite chemotherapy (Sinkovics et al. 1972b). The effect of immunotherapy on sarcomas is marginal, but it may delay progression of disease (Sinkovics et al. 1977a,b). New modalities of immunotherapy (transfer factor, immune RNA, and interferon) and better microbial products for nonspecific immunostimulation are promising, but remain highly investigational (Sinkovics et al. 1978). Results of treatment in adults lag far behind those achieved in children (Curnes et al. 1977, Malek and Kelalis 1977, Raney et al. 1978), so new modalities must be tested.

Since human interferon exhibits cell growth regulatory activity and thus inhibits the growth of lymphoma and osteosarcoma cells, it may be used to treat patients with sarcomas (for review, see Sinkovics 1978). However, interferon may reduce the growth fraction of these tumors and thus make them resistant to concurrent chemotherapy or radiotherapy. If interferon proves to be cytostatic, it may be used to arrest temporarily tumor cell growth, with release of large cohorts of tumor cells in the S and M phases of the cell cycle upon its withdrawal. Thus, tumors with increased growth fractions may be made sensitive to cell cycle-specific therapy. Unbiased clinical trials are needed.

PRIMARY SARCOMA OF THE PROSTATE

The brief case histories of three patients (Table 6) illustrate the malignancy of primary sarcoma of the prostate in the adult patient. Combination chemotherapy applied against locally invasive and metastatic tumors offers little hope for meaningful remission. Thus, early radical resection, radiotherapy, and combination chemotherapy, even in an adjuvant fashion, are recommended, but only prospectively randomized trials can determine the optimum treatment modality. The lymphocytes of patient 30 were selectively cytotoxic to cultured allogeneic rhabdomyosarcoma cells; no blocking effect of the serum could be demonstrated (Sinkovics et al. 1972a).

Table 6. *Data on Patients With Sarcomas of the Prostate*

Patient	Clinical Data	Outcome
30	Leiomyosarcoma '72. Lung, bone metastases. XRT, VCR, Act-D.	Death 1 year
31	Myxoid liposarcoma '73. Sacral root involvement. VCR, CTX, Adria, DTIC.	Death 1 year
32	Leiomyosarcoma '73. Cystectomy with ileal loop. Bilateral lung metastases. VCR, CTX, Adria, Act-D, MeCCNU, DTIC, XRT, HU, VCR, Ara-C, ↑MTX, LV, Cis-plat.	Death 3 years

Abbreviations: HU = hydroxyurea, MTX = methotrexate, LV = leucovorin, Cis-plat = cis-dichlorodiammineplatinum.

SARCOMAS ARISING IN SOFT TISSUE OF THE PELVIS OTHER THAN OF THE GENITOURINARY OR GASTROINTESTINAL TRACT

The extremely poor prognosis for patients with soft tissue sarcomas of the pelvis, other than of the genitourinary or gastrointestinal tract, is indicated in Table 7. Most of these patients received vigorous treatment. Especially malignant were two epithelioid sarcomas. Patient 37's disease advanced so rapidly, with dyspnea and fever, that he was treated for pneumonia of unknown etiology until a pleuropneumonic aspirate revealed malignant cells. He died with lymphangitic intrapulmonary spread of this sarcoma. Despite four courses of chemotherapy with vincristine, cyclophosphamide and Adriamycin, patient 36's disease rapidly disseminated and failed to respond to MeCCNU and actinomycin-D. The perineal primary tumor appeared to be an epithelioid sarcoma, but postmortem examination indicated a giant cell soft tissue tumor.

Patient 41 had huge, locally recurrent tumors without known distant metastases (Figure 3). He had already been treated extensively with combination chemotherapy including Adriamycin. During the preterminal phase of his disease, illustrated in the photographs, he received investigational phase I agents. Patient 47 had huge, locally recurrent (Figure 4), and widely metastatic tumors.

Patient 44, who had large, inoperable intraabdominal tumors, achieved partial remission on CyVADIC chemotherapy and then underwent surgical resection of residual smaller tumors. She received postoperative radiation to the left lower abdomen and remains clinically tumor free. Patient 54, after resection of a large, high-grade retroperitoneal sarcoma with intraabdominal spread, remains clinically tumor free two years after initiation of chemoimmunotherapy with vincristine, cyclophosphamide, Adriamycin, actinomycin-D, dacarbazine, BCG, and sarcoma viral oncolysates.

Table 7. *Data on Patients With Sarcomas Originating in Soft Tissues of Pelvis Other Than Genitourinary or Gastrointestinal Tracts*

Patient	Sex	Birthdate	Clinical Data	Outcome
33	F	1943	Alveolar soft part '68. Recurrent, invasive. CTX, Adria, DTIC, MeCCNU, Act-D, 5FU, Bleo, Cis-plat, BCG, X-irradiated sarcoma cells, Transfer factor (Sinkovics 1974). PR.	Death 1978
34	F	1928	Angiosarcoma '70. Recurrent, invasive (bones), metastatic (lungs). XRT, VCR, CTX, Adria, DTIC, MeCCNU, Act-D, VLB, Mithr, Bleo, Ara-C, 5FU, MTX.	Death 1976
35	F	1942	Botryoid '73. Recurrent, invasive, inoperable. VCR, Act-D, CTX, Adria, DTIC.	Death 1976
36	M	1957	Epithelioid (vs. giant cell tumor) '75. Widely metastatic. XRT, VCR, CTX, Adria, MeCCNU, Act-D (Sinkovics and Mackay, in press).	Death 1976
37	M	1951	Epithelioid R inguinal canal '76. Metastatic to lymph nodes and lungs (Sinkovics and Mackay, in press).	Death 1976
38	F	1938	Hemangiopericytoma '77. VCR, CTX, Adria, DTIC, XRT.	Alive with minimal residual tumor 1978
39	F	1912	Leiomyosarcoma locally invasive '76. VCR, CTX, Adria, DTIC, BCG.	Progression 1978
40	M	1901	Leiomyosarcoma '74. Liver, lung metastases. Resections. VCR, CTX, Adria, Act-D, MeCCNU, DTIC, Cis-plat, Adria.	Alive with minimal residual tumors 1978
41	M	1911	Myxoid liposarcoma '72. Locally invasive. Resections. Rapid recurrences. XRT, VCR, CTX, Adria, DTIC. PR, progression.	Death 1978
42	F	1901	Malignant fibrous histiocytoma '75. Locally invasive. Recurrent after resections. XRT, VCR, CTX, Adria, DTIC, MeCCNU, Act-D. Hypogastric artery occlusion with Gelfoam.	Death 1976
43	F	1927	Malignant fibrous histiocytoma '75. Locally invasive. Recurrent after resection. Lung metastases. VCR, CTX, Adria, Act-D, DTIC, Ara-C, 5FU, MTX.	Death 1976

Table 7 *(Continued)*

Patient	Sex	Birthdate	Clinical Data	Outcome
44	F	1918	Malignant fibrous histiocytoma. Locally invasive. Chest x-ray: "nodular densities." VCR, CTX, Adria, DTIC. PR. Resection, XRT.	Alive with minimal residual tumors 1978
45	M	1908	Neurofibrosarcoma '73. CLL. Radical orchiectomy. Chlorambucil, prednisone.	NED for sarcoma 1978
46	F	1953	Rhabdomyosarcoma '76. Widely metastatic. XRT, VCR, CTX, Adria/Act-D, DTIC.	Death 1977
47	M	1944	Synovial '72. Locally invasive. Recurrent after resection. Widely metastatic. XRT, VCR, CTX, Adria, DTIC, Cisplat, VM26.	Death 1977
48	M	1956	Extraosseous Ewing's sarcoma in pelvis (prostate) '77. XRT, VCR, CTX, Adria, DTIC. PR, progression. MeCCNU, Act-D. Progression.	Death 1978
49	F	1908	Leiomyosarcoma, L ovary '76. 20 mitoses per 10 HPF. Metastases to lungs, liver. XRT, VCR, CTX, Adria, DTIC, BCG.	Death 1978
50	M	1905	Unclassified (leiomyo- or neurofibrosarcoma) '69. Recurrent after resection and metastatic (lungs). Hypoglycemia. XRT, VCR, Act-D, CTX, Adria, DTIC, MeCCNU.	Progressing 1978
51	F	1927	Leiomyoma uteri '73. Hysterectomy. Leiomyosarcoma in pelvis '76. Pleomorphic with high rate of mitoses: grade 3. Intraabd. masses involving small bowel, mesentery, abd. wall. VCR, CTX, Adria, DTIC, BCG. Progression. ↑Adria, DTIC, ↑Act-D, ↑MTX, LV. Repeated resections.	Progressing 1978
52	F	1920	Leiomyosarcoma, retroperit. '76. Metastases in small intestines, lungs, liver. VCR, CTX, Adria, DTIC, Act-D (high dose).	Death 1978
53	M	1953	Synovial sarcoma, R sacroiliac joint '75. Excision, XRT, VCR, CTX, Adria/Act-D, DTIC. Pulmonary metastases. Excisions. Adria, Cis-plat, XRT. Pelvic recurrence.	Death 1978

Table 7 *(Continued)*

Patient	Sex	Birthdate	Clinical Data	Outcome
54	F	1925	Liposarcoma with intraabd. spread '76. Recurrent sarcoma 20 lbs grade 3 '76. VCR, CTX, Adria/Act-D, DTIC. BCG, sarcoma lysates. Sept. '76-Oct. '78, 22 courses.	NED 1978

Abbreviations: 5FU = 5-fluorouracil, Bleo = bleomycin, VLB = vinblastine, velban, and vinca-leukoblastine, Mithr = mithramycin, CLL = chronic lymphocytic leukemia, HPF = high power fields.

These sarcomas clearly require multimodal treatment, with repeated surgical excisions if necessary, followed by radiotherapy and combination chemotherapy. The optimal mode of chemotherapy is not known, but temporary remissions have occurred when regimens containing Adriamycin were administered.

Adenocarcinomas coexist with sarcomas of the genitourinary (or other intraabdominal) organs more frequently than would be expected by chance alone. Our records reveal two cases of carcinoma of the prostate with leiomyosarcoma of the intestine, two cases of carcinoma of the breast with mixed mesodermal sarcoma of the uterus (one of which also involved carcinoma of the endometrium), one case of carcinoma of the breast with leiomyosarcoma of the uterus, and one case of carcinoma of the endometrium with mixed mesodermal sarcoma of the uterus and invasive intraabdominal leiomyosarcoma. This association should be analyzed further.

PRIMARY SARCOMAS OF THE FEMALE INTERNAL GENITAL ORGANS

Leiomyosarcomas of the uterus behave in a wide variety of ways, and it is extremely difficult to predict their behavior on the basis of histologic criteria. More than 10 mitoses per 10 high power fields are considered a sign of malignancy. Patients 55–58 (Table 8) received little or no chemotherapy and all four died with metastases. Of eight patients who received adequate chemotherapy, three are alive. The case histories of patients 59, 62, and 63 are shown in Tables 9 and 10. The case history of patient 60 demonstrates the resistance of this tumor to chemotherapy (Table 11), while that of patient 61 demonstrates the difficulty of predicting the clinical behavior of these tumors based on the initial tissue obtained at hysterectomy (Table 12).

Gynecologists seldom refer patients with mesodermal or stromal sarcomas of the uterus to medical oncologists, and the few patients who receive chemother-

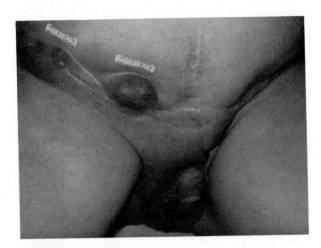

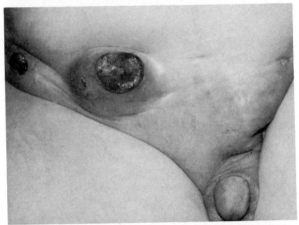

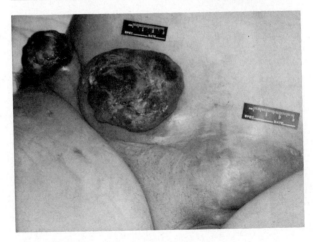

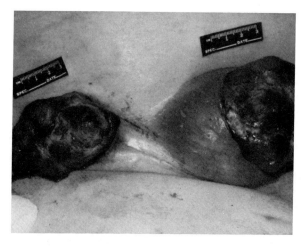

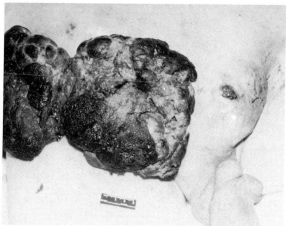

Figure 3 (see also facing page). The growth rate of the pelvic liposarcoma of patient 41 is illustrated in pictures taken approximately three to four weeks apart of tumors invading the abdominal wall after resection and radiotherapy.

apy rapidly succumb nonetheless (Table 13). As stated earlier, these tumors may coexist with adenocarcinomas of the breast or endometrium.

The natural history of uterine sarcomas is influenced by the stage of the tumor at the time of diagnosis. The five-year survival rate for patients with stage I tumors, including all three tumor types (mixed mesodermal sarcoma, leiomyosarcoma, and endometrial stromal sarcoma), is 54%. In contrast, patients with tumors in stages II–IV at the time of diagnosis have a five-year survival rate of only 11% (Salazar et al. 1978). Of the three tumor types, mixed mesodermal sarcoma appears to be the most malignant, with 29% and 22% two- and five-year survival rates, respectively. In contrast, the two- and five-year survival

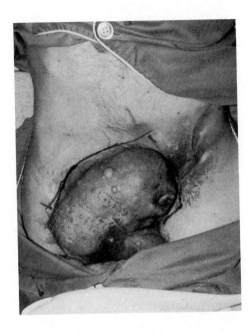

Figure 4. Synovial sarcoma of patient 47 growing through the abdominal wall after resection, radiotherapy, and chemotherapy.

Table 8. *Data on Patients With Leiomyosarcoma of the Uterus*

Patient	Clinical Data	Outcome
55	Hysterectomy '57.	Death 1964
56	Metastases '68.	Death 1968
57	Uterine tumor present 15 years. Began to grow in '67. Hysterectomy.	Death 1968
58	Hysterectomy '66. CTX.	Death 1967
59	Hysterectomy '66. Recurrence '71. Resection, chemotherapy, XRT.	NED 1978
60	Hysterectomy '66. Lung metastases '70. Chemotherapy.	Death 1972
61	Hysterectomy '69. Recurrence and lung metastases '73–74. Chemotherapy.	Death 1976
62	Cesarean delivery and hysterectomy '71. Moving strip radiotherapy, VCR, Act-D, CTX.	NED 1977
63	Hysterectomy '71. Lung metastases '71–72. Resections. VCR, Act-D, CTX, Adria, DTIC, MeCCNU.	Alive with minimal residual tumor 1978
64	Hysterectomy '75. Recurrence and lung metastases '76. XRT, Adria, DTIC.	Death 1977
51	3 resections for local recurrence. VCR, CTX, Adria, DTIC, Act-D, ↑MTX, LV.	Progression 1978

Table 9. *Patients 59 and 62, With Leiomyosarcoma of Uterus*

Patient 59	
1961	Hysterectomy for uterine leiomyosarcoma.
1971	Retroperitoneal leiomyosarcoma.
	Lymphangiogram: extensive disease.
	Inferior vena cavagram: displacement.
	Resection, VCR, Act-D, CTX 2½ years.
1974	Recurrence excised.
	Adria 80 mg, DTIC 400 mg × 5, 10 courses.
	MeCCNU 120 mg, DTIC 300 mg × 3, 5 courses.
1975	Recurrence excised.
	5,036 rads, 25 MeV to abdomen.
1978	NED (ultrasound, chest x-ray, liver scan negative).
Patient 62	
1971	3rd pregnancy delivered by cesarean section because of pelvic mass: "cellular leiomyoma."
	Hysterectomy, salpingo-oophorectomy, omentectomy, resection of sigmoid colon: well-differentiated leiomyosarcoma in uterus invading cul de sac, omentum, and sigmoid colon.
	XRT moving strip, 2,800 rads.
	VCR, Act-D, CTX for 6 months.
1978	NED.

Table 10. *Patient 63, With Leiomyosarcoma of Uterus*

1963: Uterine leiomyosarcoma; hysterectomy;
1966: recurrence; 1968: metastatic to both lungs;
1968–71: resections; 1972: recurrences.

VCR Act-D CTX	Adria DTIC	XRT 1492 rads HU	MeCCNU DTIC	MeCCNU	—
↓↑	↓↑	↓↑	St ↓	↓	St
Oct. '72– March '73	March '73– June '73	July '73– Aug. '73	Sept. '73– Apr. '76	Aug. '76– Feb. '78	Apr. '78

↓ Decrease in tumor size (partial remission), ↑ increase in tumor size, St = stable small residual disease.

rates for leiomyosarcomas are 56% and 38%, respectively, and 58% and 39%, respectively, for endometrial stromal sarcomas (Salazar et al. 1978).

The primary treatment for patients with these sarcomas is total abdominal hysterectomy and bilateral salpingo-oophorectomy, with or without radiotherapy. Patients with residual, recurrent, or metastatic pelvic sarcomas receive chemotherapy with vincristine, actinomycin-D, and cyclophosphamide in addition to surgical resection and radiotherapy. In a series of 38 patients with primary pelvic sarcomas, 14 were tumor free for 10 to 72 months (Smith et al. 1975, Wharton 1978). No synergism between Adriamycin and dacarbazine could be demonstrated in the case of gynecologic sarcomas (Omura and Blessing 1978).

Table 11. *Patient 60, With Leiomyosarcoma of Uterus*

1966 Hysterectomy for leiomyosarcoma of uterus.
1969 Lung metastases.

VCR CTX	XRT Act-D	Act-D	Adria* DTIC	VCR Act-D CTX	↑MTX† LV	Cycloleucin MeCCNU
↑	↓↑	↑	St ↑	↑	↑	↑
Feb. '70– Aug. '70	Aug. '70– May'71	Aug. '71– Oct. '71	Oct. '71– May '72	June '72– Aug. '72	Sept. '72– Jan. '73	Aug. '73– March '74 Death

* 910 mg in 9 courses.
† Escalating from 800 mg to 12,495 mg in 6 courses.
↓ Decrease in tumor size, ↑ increase in tumor size.

Thus, the optimal treatment for patients with these tumors is not known. Complete or near complete surgical resection, followed by external beam radiotherapy, adjuvant chemotherapy, or both, appears to be justified, but prospectively randomized trials are needed to determine optimum management.

SARCOMAS OF EXTERNAL GENITALIA

Kaposi's sarcoma occurs in the external genitalia. It often appears in multifocal fashion, and may be confined to the skin or may involve the mucous membranes and visceral organs. Excised lesions frequently recur. Kaposi's sarcoma is radiotherapy- and chemotherapy-sensitive (Sinkovics 1976, Sinkovics et al. 1975). Low-dose radiation (800 to 1000 rads) is often effective in eradicating selected lesions. Among the chemotherapeutic agents, vincristine and actinomycin-D,

Table 12. *Patient 61, With Leiomyosarcoma of Uterus*

1969	Hysterectomy for leiomyoma. Revised (1973) leiomyosarcoma grade 2.
1973	Pelvic recurrence: leiomyosarcoma grade 3. Resection.
1974	Pelvic recurrence. Pulmonary metastases.
1974	Referred to MDAH. VCR, CTX, Adria, Act-D 12 courses. PR, stabilization, regrowth.
1975	MeCCNU, DTIC: progression. MeCCNU, DTIC, Act-D: progression. XRT to pelvic tumor. ↑MTX, LV: progression. XRT to lung metastases. Adria, Cis-plat: progression.
1977	Death

Table 13. *Data on Patients With Mixed Mesodermal Sarcoma of Uterus*

Patient	Clinical Data	Outcome
65	Hysterectomy, R oophorectomy '69. Chest wall and lung metastases '70–71. Chest wall resection, XRT, chlorambucil, Act-D, VCR, MTX.	Death 1972
66	Hysterectomy '76. Two associated unrelated malignancies: endometrial carcinoma and breast carcinoma. Epithelial cell metastases '77. XRT, progesterone, diethylstilbestrol.	Alive with tumors 1978
67	Hysterectomy '76. Lung metastasis. CyVADIC. Tumor decreasing.	Sudden death at home 1976
68	Radium implant. Radical hysterectomy '76. Widespread intraabdominal metastases '78. VCR, CTX, Adria, DTIC.	Stable 1978

vincristine and dacarbazine, vinblastine, bleomycin, the nitrosoureas, and Adriamycin are highly effective and induce objective tumor responses in about 70% of patients treated. Currently an elderly man (patient 69) is receiving chemotherapy with actinomycin-D for Kaposi's sarcoma of the scrotum (Figures 5 and 6).

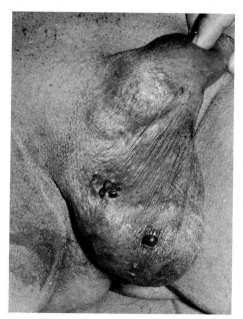

Figure 5. Kaposi's sarcoma of the scrotum in patient 69 to before resection.

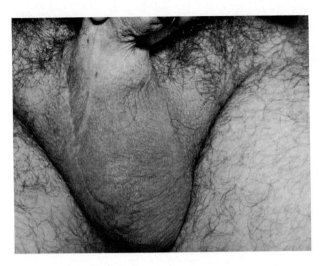

Figure 6. Within three months of surgery the tumors recurred, necessitating chemotherapy.

REFERENCES

Axelrod, R., H. J. Naidech, J. Myers, and A. Steinberg. 1978. Primary osteosarcoma of the kidney. Cancer 41:724–727.

Curnes, J. T., C. B. Pratt, and H. O. Hustu. 1977. Five-year survival after disseminated paratesticular rhabdomyosarcoma. J. Urol. 118:662–665.

Krutchik, A. N., C. Sullivan, J. G. Sinkovics, and A. Ayala. 1978. Chemoimmunotherapy of sarcomatoid renal cell carcinoma. Med. Pediatr. Oncol. (in press).

Malek, R. S., and P. O. Kelalis. 1977. Paratesticular rhabdomyosarcoma in childhood. J. Urol. 118:450–453.

Narayana, A. S., S. Loening, G. W. Weimar, and D. A. Culp. 1978. Sarcoma of the bladder and prostate. J. Urol. 119:72–76.

Niceta, P., R. W. Lavengood, M. Fernandes, and P. J. Tozzo. 1974. Leiomyosarcoma of kidney. Urology 3:270–277.

Omura, G. A., and J. A. Blessing. 1978. Chemotherapy of stage III, IV and recurrent uterine sarcomas: A randomized trial of Adriamycin (AD) *versus* AD + dimethyl triazeno imidazole carboxamide (DTIC). (Abstract) Proc. Am. Assoc. Cancer Res. 19:26.

Raney, R. B., D. M. Hays, W. Lawrence, E. H. Soule, M. Tefft, and M. H. Donaldson. 1978. Paratesticular rhabdomyosarcoma in childhood. Cancer 42:729–736.

Richaud, C., M. Olmer, M. Hermanowicz, J. F. Duvinage, and R. Choux. 1977. A report of two cases of renal sarcoma. J. Urol. Nephrol. (Paris) 83:662–667.

Salazar, O. M., T. A. Bonfiglio, S. F. Patten, B. E. Keller, M. Feldstein, M. E. Dunne, and J. Rudolph. 1978. Uterine sarcomas: Natural history, treatment and prognosis. Cancer 42:1152–1160.

Sinkovics, J. G. 1974. Improved response to conventional treatment and immune reactions to sarcoma antigens of patients with sarcomas, *in* Interaction of Radiation and Host Immune Defense Mechanisms in Malignancy. Brookhaven National Laboratory, U.S. Atomic Energy Commission, National Technical Information Service, Springfield, Virginia, pp. 331–339.

Sinkovics, J. G. 1976. Discussion of Kaposi's sarcoma, *in* Neoplasms of the Skin and Malignant Melanoma (The University of Texas System Cancer Center M. D. Anderson Hospital and Tumor Institute Twentieth Annual Clinical Conference). Year Book Medical Publishers, Chicago, pp. 543–547.

Sinkovics, J. G. 1978. Immunotherapy of human tumors. Pathobiol. Annu. 8:241–284.

Sinkovics, J. G. 1979. Medical Oncology, an Advanced Course. Marcel Dekker, New York (in press).

Sinkovics, J. G., N. Ahmed, M. J. Hrgovcic, J. R. Cabiness, and J. R. Wilbur. 1972a. Cytotoxic lymphocytes. II. Antagonism and synergism between serum factors and lymphocytes of patients with sarcomas as tested against cultured tumor cells. Tex. Rep. Biol. Med. 30:347–360.

Sinkovics, J. G., J. R. Cabiness, and C. C. Shullenberger. 1972b. Monitoring *in vitro* of immune reactions to solid tumors. Front. Rad. Ther. Oncol. 7:99–119.

Sinkovics, J. G., V. Lanzotti, C. Plager, N. Ahmed, D. K. King, L. T. Campos, and F. Gyorkey. 1975. Kaposi's sarcoma: Chemotherapy, virology and immune reactions, *in* Abstracts of the Fifteenth Interscience Conference on Antimicrobial Agents and Chemotherapy, American Society of Microbiology, Abst. #240.

Sinkovics, J. G., and B. Mackay. 1979. A multidisciplinary approach to the understanding and treatment of human sarcomas, *in* Major Problems in Pathology, vol. 10, Sarcomas, B. Mackay, ed. W. B. Saunders, Philadelphia (in press).

Sinkovics, J. G., C. Plager, M. J. McMurtrey, J. J. Romero, and M. M. Romsdahl. 1977a. Immunotherapy of human sarcomas, *in* Management of Primary Bone and Soft Tissue Tumors (The University of Texas System Cancer Center M. D. Anderson Hospital and Tumor Institute Twenty-First Annual Clinical Conference). Year Book Medical Publishers, Chicago, pp. 361–410.

Sinkovics, J. G., C. Plager, N. Papadopoulos, M. J. McMurtrey, J. J. Romero, R. Waldinger, and M. M. Romsdahl. 1978. Immunology and immunotherapy of human sarcomas, *in* Immunotherapy of Human Cancer. Raven Press, New York, pp. 267–288.

Sinkovics, J. G., C. Plager, and J. J. Romero. 1977b. Immunology and immunotherapy of patients with sarcomas, *in* Neoplasm Immunity: Solid Tumor Therapy, R. G. Crispen, ed. Franklin Institute Press, Philadelphia, pp. 211–219.

Smith, J. P., F. Rutledge, L. Delclos, and W. Sutow. 1975. Combined irradiation and chemotherapy for sarcomas of the pelvis in females. Am. J. Roentgenol. Rad. Ther. Nucl. Med. 123:571–576.

Wharton, J. 1978. Management of sarcomas of the uterus, *in* Abstracts of the XIIth International Cancer Congress Workshops, vol. 3, W55. UICC, p. 161.

JOANNE VANDENBERGE HILL AWARD AND WILLIAM O. RUSSELL LECTURE IN ANATOMICAL PATHOLOGY

Cancer of the Genitourinary Tract, edited by
D. E. Johnson and M. L. Samuels.
Raven Press, New York © 1979.

Pathology and Spread of Carcinoma of the Urinary Bladder

F. K. Mostofi, M.D.

*Department of Genitourinary Pathology, Armed Forces Institute of Pathology,
Washington, D.C.*

It is a singular honor for me to be the second recipient of the Joanne Vanden-
berge Hill Award and William O. Russell Lectureship in Anatomical Pathology.
I have known Bill Russell for over 30 years, having first heard of him when
he was in training. I have followed his career in Santa Barbara and through
the years he has been at M. D. Anderson Hospital. He served on the Council
of the U.S.–Canadian Division of the International Academy of Pathology and
moved up as vice-president, president-elect, president, and past president while
I was the secretary-treasurer of the organization. I have many happy memories
of our relationship during that period.

I have followed Bill's scientific work, his efforts in standardization of pathologic nomenclature, his national and international activities, and the many honors
he has received. That a lectureship has been named in his honor as a living
testimony to the contributions he has made to cancer research and pathology
in general and to M. D. Anderson Hospital in particular makes me very happy.
I am sorry that illness has prevented him from attending this meeting, for it
would have been a great pleasure to see him. I wish him a speedy recovery,
and would like to express my sincere appreciation for this great honor.

Before discussing the pathology and spread of carcinoma of the bladder, let
me say a few words about carcinoma of the bladder in general. This form of
cancer constitutes 2% of all malignant lesions, and 95% of the tumors are
epithelial.

Carcinoma of the bladder is one of the few human cancers in which a cause-
and-effect relationship has been demonstrated. We know there is a high incidence
of cancer of the bladder among workers in certain industries, that cigarette
smoking and certain food additives and drugs are carcinogenic, that environmental factors are extremely important in carcinoma of the bladder, and that there
has been a definite increase in the incidence among younger people and women.
In both of these groups environmental factors, especially smoking, play a major
role.

The opinions or assertions contained herein are the private views of the author and are not to
be construed as official or as reflecting the views of the Department of the Army or the Department
of Defense.

Although carcinoma of the bladder has many fascinating aspects, I welcome the opportunity to discuss the pathology and spread of this disease because I firmly believe that at least some of the unpredictable results and poor behavior associated with carcinoma of the bladder are due to the fact that its pathology has not been fully exploited in the management of patients with this disease. We must standardize and systematize our methods of pathological examination and reporting, apply certain modern techniques, and correlate our pathological findings with clinical behavior. The tissue we receive and the techniques we use can provide a tremendous amount of information of great therapeutic value.

There are two areas I would like to discuss: the distinction between papilloma and carcinoma, and the pathological characterization of carcinoma of the bladder.

CRITERIA FOR DIAGNOSIS OF CARCINOMA OF BLADDER

That benign papillary tumors of the urinary bladder exist is evident. The problem has been to define the diagnostic criteria so the great discrepancy in the reported incidences of papilloma of the bladder (3–40%) (Mostofi 1975) can be resolved. The World Health Organization (WHO) Panel of Experts on Carcinoma of Bladder (Mostofi et al. 1974) defined papilloma as a papillary tumor with a delicate fibrovascular stroma covered by an epithelium that is indistinguishable from normal bladder mucosa. Although the reported incidence of recurrence or malignant change in papillomas has ranged from 20% to 50%, the evidence to date indicates that most, if not all, single papillomas or low-grade papillary carcinomas in young patients will have a benign behavior and that multicentric tumors and tumors occurring in older patients should be carefully followed.

The criteria for malignancy have been defined as increased cellularity, crowding of nuclei, lack of differentiation from base to surface, polymorphism of cells and nuclei, increased mitoses, and increased giant cells. The existence of no more than seven cell layers has been suggested as characteristic of benign tumors (Koss 1975); however, we see many carcinomas that are four or five layers thick. We believe it is more important to look at the appearance of the cells than at the exact number of cell layers.

The criteria advocated by the WHO panel for diagnosing carcinoma of the bladder appear to be more liberal than those for other organs. They were designed to restrict the diagnosis of papilloma and eliminate such diagnoses as atypia and dysplasia, but in practice one is sometimes forced into using these terms, indicating the need for finding more realistic definitions of papilloma and carcinoma.

COMPREHENSIVE APPROACH TO DIAGNOSIS OF BLADDER CARCINOMA

In most instances, through his clinical examination, the urologist already suspects the patient has carcinoma and the biopsy confirms this suspicion. The

WHO panel felt that the pathologist can be of greater help if he can further refine the diagnosis of carcinoma. Description of five features of carcinoma of the bladder would provide assistance.

Pattern of Growth

There are four patterns of growth: papillary, infiltrating, papillary and infiltrating, and nonpapillary and noninfiltrating. About 70% of bladder tumors begin as papillary tumors, about 10% as infiltrating carcinomas, and about 20% as papillary and infiltrating tumors, while less than 1% are nonpapillary, noninfiltrating.

Papillary tumors have been shown to be associated with a good prognosis, infiltrating tumors with a poor prognosis, and papillary and infiltrating tumors with an intermediate prognosis. A number of papillary tumors remain so, but others become infiltrating. It is highly desirable to detect this capability before it becomes obvious clinically and microscopically, and Davidsohn's mixed red blood cell agglutination test offers a means to do so (Kovarik et al. 1968).

Histology of the Tumor

In the U.S. and western Europe, about 90% of carcinomas of the bladder are transitional, 7% are initially squamous, 2% are glandular, and about 1% are undifferentiated (a term the WHO panel applied to tumors that are neither transitional, squamous, nor glandular, but represent the basal, primitive cell). It has been traditional in some centers to designate all epithelial tumors as squamous or epidermoid carcinomas. Urologists have responded to this by omitting any reference to histology. A number of tumors that begin as transitional cell carcinomas will in later stages show squamous, glandular, or undifferentiated areas, leading to the diagnosis of squamous or adenocarcinoma or poorly differentiated carcinoma. The WHO panel has rightfully regarded the first two as basically transitional cell carcinomas with squamous or glandular change (metaplasia) and the third as an admixture of the four basic cell types. Transitional cell carcinomas carry a better prognosis than squamous or glandular tumors, and transitional and squamous carcinomas and possibly undifferentiated carcinomas are more responsive to radiation than glandular carcinomas. Proper histological designation of the tumor is also important from the epidemiological point of view. Bladder tumors associated with schistosomiasis are almost all squamous carcinoma and, though they may reveal little or no anaplasia, infiltrate the bladder wall deeply.

Grade of the Tumor

Tumor grade is another area badly in need of standardization. Broders (1926) advocated four grades, but Dart (1936) showed that the behavior of grade III and IV tumors was so close as to justify deletion of grade IV. This has also been the experience of our British colleagues (Dukes 1959). The American Bladder Tumor Registry (Dart 1936), however, categorized multiple recurrent tumors and tumors over 2.5 cm in diameter as grade II, irrespective of degree of cellular anaplasia, until about 30 years ago, but the practice persists in some quarters.

The WHO panel felt that grade should be based on degree of anaplasia, that there should be three grades, and that these could be applied to any histological type.

Depth of Infiltration

The most important single prognostic factor in carcinoma of bladder, depth of infiltration, is an area in which pathologists as a whole have been negligent. The UICC (1974) and WHO (Mostofi et al. 1974) have proposed the following categories:

Tumors without invasion of the lamina propria—PIS,
Tumors in which invasion is limited to the lamina propria—P1,
Tumors in which invasion is limited to superficial muscle—P2,
Tumors with infiltration of deep muscle (more than halfway through the muscle coat)—P3a, or perivesical tissue—P3b,
Tumors with infiltration of the prostate—P4a, or other extravesical structures—P4b.

Jewett (personal communication) has proposed that a category be created for papillary tumors that do not invade the lamina propria. The distinction is very important. As Jewett has observed, there are no lymphatic vessels in the epithelial layers and it is only with a break in the basement membrane that lymphatic invasion may occur.

Grading and pathological staging are sometimes confused. While there is an 80% correlation between grade of the tumor and depth of infiltration, the two are distinct entities.

Mode and Location of Spread

Mode and location of spread are other aspects of pathology that have generally been overlooked. The carcinoma may spread in a broad front or in a tentacular fashion. Broad front spread can be readily detected by the urologist, but not so tentacular invasion, in which the tumor infiltrates the bladder wall as individual or nests of cells.

Similarly, subjacent spread is easily recognized by the urologist, who always endeavors to get beyond the tumor by removing the uninvolved lamina propria or muscularis. However, in lateral spread the tumor undermines normal-appearing mucosa, and the urologist who tries to remove adequate uninvolved margin is misled by the normal-appearing surface epithelium. Thus, the pathologist must call attention to the location and mode of spread to alert the urologist to the possibility of incomplete removal.

Lymphatic and vascular invasions are usually recorded by the pathologist in his report. However, superficial lymphatic invasion in superficial tumors has not been generally recognized. Some years ago, Jewett and Eversole (1960) had alerted us to the existence of this phenomenon and its importance; we found it in 10% of our superficial carcinomas, in which we had previously overlooked it (Mostofi 1975).

Carcinoma in Situ of the Bladder

No discussion of pathology and spread of carcinoma of the bladder is complete without mention of carcinoma in situ. Dr. Sesterhenn and I are currently studying 208 cases of carcinoma in situ of the bladder. These fall into three broad categories: initial carcinoma in situ (82 cases), carcinoma in situ associated with obvious papillary and/or infiltrating carcinomas of the bladder (72 cases), and carcinoma in situ found on follow-up examination of a patient treated for obvious carcinoma of the bladder (54 cases).

Pathological confirmation is easily made if one sees a full-thickness biopsy specimen of the epithelial layer that shows severe anaplasia. Not infrequently, however, while the results of the cytologic examination are positive, the pathologist is confronted with a biopsy specimen that shows no epithelium or only a single layer or small clusters of neoplastic cells. Furthermore, while the diagnosis of carcinoma in situ is readily made with grade III tumors, the tendency has been to label grade I or II nonpapillary, noninfiltrating tumors as dysplasia.

We have observed that, in addition to exhibiting full-thickness changes, the carcinoma in situ may overlie or undermine normal mucosa or be scattered in single or clones of neoplastic cells through a normal mucosa. Whether or not this represents de novo tumor formation or spread has not been settled.

Carcinoma in situ can spread continuously along the surface and thus extend into prostatic ducts, the urethra, or the ureters. It may also become implanted in or break through the basement membrane, in which case it becomes an infiltrating carcinoma.

We have neglected to record the presence of carcinoma in situ in association with papillary or infiltrating carcinomas of the bladder, which may well explain some of the unpredictable and frustrating results we have had in treating these patients. Calling attention to the existence of carcinoma in situ in such instances will warn the urologist that he is dealing with a more serious and extensive neoplastic change in the vesical mucosa than he would have assumed on the basis of a single obvious tumor.

Our preliminary studies indicate that not all carcinomas in situ rapidly progress into aggressive infiltrating tumors. A number either disappear or remain stable.

CONCLUSIONS

A simple pathological diagnosis of carcinoma, even including grade, does not give the urologist the information a comprehensive examination of the specimen could provide. Pathological diagnoses should include the pattern of growth, histology, grade, depth of infiltration, and mode and location of spread of the tumor. There is a need to recognize carcinoma in situ when the tumor cells do not show marked anaplasia and to record the existence of carcinoma in situ found in association with papillary or infiltrating tumors.

REFERENCES

Broders, A. C. 1926. Grading and practical application. Arch. Pathol. 2:376–381.

Dart, R. O. 1936. Grading of epithelial tumors of urinary bladder. J. Urol. 36:651–668.

Dukes, C. E. 1959. The Institute of Urology scheme for histological classification of epithelial tumors of bladder, *in* Tumors of Bladder: Neoplastic Diseases at Various Sites, D. M. Wallace, ed. Vol. 2. Williams and Wilkins, Baltimore, pp. 105–115.

Jewett, H. J., and S. L. Eversole. 1960. Carcinoma of the bladder: Characteristic modes of local invasion. J. Urol. 83:383–389.

Koss, L. G. 1975. Atlas of Tumor Pathology. 2nd series, fasc. 11. Tumors of the Urinary Bladder. Armed Forces Institute of Pathology, Washington, D.C.

Kovarik, S. L., I. Davidsohn, and R. Stejskal. 1968. ABO antigens in cancer. Arch. Pathol. 86:12–21.

Mostofi, F. K. 1975. Pathology of malignant tumors of urinary bladder, *in* The Biology and Clinical Management of Bladder Cancer, E. H. Cooper and R. E. Williams, eds. Blackwell Scientific Publications, London, pp. 87–109.

Mostofi, F. K., L. H. Sobin, and H. Torloni. 1974. International Histological Classification of Urinary Bladder Tumors, No. 10. WHO, Geneva.

UICC. 1974. TNM Classification of Malignant Tumors. 2nd ed. UICC, Geneva, pp. 79–83.

Author Index *

See also List of Contributors, pp. *xiii-xv*.

Subject Index